DR. ATKINS' NUTRITION
BREAKTHROUGH

DR. ATKINS' NUTRITION BREAKTHROUGH

How to Treat Your Medical Condition Without Drugs

by
ROBERT C. ATKINS, M.D.

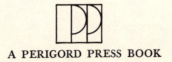

A PERIGORD PRESS BOOK

WILLIAM MORROW AND COMPANY, INC.
New York   1981

Grateful acknowledgment to:

The Bradford Foundation for permission to quote from *The Metabolic Management of Cancer* by Robert Bradford and Michael Culbert. Copyright © 1979 by the Robert W. Bradford Foundation.

And to Harold W. Harper, M.D., for permission to reprint his Harper Health Indicator Test, copyright © The Health Corps, from *How You Can Beat the Killer Diseases*, published by Arlington House, Westport, Conn., 1977.

Library of Congress Cataloging in Publication Data

Atkins, Robert C
    Dr. Atkins' nutrition breakthrough.

"A Perigord Press book."

    Bibliography: p.
    Includes index.
    1. Diet therapy.   2. Orthomolecular medicine.
I. Title. II. Title: Nutrition breakthrough.
RM217.A85   615.8′54   80-39910
ISBN 0-688-03644-9

Printed in the United States of America

5 6 7 8 9 10

BOOK DESIGN BY MICHAEL MAUCERI

This book is dedicated to the pioneers of Nutrition Medicine, who risked their professional standing to develop the methodology that led to the Nutrition Breakthrough, namely, that a substantial number of degenerative and recurrent medical problems may be more effectively and safely treated by substances normally found in our bodies than by the pharmaceuticals that can place our health in jeopardy.

PREFACE

This is a book about the management of common conditions that usually require a doctor's attention. But don't expect a recounting of the way these conditions are customarily treated by my medical colleagues.

You will find that the therapies discussed here represent an alternative to orthodox medicine—a little-used and poorly understood approach known as nutrition medicine.

Despite the relative unfamiliarity of nutrition medicine, most of these therapies are being used in medical practice on an increasingly wide scale, and they often represent a far safer alternative to the drug-oriented system around which orthodox medicine has developed. That they are *safer* has long been accepted by the medical profession, but the fact that the science has now progressed to the point where they are *effective* is the real news—the breakthrough you will be reading about.

The diet and nutrition breakthroughs presented here have been developed in three ways. Primarily they are the techniques I have been using, and currently use, in my medical practice. Secondly, they have been reported upon in scientific journals and at scientific meetings. And finally, they are being used by those colleagues of mine who, like me, have committed their medical practices to nontoxic, nonpharmaceutical methods of treating the whole patient.

If, as you read this book, you feel it affords a mandate for self-diagnosis and self-treatment, you will have missed the point. All my patients, and the patients of my colleagues, succeeded in large part because they were treated by a responsible, caring physician

7

who sought a complete diagnosis on each patient and who knew the strengths and limitations of both the orthodox and the alternative therapies he would be using.

Any self-treatment, particularly when combined with self-diagnosis, can be hazardous. For example, a person with impaired heart or liver or kidney function may be at risk when he tries a technique that is easily tolerated by healthier individuals. Even the relatively safe Nutrition Breakthrough techniques I will be teaching you can carry that risk for certain individuals.

For these reasons I urge you to find a doctor who is sympathetic to the idea of using good nutrition before drug therapy. Allow him to know your medical status thoroughly, and give him the responsibility to make those medical decisions appropriate to your condition.

Let this book serve merely as a guide to show you what is possible now on a limited scale and what has enough merit soon to be practiced throughout our community.

—ROBERT C. ATKINS, M.D.

CONTENTS

BOOK ONE

BOOK ONE

Chapter 1

WHAT THIS BOOK WILL REVEAL TO YOU

Several months ago, I sat down to study the records of twelve new patients with a dozen different problems. All twelve had been placed on the same diet and the same vitamin formula for their first two weeks in my care.

When they came back for their second visit, their reports were astonishingly good.

The diabetic had stopped spilling sugar after four days and discontinued his insulin. The secretary who'd been tortured by migraines had not had a headache—or an aspirin, for that matter—in ten days. The student whose anxiety had been so debilitating that he'd dreaded getting up in the morning felt so "together" that he had stopped taking his tranquilizers. And the hyperactive kid's mother reported that her son was much easier to live with—and much happier, too.

The depressed middle-aged man who had been on large doses of antidepressants to combat a "sinking, empty feeling of nothingness" noticed his mood lifting and decreased his dosage. He was actually cheerful when he came in for follow-up.

The tall, stately white-haired lady reported less arthritis pain and showed me how much more freely her hands now moved. She was especially pleased to get off the anti-inflammatory medication that had irritated her stomach.

The asthmatic teenager proudly showed me a blister from playing tennis *without* the aid of her potent, multidrug asthma remedy. The tense, wiry schoolteacher who'd had insomnia for years was astonished that she had gone a whole week without a sleeping pill, and the dental student who had come in feeling tired all the time couldn't get over how much pep and energy he now had. The corporate executive, whose heartburn had had him gulping antacids every two hours, just radiated delight when he reported twelve days without pain—and without antacids.

And the young mother, who had seen eight doctors before coming to me, was often so dizzy she wouldn't go out alone and couldn't imagine driving. On her second visit, she gave me a jubilant thumbs-up when I asked about her symptoms. Not a single dizzy spell since the third day of her regimen.

The last patient, whose severe hypertension had required that he take three different blood pressure medications, came back so much improved that we eliminated two of the drugs completely on his second visit.

These twelve patients were astonished at how easily they adapted to my recommendations, and even more surprised at how well they felt. All were relieved to need less medication—or none—some for the first time in years.

By the third visit I had gone back to my usual method, tailoring the regimen to the individual, and they all continue to do well.

It is obvious, of course, that the same eating pattern and vitamin formula will not necessarily be right for everyone. But these twelve cases do indeed prove the points I set out to make:

- These patients must have had *something* in common if they all showed improvement on the same initial regimen.
- The basic diet and vitamin formulation somehow helped to combat this common factor and began to reverse its destructive trend.

The Common Factor Was Right Here at Home

You may have begun to wonder what a hypertensive, a diabetic, an asthmatic, an insomniac, and the rest have in common.

All these patients were victims of their food consumption patterns —the so-called civilized Western diet. It should come as no surprise that their health improved when they adapted to a more favorable eating pattern. This is especially so because our society's diet is *anti* blood sugar control, and it is our blood sugar control mechanism that is most likely to go out of kilter, both as a result of our diet and as a result of the drugs we may ingest.

Interestingly enough, I first developed the Atkins Diet—which does, of course, control blood sugar—as a lifetime treatment for obesity. But many years' experience and over fifteen thousand patients have demonstrated that this diet, combined with the appropriate vitamin and mineral supplements, can do much more than restore my patients' weight to normal. In case after case it restores their health to normal, too.

Our Balanced Diet Is Unbalanced

On the face of it, there's nothing wrong with a good balanced diet that includes all the food groups. Just like Grandma used to recommend. And for the most part, this is what my patients were eating.

Unfortunately, the civilized Western diet's refined, processed foods and the proportions in which we eat them pave the way for susceptible people to "lose their balance." They no longer obtain the right nutrients in the right proportions. As night follows day, they succumb to the nonbacterial, nonviral chronic conditions that seem to go hand in hand with advanced cultures. All because the goodness and balance Grandma associated with the proper mix of foods have been refined out.

If You Have Chronic Complaints, You Are Not Alone

Recently, during a lecture, I told the story of a woman in her sixties who had a multiplicity of complaints: disconcerting irregular heartbeat, headaches, heartburn, stiff joints, and insomnia. On top of that, she was considerably overweight. For these conditions she took six or seven medications every day.

As I described her case, a woman halfway back in the auditorium could contain herself no longer. "It sounds like you're describing me!" she burst forth. The audience laughed good-naturedly, and when they finished, I reassured her, "Don't feel that I'm singling you out. I'll bet most people in this room feel the same way."

It wouldn't surprise me if at times you feel that I am describing you, too.

You Don't Have to Be an Atkins Office Patient to Improve Your Health

I believe that perhaps you, like the twelve patients I mentioned earlier, can probably improve your health by working with nutritional techniques to restore your body's balance. And it is just this fundamental balance—blood sugar control and insulin regulation—that my basic diet achieves. Once a patient's metabolism is stabilized, it is far easier for nutrients to do a therapeutic job. Then we can start eliminating, one by one, the drugs that have been needed. We'll have gained this: Instead of blocking symptoms with drugs, we'll build health with nutrients.

All We Know Is What They Want Us to Hear

I am increasingly distressed by what appears to be an industrial conspiracy. Many government agencies are party to it, too. The truth about nutrition is hidden not only from the public (who, after all, are the patients), but from our physicians—the very front-line practitioners to whom we all entrust our health and well-being.

The food industry (with the government's blessing) knowingly brings us the partitioned, less-than-optimum diet that hastens the development of our modern illnesses.[1] Then the drug industry profits from the sickness our diet engenders. The voice of better nutrition is silenced.

Nutrition is not profitable enough.

Who loses? All of us. Because all of us must eat.

It's Not Too Late to Do Something Positive

It is time for a nutrition revolution.

We are already seeing the beginnings of it. The health-food movement is gaining momentum, and consumers are demanding more and more whole foods without additives. As a result, the "All Natural" banner is increasingly common on supermarket packages. It's a selling point these days. But don't be misled. "All Natural" does not guarantee the healthfulness of the product. It does show that food purveyors are aware of what the public wants to hear and are willing to exploit that demand.

Sugar is now decried as a dietary evil, and there is increasing mistrust of both the food and the medical establishments. (Let's be fair—if physicians are misled from the first day of their medical training, how can they be blamed?)

All the same, things may not be moving fast enough.

Old Habits Die Hard

Our eating habits seem to continue in the same destructive direction. We still feed our children sugar-coated junk and sugar-laced soft drinks. We unknowingly eat foods with disguised sugar. (More about this later.) We eat gummy white bread ridden with "dough conditioners," stabilizers, enhancers, and other chemicals. We have no idea what the long-term effects of these substances will be.

It's like the old saw about the weather. We all talk about it, but none of us takes any definitive action. Unlike the weather, however, our food supply and our diet are matters we can take in hand. We *can* do something about the way we eat. It's time we did.

Positive Measures That Could Improve Your Health

This book will show you further applications of the Atkins Diet. It will explain how you may prevent or reverse some of the ravages our current eating pattern has visited upon us all, and how simple dietary techniques can improve your health and overcome so many major problems and nuisance complaints. And as a bonus, you'll reach and maintain your ideal weight.

There is no time like now to get started.

Although there is still much to learn, I can show you how to use what we do know to assess your health and to devise a program that fits your way of life and medical profile. Don't assume that I'm asking you to bypass your doctor, for only he can assess your diagnosis and evaluate the potential risks of discontinuing any medications you may now be taking. I propose to show you what can be done under the guidance of a nutritionally oriented doctor.

Best of all, though you will change your diet and add supplements to it, you'll enjoy what you eat. Most of you will be able to have juicy spare ribs, lobster with butter, eggs Benedict, sour cream, caviar, nuts, and other foods that are not usually thought of as therapeutic or dietetic.

All this in your diet, while treating and preventing the diseases of our culture. The man-made diseases. And without drugs.

Chapter 2

WHAT IS WRONG WITH DRUGS

When I first started to practice medicine I'm sure I wrote at least as many prescriptions as the next doctor.

If a patient suggested that she retained fluid, I would reach for my prescription pad and prescribe a diuretic (water pill) without a second thought.

And if I noticed a slight elevation in blood pressure, the answer was simple. Out came the pad and a prescription for the latest anti-hypertensive.

What about the patient with a stressful occupation who complained of "nerves"? He, too, received a prescription. This time for a generous helping of tranquilizers.

After all, I wanted to help my patients. And I certainly wanted to show them my concern for their welfare.

Rarely did a patient leave my office without a prescription in hand for one of modern medicine's latest miracles.

I Stopped Thinking Drugs

After I had supervised a few thousand patients on the Atkins Diet, a growing suspicion sneaked across the border of doubt, and I recognized a startling fact.

Not only did my patients lose weight, but one after another they lost their illnesses.

Instead of prescribing *more* drugs as I might have in the past, I was helping eliminate the need for them. I found myself encouraging my patients to decrease their medications. It seemed that I had come across something much more powerful than drugs. Nutrition.

That set me thinking. I began to suspect that the drugs I once prescribed so blithely were not at all what their manufacturers and my professors claimed. It dawned on me that drugs masked disease symptoms without tackling their underlying causes.

A classic example of this masking without actually curing (and thus producing a false sense of security) is the way hypertension is treated with traditional pharmaceuticals. The patient relies only upon medication to keep his pressure down.

The case of Joe T. makes my point very well.

Joe T. had intermittent high blood pressure in his teens. His doctor said not to worry; wait and see. He noted that Joe's fluctuations coincided with his stress levels. (This is known as labile hypertension.) When Joe went on to become an airplane mechanic, an airline doctor noticed his blood pressure, too. This time, however, it was higher than it had been in high school, so Joe was put on a diuretic (the "water pill" is also used in blood pressure control) and another drug.

From time to time, the airline doctor would tell Joe to stop his medication—and every single time he did, his pressure climbed back to pretreatment levels or beyond. Joe's blood pressure seemed to be on an upward spiral.

One must not jump to the conclusion that Joe's ever-climbing pressure was due solely to the drugs. I would guess that it was Joe's innate susceptibility to hypertension, all other things—like diet—being equal.

In any event, Joe didn't much like the medication, because of its side effects. Aside from mild depression and an "out-of-it" feeling, Joe had trouble with his sex life. His wife was not wild about that, to say the least. So Joe kept trying to swear off his pills. And each time he did, he got such painful headaches he couldn't go to work. It was obvious that Joe had to have *something* to control his blood pressure.

Until he came to me, that something meant drugs.

Joe's high blood pressure wasn't *cured* by the pharmaceuticals. The drugs were merely controlling or blocking the imbalance that allowed it to exist. The hypertension was simply there. And it returned (sometimes worse than ever) when the drugs were withdrawn.

Joe and his wife were fairly desperate when he first visited my office. We decided to try my basic diet for several weeks before even thinking about tinkering with dosage reduction.

After four weeks of rigorous adherence to the Atkins Diet, Joe's blood pressure (granted, he still took his pills) was lower than it had been the first time he came in. That was our cue. We decided to reduce his dosage by one fourth and watch carefully.

When Joe came in the next week, his blood pressure had gone down a few points more—even though his dosage had been reduced. From that point on, in a careful stepwise manner, we got Joe off his antihypertensives.

Joe no longer takes any medications. He says he never even needs an aspirin. He is ecstatic because he doesn't have the "draggy" feeling and because he is once more sexually active. His wife is ecstatic too—especially because Joe now feels so well that he participates more than before in family activities.

It is evident that Joe's drugs blocked the symptoms, but they didn't cure the disease.

Joe's case brings up another interesting point: side effects. His dragged-out feeling and sexual difficulties were not all in his head. The drugs Joe took acted on metabolic pathways *in addition to* those that merely reduce blood pressure. The drugs threw his whole system out of whack.

We Just Don't Know Enough About Drugs

Joe's discarded drugs are not the only ones that can cause unwanted side effects. Most can do that. Obvious side effects, however, are not the worst of the picture. A drug is a substance *foreign to the body* which works by interfering with one of the body's enzymatic reactions. Its main purpose is to block one or more physiologic functions. In so doing, it compromises the integrity of the body's metabolic pathways, which are the natural routes for the transformation of food into energy.

Some of these effects are subtle. They are not quite obvious enough to be classified as "adverse side effects," and they may not be obvious enough to have been studied in the laboratory before the drug hit the market. But that these effects are subtle doesn't mean we can make light of them. The truth of the matter is that we physicians (and the researchers, too, I fear), have relatively little idea what the long-term metabolic effects of most drugs are—other than those that are grossly obvious.

Drugs Are Biochemical Invaders

Doctors think twice before they order an invasive technique. No one would dispute that surgery is invasive. And so are most forms of instrumentation, X rays, injection of dyes, and other diagnostic procedures.

How many doctors realize that drugs are invasive?

Drugs May Not Always Be Indicated

Those of you who follow politics have probably seen this strategy: An aggressive political power creates an imaginary enemy, which in turn provides the excuse for attack, or invasion.

Warrior physicians have learned that same strategy. And they apply it often. Just reflect upon the imaginary swine flu epidemic of the 1976–1977 winter.

On a level closer to home, I have seen many patients treated for imaginary diseases. Like some cases of hypertension. For example, it is common for blood pressure to go up on a first visit to a strange doctor's office. But this doesn't always mean the patient has or will develop high blood pressure. Joe T.'s high-school physician was practicing good medicine when he took a wait-and-see attitude. As the second physician on a case, I have often taken nonhypertensives *off* blood pressure medication.

Prevention: Indication for Invasion

There is no question that prevention is the best medicine. But all too often, the physician invades in its name. And a little invasive prevention can add up to lots of side effects.

Sue K., a patient I saw recently, had had a seizure fourteen years ago. Her physician certainly didn't want this to occur again, so he prescribed a potent anticonvulsant drug as insurance.

During the fourteen years, Sue had *no other seizures*, even on those occasions when she forgot a dose or two. Yet her doctor insisted that she continue taking her medication. He told her dire tales of what might occur if she discontinued her drug. He did *not* tell her that the type of seizure disorder she had had fourteen years ago usually involves mild seizures that leave no lasting effects in the majority of instances. Can a patient who knows less than the whole story give an informed consent? Do today's patients have to put up with the "just take it" mentality?

By the time Sue K. visited me, her gingivae (the gum tissues surrounding her teeth) were an unsightly red and overgrown. Her blood sugar was elevated (a common side effect of this drug), and because of the drug she proved to be deficient in the key vitamin folic acid.

All in the name of prevention. And it is particularly unfortunate in this particular case because diets (such as those I frequently recommend) were proven effective in the management of seizure disorders as early as the 1920s.[1]

It's Not Solely the Doctor's Fault

In the interest of a balanced view, I must make an additional point about Sue's "preventive" treatment. Her doctor is probably not the only one to blame.

The legal system shares much responsibility for her life sentence to medication. Again and again, physicians have seen lawyers accuse and indict at the slightest excuse. Suppose Sue had had a seizure worse than could be reasonably expected? That would provide just the excuse for a malpractice suit.

Every time a doctor treats a patient, he stakes his career and his malpractice coverage on his judgment. He knows he is at the mercy of a legal system with neither understanding of nor sympathy for his decisions.

It is unfortunate—and, even more unfortunately, understandable —that so many physicians feel they must practice "self-defensive medicine." And since the safe move is to stick with the majority, this can mean prescribing drugs—unnecessarily.

Some Diseases Don't Respond to Drugs

Most viruses—such as those that cause colds—are not susceptible to antibiotics. But many doctors are undeterred by that fact, though they are well aware of it. How many times has your doctor "treated" your cold with antibiotics, knowing full well that it won't respond? His rationale is that he's preventing complications, but he may in fact be causing them.

Although antibiotics certainly have their place in treating *susceptible* infections, it is also true that chronic diarrhea and monilia overgrowth, not to mention allergic reactions, are associated with their use. Further, overuse of antibiotics may bring about bacterial resistance—which makes the antibiotic that caused the resistance useless against that "bug."

Later in the book, I will talk about how I help my patients over-come the common cold and other viruses. With vitamins, not drugs.

Is Prevention Worth the Risk?

Ideally, any treatment should be defensible if the probable benefit outweighs the possible risk. This is known as the benefit-to-risk ratio. In other words, will the treatment do more good than harm?

I maintain that, in many cases, the ratio is almost impossible to assess. We always seem to learn a little too late about the more subtle effects of drugs, particularly those effects accrued over the long term.

Let's face it: Drugs for long-term use in humans are cleared for sale after short-term studies. A careful study carried out for two years cannot hope to predict the effects of a prescription filled for twenty-five years.

For example, in our zeal to eradicate the medical problem called "high cholesterol," the pharmaceutical industry, with the enthusiastic support of many in the medical profession, in 1960 made the cholesterol-lowering drug triparinol (MER-29) a best-selling pre-scription. By April 1962, because of an alarming incidence of cataracts and impotence among its users, an embarrassed FDA had to remove it from commerce.

Have we learned from this? Perhaps. But we now have clofibrate, the present leader among cholesterol-lowering drugs. Unfortu-nately, it may cause cardiac irregularities, decreased sex drive, gallstones, breast tenderness, weight gain, and even a tumor of the liver.[2]

This is the more distressing when you consider what we now know. Niacinamide, lecithin, vitamin C, and PABA (para-amino-benzoic acid) can do a much better job on cholesterol levels, with virtually none of the risk. (I'll expand upon this at length later, for those of you who want to reduce *your* cholesterol levels.)

Worse still, clofibrate has been proven to *shorten* life-span.[3] Can its possible benefits justify the risks?

A New Look at Aspirin

One of the most recent recommendations for the use of aspirin is as an anticlotting agent (in selected patients) to prevent heart at-tack. Yet the side effects of aspirin—not the least of which may in-clude increased susceptibility to prolonged bleeding—include gastric bleeding, ringing in the ears, and nausea. If it were developed today and submitted to the FDA for marketing approval, it is doubtful that aspirin would be cleared.[4] If we need an anticlotting agent, why not use vitamin E? It surely is safer. (More about this later, too.)

A New Look at The Pill

Where could you find a more spurious excuse to invade than in the case of the oral contraceptive, popularly known as The Pill? Available in a variety of formulations, The Pill is a best seller despite the fact that it might contribute to cancer, thromboembolism,[5] premature heart disease, diabetes, depression,[6] gallbladder disease, loss of menstrual function after discontinuation, emotional problems, weight gain, and a plethora of other discomforts and problems. Further, The Pill has nutritional side effects. It may cause deficiencies of key vitamins and minerals—vitamin B_6, folic acid, and zinc, to name a few.[7]

And yet The Pill is a treatment for something that could hardly be called a disease.

This pharmaceutical invasion has characterized the modern era of medicine. Most of us see it as just the way things are done. But I wonder if it is not simply an era that will soon be drawing to a close.

Chapter 3

WHY NUTRITION IS BETTER

Arthritis or headache? Take ANACIN. Tummy trouble? PEPTO-BISMOL or TUMS. Sinus, cold, or allergy symptoms? Take DRISTAN for "Fast, Fast, Fast Relief." Menstrual cramps? Rely on MIDOL. Tense, not coping? Cope again with COPE. Can't sleep? "Take SOMINEX tonight and sleep, sleep, sleep." Coughing? NYQUIL, of course. How about EX-LAX for "irregularity," and ALKA-SELTZER for "the blahs"?

The litany sounds familiar. And why shouldn't it? This is just a sampling of the messages you are likely to hear when you turn on your TV. Our magazines are awash with drug plugs, and you cannot drive very far without your car radio exhorting you to try this miracle remedy for that down-dragging symptom.

So it's not just our doctors who are deluged with drug advertising. You are too. You may be so inured that you don't notice anymore, but drug ads flood the media and *you* are their target.

It's an atmosphere that fosters pill-popping. No matter what the problem, someone somewhere has just the pill to cure it. It is hard to escape the "pills cure all" mentality when both the public and the physicians who treat them have been lifetime targets of persistent, convincing drug advertising. What is a poor consumer to do?

John Q. Public may hear a commercial and recognize his own problem in it. Since he doesn't want the expense of a doctor's office visit, he will go to a drugstore and buy the product. If, after using the advertised wonder drug for a while, he isn't any better, John Q. will visit his doctor. And to what end? Right! John's doctor will write a prescription—probably for a drug not too different from those advertised to him.

John Q. did have the right idea the first time. He just went about it the wrong way.

For John Q. was taking some responsibility for his own health—trying to identify his problem and deal with it himself. But he should have turned to improved nutrition (and nutrition's "enablers," the vitamins and minerals) instead of medications.

John Q. did what big business and the advertising industry wanted him to do. Because, like his "brainwashed" doctor, John Q. Public never had a chance to learn about the alternative.

Or take the case of Sally Jessup, who got on the medication roller coaster and almost didn't get off. She was feeling worse and worse, taking more and more medication and gaining weight all the while. She did some reading, chatted with friends, and talked to her druggist. She finally decided to attack her weight problem first, thinking that maybe weight loss would improve things. And that's why she came to me.

Sally Needed Drugs to Counteract the Effects of Drugs

On Sally's first visit to my office, I knew one thing for sure. Sally was a victim of the Snowball Effect. Her case, unfortunately, is not unusual in the least.

Before her marriage, Sally had been a svelte, lithe fashion model. When she decided to have a family, she stopped her career to become a full-time wife and mother. A few years after her last child was born, Sally had to have a hysterectomy.

And that's when her trouble really began.

The doctor who performed the surgery opted to remove Sally's ovaries along with her uterus, reasoning that was one more place she would never get cancer. But since the ovaries are a woman's source of estrogens, and since Sally was too young for menopause, the surgeon prescribed estrogen tablets a few days after the operation. An accepted medical practice.

The estrogen tablets did indeed prevent menopause symptoms. But after taking them for a while, Sally began to gain weight and retain fluid. Compassionately, because Sally loathed feeling bloated, her doctor prescribed diuretics, which in turn played hob with her blood sugar levels. Mood swings, anxiety, and an insatiable appetite were Sally's response to her unstable blood sugar. So her doctor, thinking "symptom," not "cause," prescribed a tranquilizer, which was supposed to make Sally feel calmer. Instead, it raised her insulin levels (which in turn lowered the blood sugar levels) and thus aggravated her mood swings.

The tranquilizers did nothing for Sally's enormous appetite and craving for sweets, except possibly make them worse. Sally ate constantly, everything she could get her hands on. Naturally, the more she overate, the more weight she gained. And the fatter she got, the more miserable she felt. Finally, her doctor prescribed a diet pill to knock out Sally's appetite and help her eat less.

But this only made matters worse. (Diet pills also raise insulin levels.) Now Sally was more tense than ever. She cried at the slightest provocation and yelled constantly at her husband and children. The situation steadily deteriorated as the diet pills further aggravated Sally's blood sugar instability.

And although she lost weight at first, the effect stopped after a while. When her doctor suggested that she increase her diet pill dosage, Sally finally realized that she had to find an alternative.

What Sally now had was a full-blown case of the Snowball Effect. It had started with the estrogen tablets and continued with a sequence of additional medications. And after the first one, every drug was prescribed to *counteract some effect of the previous one.*

Is it any wonder that Sally was distraught?

Sally May Have an Alternative

Although Sally's major reason for coming to see me was overweight, and although her weight was indeed troublesome and unhealthy, obesity was not her main problem. She was, in fact, a healthy young woman who was on several prescriptions too many. Her problems were physical, from the drugs—including her weight problem—and emotional, from the blood sugar instability they caused.

Had Sally known better, she would have asked, "Is there any alternative?" every time her doctor tried to add a pill to her regimen. Instead, she took her doctor's prescriptions, had them filled, and accepted "just take it" as the sum total of the medical advice she needed. She placed too much of the responsibility for her health in the hands of her doctor, and not enough where it really should have been. In her own.

Her doctor met *his* responsibility in a characteristic way. By responding to symptoms with a prescription.

So neither Sally nor her doctor had looked at the root of Sally's problem. Part of it was a whole lot of medication she shouldn't have been taking in the first place, and part of it was her unenlightened eating habits.

When Sally and I sat down for our first consultation, she truly believed that her medications were the *only* answer to her problems. And up to the time she visited me, they were.

I pointed out to Sally that although there are many useful, necessary medications for which no nutritional alternatives exist as yet (digitalis, the "heart tonic," is one of them), most of her problems could be handled by a nutritional approach. I told her that drugs are blocking agents and may block more than the intended metabolic pathway.

That combinations of drugs may interact in ways not yet known—because every conceivable "safe" combination of drugs has not been tested for possible interactions.

That side effects may be worse than the condition the drug is used to treat.

Sally understood what I meant, but she still *had* to ask, "Doctor, how will I ever get along without my pills?"

Because I have treated hundreds of patients like Sally and have seen their responses to nutritional techniques, I am confident that the nutritional approach works. So I said, "Just wait. I think you'll be pleased."

And then I went on to fill her in on more of the facts.

Sally knew by now that I wasn't much in favor of pharmaceuticals. She knew that I specialized in nutrition and that I was confident that nutrition had much more to offer than weight loss (no mean benefit in itself).

She appeared surprised when I told her that vitamins can do much more than prevent deficiencies. They can often be used to treat illness and in many cases can substitute for pharmaceuticals.

Enablers and Blockers

Vitamins and minerals work differently. They were meant to be used by the body and are natural to human metabolism. Our bodies carry within them the chemical mechanisms essential to utilizing these nutrients. *Vitamins and minerals are nature's enabling agents.* They provide substances the body needs to carry out its essential functions. To sustain, build, and heal. These building blocks are virtually nontoxic and work *within* the body's pathways, instead of against them. *Nutrients enable. Drugs block.*

I pointed out that too much of anything is not good. For example, it's possible to give too much water, or potassium or iron. And it is certainly possible to take too much of the fat-soluble vitamins (A, D, E, and K) which are stored by the body. But it's not likely, because the great quantities required to constitute an overdose are seldom taken. In general, vitamins are not likely to be toxic; and the reverse is true of drugs, even though their toxicity may be very subtle. Almost unnoticed in most cases because, among other reasons, their side effects are often delayed, sometimes until long after the drug has been discontinued.

Sally was amazed at how narrow the range between therapeutic and toxic effects (and doses) can be. She had not realized that too much of a diuretic or tranquilizer could have unbargained-for, and potentially serious, side effects.

But after telling Sally about the toxic potential of pharmaceuticals, I pointed out that for vitamins the range between therapeutic and toxic doses is far wider—somewhere on the order of 1 to 10,000 for some of the B vitamins, which means that the toxic dose is 10,000 times greater than the therapeutic dose.

"Do you really mean that I could control my symptoms with vitamins? And that I'd be doing it far more safely?" she asked with some skepticism.

"It seems hard to believe, I know, but in the next few weeks, you'll see for yourself that vitamins and minerals are important," I answered. "But don't forget that a revamping of your diet is the cornerstone of what we're about to do—and that it's crucial to your success."

This academic discussion seemed to do the trick for Sally. She told me that she now understood some of the principles behind the nutritional approach and was ready to try giving up her medications. In fact, she handed over her bottle of diet pills, and I ceremoniously filed it in my wastebasket.

Sally followed my diet instructions implicitly. She also took her vitamins as prescribed.

The very first week she eliminated her diuretics and tranquilizers (the carbohydrate-restricted diet and vitamin B$_6$ helped here). She also eliminated about eight pounds.

Week after week her weight loss continued and her health improved. She was delighted to find her ankles trim again—a sign that she was no longer retaining water. Her temperament changed quite dramatically. Her kids were relieved not to be yelled at anymore, and her husband once again looked forward to coming home at the end of the day.

Most significantly, I believe, Sally's new feeling of well-being convinced her that nutrition provided a better way.

Sally's Is Only One Success Story

Sally is not unique. Most patients whom I see have more than one complaint. (Many, however, are not as inherently healthy as Sally, but have a mixture of serious and not-so-serious conditions.) Many of their problems hinge on other problems, as did Sally's. And many of my patients are as successful as she was.

But Sally *is* unique; she is an individual. And if I don't regard my patients as individuals—and treat them accordingly—then I can't treat them successfully.

For as Dr. Roger Williams, the man considered by many the patriarch of modern nutrition medicine, pointed out, every person is biochemically unique.[1] He has individual needs and individual ways of making use of the nutrients he takes in. One could say we are all idiosyncratic in that we are all deficient in different areas, and—most important of all—there is room for improvement in all of us.

And this is why nutrition medicine works so well. Why it can work better and do more than allopathic (drug-oriented) medicine.

In other words, a drug is safe only within a narrow dosage range. If you give too much, you poison the patient. If you give too little, you may cause subtle metabolic effects but no therapeutic effect.

But nutrition gives the doctor the option of tailoring the dosage over a wide range, to arrive at the exact dose that best suits the patient. Perhaps if more doctors were aware of the effectiveness of nutrition therapy, they, too, would appreciate its many advantages. Because with nutritional techniques, side effects are not usually a cause of concern. And the doctor has more latitude in arriving at the appropriate dosage level.

In the next few chapters I will give you the background you need to make an assessment of your own case, to take more responsibility for your health, and to do what you have to do with the help of your doctor. I will also give you the information you may need to help your doctor help you.

Chapter 4

WHY MY REGIMEN WORKS

We all give lip service to the harmfulness of our junk-food diet. We may even try to mend our ways. But somehow, real change seems always to be just around the corner.

Perhaps we don't change our habits because we have not grasped the full significance of the biochemical havoc our junk-food, supermarket, fast-food diet can wreak.

If you like to browse through the latest nutrition books, you may be struck by the plethora of words implicating dietary fiber—or, more precisely, the lack of it—as the problem with our modern eating patterns. There is no shortage of advice exhorting you to save your life by incorporating this miraculous substance in your diet. Many of these suggestions are indeed sound. Some, on the other hand, merely counsel you to add fiber to whatever else you eat.

What's Behind the Furor over Fiber?

The fiber hypothesis is based upon some highly astute observations which, however, were purely circumstantial. Most studies supporting this theory were epidemiological (based on observing the prevalence of illnesses in various populations) and did nothing to prove directly the causative link between fiber and the conditions in question.

Much of the basic work on fiber was carried out by three eminent British researchers, Drs. Burkitt, Cleave, and Trowell, who studied the changing patterns of illness in emerging (pre-Westernized) cultures.[1]

These scientists noticed that many illnesses that we in our society take for granted are virtually unheard of in those developing nations where the prevailing diet remains primitive. For example: colitis, ileitis, irritable bowel syndrome, diverticulitis, appendicitis, hiatus hernia, gallstones, hemorrhoids, varicose veins, gout, osteoarthritis, rheumatoid arthritis, osteoporosis, multiple sclerosis, pernicious anemia, and others—not to mention obesity, diabetes, and heart disease.

Many of the conditions on this list are probably what you would expect to find in any doctor's office on a typical day. But the physician of one hundred years ago rarely saw the so-called commonplace diseases of today, because they simply were not that routine.

When the British scientists tabulated their data, they were unable to escape the conclusion that as a society's technologic abilities advance, its dietary pattern changes, and certain once-rare diseases begin to occur more frequently. The incidence of previously rare diseases seems to increase more or less in proportion to the degree of refinement of staple foods in the diet. Burkitt, Cleave, and Trowell thus concluded that the fiber lost in refining foods was the health-giving factor somehow responsible for the previous rarity of the "new" diseases.

The *Journal of the American Medical Association* carried a brilliant essay by Dr. Burkitt in which he put forth his findings and offered his conclusions. So broad was the impact of this essay that several best-selling books heralding the "age of fiber" went rapidly to press and into the hands of the public.

Is Fiber the Whole Story?

Quite another conclusion can be drawn from the same type of observations. For example, Henry Schroeder, M.D., of Dartmouth Medical College, placed the emphasis in a different area.[2] Schroeder pointed out that the same milling process that eliminates the fiber also eliminates many of the *micronutrients* (vitamins and minerals) essential to our health. Since wheat is the mainstay of our diet, we should obtain from it its maximum nutritional benefits. Schroeder pointed out this is virtually impossible when we consume refined wheat from which the bran and germ have been removed. Sixty-seven percent of folic acid, 71 percent of vitamin B_6, 86 percent of vitamin E, 89 percent of cobalt (the mineral essential to vitamin B_{12}), 78 percent of zinc, 85 percent of magnesium, and 86 percent of manganese are lost when we blow away the chaff (bran) and strain out the germ of wheat. The enrichment process replaces only the vitamin B_1 (thiamine), vitamin B_2 (riboflavin), and vitamin B_3 (which we did not mention above because, though they are also refined out, the milling industry sees fit to replace them). Yet all the other vitamins—which include vitamin E and the B complex factors—and essential trace minerals remain unrestored, along with all the yet-undiscovered nutrients that are doubtless part of the bran and/or germ of wheat.

Virtually all the evidence concerning disease prevalence could support either school of thought, since the milling process has removed *both* the fiber and the micronutrients. As a matter of fact, such data support *any* conclusion derived from factors that occur in advanced but not in primitive cultures—such as the number of television sets, electric can openers, and supermarkets.

The real test of the hypothesis would be to find out which works better—replacing the lost fiber or replacing the lost micronutrients.

Fiber has indeed proven itself useful in solving some problems of the large intestine, just as we would expect. But despite the exuberant claims, it has demonstrated very little effect in controlling major illnesses that do not involve the digestive tract. On the other hand, vitamin therapy does work. Entire schools of medical thought have evolved around it. A large part of this book will show just how nutrition medicine relies on those very vitamins and minerals we currently process out of the foods we most often consume.

I must conclude that though the epidemiological observations upon which the fiber enthusiasts base their conclusions are logical and possibly correct, factors other than the mere presence of fiber must be involved.

There Is Another Theory Too

In all the debate between the fiber enthusiasts and micronutrient advocates, a third problem inherent in our fiberless diet tends to be overlooked. That is the effect of concentrated carbohydrates on our blood sugar levels. American medical leaders as far back as 1923, when Nobel Prize-winner George R. Minot, M.D., first worked out the cause and treatment of pernicious anemia, pointed out that some headache patients are "benefited by a reduction particularly of carbohydrate. . . ."[3]

More recently, H. J. Roberts, M.D., described a large number of patients who suffered from such seemingly diverse conditions as headache or migraine, spontaneous muscle cramps, restless legs, recurrent water retention, obesity, and the sleeping disorder narcolepsy.[4] He was able to show that the denominator common to all these patients was relative hypoglycemia (low blood sugar), which he found in 226 of 421 patients (another 155 had clinical evidence of hypoglycemia but did not have abnormal glucose tolerance test results).

Other clinicians such as E. M. Abrahamson, M.D., co-author of the 1951 best seller *Body, Mind and Sugar*, pointed out that asthma and allergy, as well as arthritis, were associated with this hypoglycemic curve.[5] Others add peptic ulcer to the list.[6] More recently, gout has been included.[7] It is significant that the nutrition-oriented psychiatrist finds the glucose tolerance curve abnormal in a majority of his patients—notably among alcoholics, schizophrenics, children with some behavior disorders, and adults with "nonspecific" disorders.

What Does All This Mean?

All of these correlations indicate that the mechanism for balancing blood sugar is askew in a variety of prevalent and sometimes serious conditions.

Perhaps this is another way of saying that there may be something directly harmful about sugar.

John Yudkin, M.D., professor of nutrition at Queen Elizabeth College, University of London, England, reports that results of all studies combined demonstrate a greater correlation between sugar intake and heart disease than between fat intake and heart disease.[8] He notes that patients who develop coronary heart disease and related vascular diseases have been consuming more sugar than people who do not develop these conditions. More recently, Dr. Yudkin's research has shown that the sugar-sensitive individual, when he consumes sugar, develops an increased clumping of his blood platelets.[9] This platelet adhesiveness has been gaining recognition as a factor closely correlated to the incidence of heart disease.

All of the conditions that I have mentioned as being associated with high blood insulin levels could be quite appropriately considered conditions caused by sugar. Sugar is that concentrated carbohydrate which, more than any other part of our diet, causes insulin levels to go haywire.

Where Does the Problem Lie?

So one school of thought would have you believe that lack of fiber is the root of all evil, and another that lack of vitamins and minerals is the real problem. The third school would tell you that sugar is the main villain. I maintain that they're all valid, some more so than others.

If food were refined to the point where no fiber is left, then surely micronutrients would be refined out, too. I cannot dispute the importance of fiber, and I certainly wouldn't underrate the necessity of micronutrients, either. In my view, sugar comes into the picture not only because the excess of it may give rise to blood sugar instability and problems with the insulin mechanism, but because sugar itself is highly refined and as such takes the place of other, more nutrient-filled sources of calories in our diet. In fact, United States government figures indicate that, by now, three quarters of our carbohydrate intake is from sources classified as refined, and that despite growing concern over nutrition, the proportion is still climbing.[10]

It follows, then, that the composition of your diet should be your single most important nutritional consideration. Supplements are of course valuable. But they are nowhere near as important as a diet that supplies the nutrients nature intended us to have.

How Nutrition Works

To understand how good nutrition improves health, we must know a bit about how we extract energy from food. The delicate balance between the body's energy-extracting and energy-storing functions depends upon a process called metabolism.

Metabolism involves a series of biochemical reactions, each of which is a step toward energy release. These reactions depend upon enzymes, different ones for different reactions.

Many people think an enzyme is a mysterious, complicated thing. But that is not so. An enzyme is simply a protein (that usually incorporates a vitamin and one or more minerals) produced by living cells to bring about chemical reactions. Specifically, an enzyme is neither altered nor destroyed during the chemical process it promotes, and it is responsible for starting in motion a chain of biochemical events. Thus, enzymes are called "organic catalysts." Each individual reaction in the metabolism depends upon an individual, unique enzyme—one that is especially suited to the chemical reaction it governs.

Enzymes are absolutely essential to metabolism. And this is where our nutritional status becomes critical. For if the body is to manufacture enzymes, it must have the appropriate raw materials with which to build them.

Trace minerals and vitamins—essential to the formation of enzymes—*must be supplied by the diet or by dietery supplements*, for without the appropriate enzyme a reaction cannot occur. Enzymatically controlled reactions occur as a series of steps leading to energy release. This sequence is called a metabolic pathway.

When an essential ingredient for making an enzyme is in short supply, a metabolic pathway may be partially blocked by being limited in the rate at which its reactions can progress.

Think of it as traffic funneled into a single lane during superhighway reconstruction. Just as the traffic slows down and backs up, so may metabolic traffic, and not enough energy arrives at its destination to accomplish the full potential of the reaction.

How Our Diet May Shortchange Our Energy Requirements

When certain vitamins and minerals essential to our production of enzymes are refined out of our food, the effect is to deny us the means to make proper use of what we eat. This leaves biochemical roadblocks in our network of metabolic pathways. For example, most vitamin B6 (pyridoxine) is eliminated when wheat is refined to make white flour. (And, unfortunately for us all, it is not restored in the enrichment process either). This reduces our efficiency in metabolizing those very foods that are made with refined white flour.

But don't think that taking a vitamin B6 pill is sufficient to undo the damage—for trace minerals have also been removed from the wheat, as have other vitamins.

Theoretically, the solution would be to eat unrefined whole wheat products. But wheat is only one case in point. Other partitioned foods include most flours, as well as white rice, cornstarch, corn sugar (dextrose) and degerminated cornmeal. (That's what is in the supermarket—the good stuff that's undegerminated is in the health-food store.) They've all been stripped of essential nutrients in refining.

How Does White Sugar Fit In?

White sugar is the worst of all. And not only is it the worst, it's what we get the most of.

In the first place, sugar is devoid of nutrients as a result of the refining process. It is concentrated and provides a dense source of carbohydrate that nature never intended us to have. It's human, of course, for us to enjoy sweets—study after study has shown that human infants select sweetness over other taste sensations, almost without exception.

Secondly, in being almost devoid of nutrients (nutritionally, it's a total loss), sugar lacks the one major element necessary to our making good use of it. Chromium, the mineral that's essential to the glucose tolerance factor—a newly discovered chemical entity essential to the action of insulin on glucose—is missing from refined sugar. So the stumbling block here is that we lack the tools we need to deal with the incredible quantities of refined carbohydrates (and especially sugar) in our society's diet.

Consider our concentrated, sugar-bathed, partitioned foods from this vantage point: Surgeon-Captain T. L. Cleave, the eminent British physician-essayist, acknowledges that man has always had a taste for sweets.[11] And he concedes that this taste is normal, but states unequivocally that man was not meant to eat concentrated (thus, refined) sweets.

He gives the following as an example—which I quote simply because I can't improve upon the way Dr. Cleave says it:

> Let us suppose that you take sugar in its natural form [for example] the ordinary apple. . . . You would need to eat twenty apples a day to get the amount of sugar we get per day in combinations of foods containing refined table sugar. Or you could eat a three-pound sugar beet to get that amount of sugar, but the beet would have to be about the size of a child's head. Either way, eating the twenty apples or the sugar beet would be difficult if not impossible, and if by chance you did manage, you would be eating very little else.

The message is clear. Too much of what we eat is partitioned and unnaturally concentrated.

Dysnutrition: Our Society-Wide Health Problem

When you stop to think about it, it would be surprising if our thoughtless dietary excesses did not have some effect upon us. Just take a close look at the baking-supplies aisle in any supermarket. In addition to white flour and white sugar (a good three brands each in most stores), you will see hosts of mixes. And what do these mixes contain? As though the white flour and white sugar weren't bad enough, they're chock-full of such goodness as chemical emulsifiers, stabilizers, preservatives, flow agents, anti-caking powders, and some antioxidants. (Some people's bodies are incapable of handling these substances, and allergic reactions occur which take the form of hives, nervousness, irritability, depression, and hyperactivity in children, to mention a few.) When you remove the ingredients that are artificially concentrated (the white flour and white sugar) what is left are the ingredients for a respectable—and highly profitable—chemical soup.

If this is what we're offered as food, we have to make considerable effort to achieve a good diet. And most of us don't.

But because our schools, the food industry, and the government haven't taught Americans what and how to eat (and indeed, this is true in most Westernized nations), we just don't know enough to help ourselves. Thus we have left ourselves open to victimization by industrial avarice, which preys on our taste for sweets—the satisfaction of which results in dire nutritional consequences.

Simply put, our disease pattern is the result of society-wide dysnutrition. By dysnutrition, I mean that condition in which *specific nutritional requirements are undersupplied by a diet that is otherwise plentiful* and in some ways oversupplied. (Dysnutrition should be differentiated from malnutrition. In current usage, malnutrition is used to describe "starving" people.) Even obesity, which some call overnutrition, is really an example of dysnutrition. Dysnutrition implies *specific* nutritional imbalances which can be corrected only with *specific* nutrients.

Dysnutrition is the result of the diet that most of us now consume, and it underlies most of our nonbacterial, nonviral diseases. It is becoming harder and harder to deny that dysnutrition is at the root of our man-made diseases, such as hypertension, diabetes, headache, and hypoglycemia. Even though in a sense we are all to blame, dysnutrition is one condition that we as individuals can remedy if we choose to.

We can start right now to remedy the adverse effects our diet produces. But we can't expect miracles. It took our diet a hundred years or so to evolve to its present state—the most recent change being the deluge of refined carbohydrates. We've lived on this diet most or all of our lives, so we can't expect to undo the damage in a trice.

Nonetheless, the nutritional techniques you are about to begin may be so dramatically corrective that you may start feeling better within a few days, and gradually the improvement will grow until, if you are like most of my patients, you will feel better than ever.

Where Do We Begin?

My patients gain their initial insight into the benefits of a nutritional overhaul when they are first placed on my basic vitamin-and-mineral formula (see page 319) combined with one of the basic blood-sugar controlling diets (see page 270). For I have found the most useful approach in all of nutrition is to stabilize the blood sugar.

Blood sugar control depends upon control of insulin release, and that is what the basic diet is all about. Don't underestimate the importance of insulin: More than any other hormone, it is directly involved in governing the energy-releasing process. One of insulin's major functions is to ensure us a steady energy supply, despite the fact that we may eat only three or four times a day. It does this by inhibiting the immediate release of energy and converting the food we eat into stored energy.

The Role of Insulin

Insulin starts the process of carbohydrate (sugar and starch) metabolism by converting blood glucose (sugar) into a form the body can use. For example, it converts glucose to glycogen (muscle sugar) for energy storage in muscles and the liver, and excess glucose to fat for storage in our "fatty deposits." This is why insulin is sometimes called the fattening hormone.

Whereas the regulatory mechanism that governs insulin release is not yet fully understood, we do know that when insulin secretion is stimulated by large amounts of artificially concentrated carbohydrates (especially over a period of years, as in the typical Western diet) the body may overreact, and the excessive response may persist. When this occurs, we call the condition hyperinsulinism.

When sugar enters the bloodstream, insulin is mobilized to bring the level down. And in a susceptible individual—one whose mechanisms are askew—an overreaction would push blood sugar levels down too low or too rapidly, resulting in hypoglycemia (low blood sugar).[12]

Hypoglycemia has many symptoms, some of which include mood swings, depression, irritability, fatigue, hunger, headaches, muscle weakness—the list could go on and on. It is of utmost importance to keep in mind that the average American consumes over 150 pounds of sugar per year as opposed to only 10 pounds 140 years ago.

The body is not capable of handling this amount of sugar. And so it starts to compensate by secreting more insulin to bring the blood sugar level down.

But let's look at what happens next. The individual who feels the adverse effects of hypoglycemia usually wants more sugar in order to bring his blood sugar level back up and relieve his symptoms. The ingested sugar prompts a further secretion of insulin, and so the cycle begins again. Soon the pancreas becomes so sensitized that even a small amount of any simple sugar (glucose from any source) triggers it to secrete insulin. The hyperinsulinism, if untreated, will probably be present for the rest of that individual's life. But other factors (perhaps an insulin antagonist, perhaps the other hormones known as counter-regulatory hormones, or perhaps a shortage of insulin receptors [13]) become operative and may in many patients render the insulin ineffective. In these people the hypoglycemia (low blood sugar) becomes hyperglycemia (high blood sugar) which is commonly known as diabetes. After this stage of high blood sugar and high insulin has persisted long enough, a later stage of diabetes develops in which, as though the pancreas were exhausted, the insulin levels begin to fall and the patient enters the stage known as insulin dependent diabetes.

Most doctors are coming to feel, and I must agree with them, that diabetes and hypoglycemia are so closely related that we must refer to them together as "blood sugar disorders." A significant percentage of patients with hypoglycemia in early life will develop diabetes in later life.

Although all the evidence isn't in, we do understand that when insulin levels are regulated, many patients whom we would otherwise expect to become diabetic do not. Hypoglycemics become controlled and rarely progress to diabetes. Further, other conditions such as hypertension, certain arthritic conditions, certain metabolic imbalances, and other problems would be more likely to develop in an individual with uncontrolled blood sugar. These may be nipped in the bud if blood sugar control is maintained.

By controlling blood sugar, we control the major factor underlying our current disease pattern.

What Insulin Regulation Involves

That is the *why*, but not the *how*. Just to say that a diet that regulates insulin is beneficial, without saying what is *in* the diet, won't help you very much.

To understand the basic principles that underlie the diets for blood sugar control, you must first understand my system for classifying carbohydrates.

I have mentioned that carbohydrates can be refined or unrefined; we can also delineate carbohydrates by molecular makeup. Carbohydrates can be subdivided into two groups: sugars (the simple carbohydrates) and starches (the complex carbohydrates). Add to these distinctions the criteria of refined and unrefined, and note that we can then differentiate four groups of carbohydrates by complexity and refinement.

THE FOUR BASIC CARBOHYDRATE SUBGROUPS

I COMPLEX—UNREFINED	II SIMPLE—UNREFINED
All vegetables All whole grains All whole cereals Nuts Seeds Legumes Greens	All fruit Milk, yogurt, buttermilk Raw honey Sugar cane, molasses
III COMPLEX—REFINED Flour Cornstarch White rice Potato starch Bread, crackers Pasta, etc.	IV SIMPLE—REFINED Sugar Honey Corn syrup, dextrose Fructose Lactose (powdered skim milk) Glucose Maltose (barley malt) Maple syrup Sorbitol

Since we have agreed that wholeness is important and that sugars may have untoward metabolic effects upon us all, you can see that the carbohydrates in quadrant IV are the least desirable, since they provide the greatest stimulus for insulin release, and conversely those in quadrant I are best because they provide the least stimulus. Refined carbohydrates do not belong in the diet; unrefined ones do. There are some people—the overweight in particular—who should avoid virtually all carbohydrates in order to lose weight and progress toward their optimum health. The foods in quadrant I cover the entire spectrum from whole grains to leafy greens. The grains provide the carbohydrate energy we sometimes need to prevent the weight loss that usually occurs when total carbohydrate intake is restricted. The leafy vegetables—the salad greens—provide unabsorbable (unavailable) carbohydrate and some of the bulk necessary for normal bowel function.

What I have learned from working with my patients (and what makes my diets unique) is that the quadrant II carbohydrates, which are principally sugar and are simple rather than complex, even if unrefined, *induce a greater insulin response* than do starch-derived carbohydrates. Thus the latter provide much better blood sugar control. Therefore, the lion's share of carbohydrate in my dietary recommendations must always come from choices in quadrant I.

What About Protein and Fat?

I have concentrated on the carbohydrate part of most people's diets. The rest of the diet should consist of those combinations of protein and fat which occur together in nature and which traditionally constitute our main courses.

Thus, the Atkins Diets may be tailored to your own individual preferences and metabolic needs. If you eat meat, eggs, and dairy products, you may structure your diet around them. Even if you avoid meat, eggs, and dairy products, you can still make the Atkins Diets work for you by building your diet around such vegetarian proteins as nuts, seeds, and soybean products.

It is possible to enjoy a diet while you get the results you want. Overcome the preconception that dieting represents torturous restrictions. The Atkins Diet is luxurious. It is an easy diet, a "fun" diet, and it does not require that you skimp on food.

I devised it because I learned from my patients that they didn't like to be on a diet. Most people, and I am no exception, enjoy eating and will not stick to a diet that's difficult to follow. The real success of any diet in the long run is based on the degree to which the dieter will be satisfied by what he is permitted to eat.

I also favor this diet because it does not, like so many plans in current fashion, restrict foods for the wrong reasons. Eggs, meat, butter, and salt are but a few examples of what a "therapeutic" diet may deny you. Even though in some cases the restrictions are appropriate, I think these cases are far less common than is popularly believed. The exclusion of eggs, salt, fat, and dairy products does nothing to make a diet more pleasant.

The Atkins Diet is effective because it *specifically* corrects the dysnutrition caused by our twentieth-century diet.[14] That diet is under increasing indictment as the cause of so much twentieth-century illness, which has in turn given rise to an epidemic of prescription writing and pill-popping—all to correct conditions which seem to originate in our eating patterns.

The Role of Vitamins and Minerals

In addition to helping his patients control their blood sugar, the nutrition doctor must work with micronutrients and use them in place of pharmaceuticals when necessary. It is worth noting that many cases of blood sugar disorders are caused by deficiencies of specific enzymes, deficiencies that can be corrected by administering the specific vitamin and/or trace mineral that can overcome the specific metabolic impediment.

Thus, dysnutrition can be corrected when the nutrition doctor uses vitamins and minerals much in the way his traditional counterpart uses pharmaceuticals.

Because the vitamins and minerals have such wide potential dosage ranges, my patients work with a variety of doses until we find just the right combination. It's not as slow and tortuous as it sounds—and it certainly has the advantage of being almost free of adverse side effects.

In the chapters that follow, you will read about actual patients and the problems they have overcome or controlled with proper diet, vitamins, and minerals.

I will show you how my patients monitor their progress, shed drugs, and normalize weight, without adverse side effects and without a dietary regimen that is hard to stick to.

Chapter 5

IF YOU WERE MY PATIENT

Before we work out an individualized diet and vitamin scheme, there are certain preliminary steps I go through with my office patients. The information I obtain from the doctor-patient interchange and from laboratory tests provides some of the basis for my subsequent dietary advice.

Again and again I realize how much I must rely upon what a patient tells me. When what a patient says is at variance with what the lab says, I know I must look further or question the laboratory data. I have learned not to discount what my patients say.

Suppose You Were My Patient

When you call my office for an appointment, my nurse always requests the usual information—name, address, telephone number, and the name of the referring physician, if any. In addition, she asks you about your symptoms and painstakingly finds out exactly what medications you may be taking. She then advises you, in accordance with my instructions, which ones to continue and which to discontinue temporarily (because they'll affect the lab tests I'll run) and for how long. Because the first visit includes a glucose tolerance test (GTT), she will inquire whether you are following a special diet. In all cases, she will advise you to eat a "standard balanced diet" that includes a minimum of 600 calories from carbohydrate sources (150 grams of carbohydrates) for at least four days prior to your first office visit. She will further instruct that you eat and drink nothing (except water) after supper the evening before

44

coming to see me. This twelve-hour fast is essential to provide standardization for the glucose tolerance test.

When you arrive at my office for your first visit, one of my nurses will ask for a urine specimen. She will weigh you and take your pulse and blood pressure. All this for "baseline" data.

Then she will draw the blood samples which will be analyzed for all the routine studies any family doctor would require (cholesterol, complete blood count, triglycerides, uric acid, liver, kidney and thyroid profiles, minerals, and the like). In addition, blood will be taken to determine both glucose and insulin levels. This is the first (or the "fasting") sample of the glucose tolerance test—even though you haven't yet taken any glucose. These values will provide a standard of comparison against which to measure later samples.

Then my nurse will hand you a premeasured glucose drink. Blood will be drawn thirty minutes later and then every hour for the next five or six hours to check your blood sugar and insulin levels. (For a complete explanation of the glucose tolerance test, refer to my previous book, *Dr. Atkins' Superenergy Diet*, pages 76–90 paperback, pages 69–81 hardcover.[1])

The GTT is invaluable because it will tell me much more than whether you are hypoglycemic, diabetic, or "normal." It gives me a description of the timing and severity of your biochemical response to nature's primary metabolic fuel, glucose. The results provide descriptive information about your metabolism. Too often doctors ask, "Is it normal or abnormal?" and dismiss anything that falls within normal limits as being outside their province. After all, doctors treat sick people, not well ones.

I Ask a Lot of Questions Even Before I See You

Once you have taken your glucose cocktail and are comfortably seated in the waiting room, you will receive two questionnaires from my nurse.

One is a "general health" questionnaire to give me an overall health picture and a complete history. This goes into your file with your lab results and my notes.

The other questionnaire is less comprehensive, but no less important. It doesn't deal with such general problems and symptoms as chronic cough or postnasal drip. Instead, it lists those symptoms commonly associated with blood sugar disorders and provides useful data in a well-organized, easy-to-assess format. As I scan its columns, I form an impression of the likelihood of your suffering from a blood sugar disorder. I may then further question you about those symptoms which are most likely to be helped by nutritional techniques.

The number and severity of symptoms my patients check off on this sheet correlate closely with their glucose tolerance test results.

I use a questionnaire devised by Harold W. Harper, M.D., reprinted on pages 48–49 with his kind permission.[2] Why not fill it out now and learn to what extent your symptoms are caused by nutritional factors, such as unstable blood sugar or individual food allergies.

Total up your score. If it's greater than 40 points, the possibility of a blood sugar disorder is considerable. If it's greater than 80 points, it is more than probable. If your score is high—say within the 40-and-up range—and you've never had a five- or six-hour glucose tolerance test, you probably should have one as soon as possible.

At this point you and I would sit down for our first consultation. The first thing I need to understand is why you are seeking medical help. Often a patient will say, "I need to lose weight." But further questioning reveals that fatigue, recurrent depression, anxiety attacks, or intractable insomnia are far more urgent problems than are the extra pounds.

I Need to Know How You Eat

And now I do something only a nutrition-oriented doctor would think to do.

I ask you what you eat. That means a complete dietary history.

Usually I ask a number of questions. For example: What do you have for breakfast? How about lunch and supper? What do you eat at snacks? When do you snack? Where do you eat? At home, dinner parties (where you have least control), restaurants, on the run? All this helps me to understand how to personalize your diet.

And then I ask a number of other questions: Do you eat because you are hungry? Or for a pick-me-up? Or from frustration? In response to peer pressure (say, at coffee breaks), to be sociable? Does food ever mean more to you than enjoyment of eating or relief from hunger? When it does, then merely teaching you a new diet may not be sufficient. Perhaps some serious soul-searching is in order.

Are you hungry in the morning? Are you perhaps more hungry after meals than you were when you started to eat? Must you eat to fall asleep? Do you wake up at night to raid the refrigerator? Nighttime awakenings may represent nocturnal hypoglycemia. This pattern can be treated two ways: You can undergo fifteen years' psychotherapy or follow three simple words of advice: Stop eating carbohydrates.

And after you have answered all these questions, I will then ask the most important one of all.

"Is There Anything You Are Sure You Couldn't Live Without?"

Nine times out of ten, my response to the answer is not what my patients would like to hear. (If the answer isn't sweets, chocolate, baked goods, or fruit, then it's coffee, tea, or booze. And failing that, it's something very starchy like white rice, potatoes, pasta, or white bread.)

When I first started to devise diets for my patients, I always tried to show some mercy and allow small portions of favorite foods. But I soon learned that those patients who eliminated them entirely were the most successful.

It wasn't that those who indulged their cravings cheated. I'm sure that at first they had only the "sliver" or "tiny spoonful" I permitted, and only as often as I allowed. I am also confident that these patients didn't extend their indulgence to other almost-favorite foods.

Some Foods Are Addictive

The cardinal rule is this: Most hypoglycemics *are addicted to sugar*—even though sugar may be the worst thing in the world for this condition.[3] Sugar really does relieve symptoms of hypoglycemia—for a little while. But then insulin is released, rapidly using up the blood glucose, the blood sugar level goes down, and the newfound relief subsides as quickly as it was felt. The luckless sugar addict then feels even worse than before.[4]

This is the addiction cycle: If sugar made the hypoglycemic feel better in the first place, and now he feels worse, then why not take more . . . ? And so it begins—take sugar, feel better for a little while, feel worse, take sugar, and so on.

Sugar isn't the only addictive substance in our diet. Caffeine (in cola drinks—both regular and low-calorie, coffee, tea, etc.) may raise insulin levels and thereby cause blood sugar levels to drop. Caffeine, too, can be addictive.

Giving up favorite foods isn't easy, and I don't relish telling patients to do without, for example, their morning coffee. Especially

HARPER HEALTH INDICATOR TEST

Check off each symptom that you have according to its severity.

- (0) means you never have the symptom,
- (1) means it is mild when it occurs or it occurs occasionally,
- (2) means moderate or occurring at least once a week, and
- (3) means severe or occurring frequently.

Multiply the number of checks in each column by the number at the top of the column and then add the numbers in the three columns to get your total score.

0	1	2	3	
				Tired all the time
				Hungry between meals or at night
				Depressed
				Insomnia
				Wake up after a few hours sleep
				Fearful (overwhelmed by people, places, or things)
				Can't decide easily
				Can't concentrate
				Poor memory
				Worry frequently
				Feel insecure or low self-image
				Highly emotional
				Moody
				Cry easily, or feel like crying inside
				Fits of anger
				Magnify insignificant details (make mountains out of molehills)
				Eat candy, cake, cookies, or drink soda pop
				Eat bread, pasta, potatoes, rice, or beans
				Consume alcohol

			Drink more than 3 cups of coffee or cola drinks daily
			Crave candy, soda, or coffee between meals or mid-afternoon
			Can't work well under pressure
			Headaches
			Sleepy during the day
			Sleepy or drowsy after meals
			Lack of energy
			Reduced initiative
			Can't get started in the morning
			Eat when nervous
			Stomach cramps or "nervous stomach"
			Allergies: asthma, hay fever, skin rash, sinus touble, etc.
			Fatigue relieved by eating
			Suicidal thoughts or tendencies, feelings of hopelessness
			Bored
			Bad dreams
			Irritable before meals
			Heart beats fast (palpitations)
			Get shaky inside if hungry
			Feel faint if meal is delayed
			Ulcers, gastritis, chronic indigestion, abdominal bloating
			Cold hands or feet
			Trembling (shaking) of the hands
			Blurred vision
			Bleeding gums
			Dizziness, giddiness, or light-headedness
			Aware of breathing heavily
			Bruise easily
			Reduced sex drive
			Incoordination (drop or bump into things)
			Sweating excessively
			Unsocial or anti-social behavior
			Muscle twitching or cramps
			Excessive thirst
			Phobias
			Weight change
			Frequent urination
			TOTAL

since I do without it myself these days. It struck me several months ago that I really *needed* that after-meal cup of coffee—and I knew it was time to kick the coffee habit, because it had apparently become an addiction. I did, and it wasn't as bad as I thought it would be.

Food Allergy May Also Cause Addiction

Certain foods to which an individual may be allergic are addictive.

If a person has an allergy to a food, he will most likely crave it. Thus his "trigger" foods will both relieve his craving and aggravate an allergic response. A vicious cycle develops: Crave the trigger food, ingest it, feel better, feel worse, need it again.

The chapter on food allergy contains a list of foods most likely to trigger allergic responses. You may find it useful when you suspect food allergy. In the same chapter you will find information about some easy-to-perform tests that should help you identify foods that bring on allergic reactions, as well as more sophisticated tests that require both a laboratory and your doctor's cooperation.

Then We Talk About Diet

Once we have discussed your food cravings, I often ask, "Have you ever been on a diet that relieved your symptoms?" Most patients tell about a past regimen that consisted of eating very wisely. And almost all of them report that they felt better when they ate this way.

My next question opens the most important discussion: *"If you felt better, then why didn't you stick to the regimen?"* And this is how I approach the most valuable contribution that I (or any other doctor, for that matter) can make. Help a patient motivate himself.

I often tell my patients that *the easiest thing I do is to tell them what to eat. The hardest is to get them to do it.* The guidance of a physician often allows a patient to gain insight, motivation, and commitment.

Our discussions concluded, I do a physical exam—which includes an electrocardiogram, and a chest X ray if indicated. This is critical, because neither my office patients nor you should undertake a change in dietary regimen without a thorough medical evaluation.

So far, with the possible exception of the GTT and some vitamin and mineral determinations, I have done the tests that almost any family physician would do. But I've done them in a slightly different frame of reference. Instead of looking for disease to attack, I look for ways to improve your health.

Then I recommend a diet for the first week.

What the First Week's Diet Does

The first week's regimen isn't permanent, but it does do something very positive. It stabilizes the blood sugar quickly and provides the groundwork we need to devise a longer-term diet that's just right for you.

I call the first week Sorting-Out Week. In many ways, a patient's first diet week is the most important of all. Because this is the week in which we will learn which symptoms are relieved when blood sugar has been controlled.

If your mood improves, your sleep pattern gets better, your energy level goes up, or your symptoms disappear during the first week, it's obvious that something we did nutritionally is responsible for the benefit.

If, on the other hand, some of your symptoms remain unchanged while others improve or disappear, we may suspect that these remaining symptoms are not responsive to your new diet.

The most workable hypothesis is this: Those symptoms that clear up promptly on the diet were probably caused by blood sugar instability or by an allergy to a food we eliminated or by a nutritional imbalance corrected by the vitamin and mineral regimen.

In all cases, the first week sorts out those symptoms that are likely to respond to the nutritional techniques from those that *may* not. Those factors that didn't respond may be related to nutrition, certainly, but they may respond only to a longer-term regimen.

The short-term nutritional factor is usually the blood-sugar-related disorders which generally clear up in the first four to five days of your new regimen.

The Second Visit

By the second visit, we will have a lot to talk about. My first question, just to be on the safe side, will be to ask how well you followed your diet. If you are like most of my patients, chances are that you followed it well. Although the diet does seem a little strange to many people at first, most find it luxurious and easy to follow.

You will tell me which symptoms went away and which ones remain. I review any change in pulse, blood pressure, and weight, and then go over the first week's laboratory data, looking for information about your general medical condition. I'll pay particular attention to the GTT findings and closely examine the insulin levels, because when they are abnormally elevated it points rather strongly to a diagnosis of blood sugar disorder.

(Since my last book was published, testing for insulin levels has become more economically feasible, and I have discovered that a significant number of patients with seemingly normal glucose tolerance test results have abnormal insulin elevations. Thus I am forced to conclude that the incidence of blood sugar disturbances is even higher than I once thought.)

It seems appropriate to mention here that medicine is still, to a great degree, a matter of judgment. Although there is some science in terms of laboratory data and statistics, the physician *must* assess each case individually and do what he can, based upon his knowledge, experience, and intuition.

The doctor must treat the patient now on the basis of what he knows *now*. Conservatism applied at this point is callous. Many patients will happily try something that's iffy, so long as it is safe or without adverse side effects.

And this is one of the advantages of nutrition medicine. Most of the nutrition doctor's techniques are in keeping with Hippocrates' dictum "First do no harm." Direct adverse effects or toxic reactions are virtually unheard of. And although many of the techniques are not proven to the satisfaction of the establishment (more about this in the next chapter), they have been shown to work in clinical practice. The problem is that they don't lend themselves to the sacred "double blind" study so often required for "proof."

Nutrition doctors have a saying: "In nutrition, the worst thing that can happen is nothing." The nutrition doctor recognizes that harmful outcome is a remote possibility indeed.

The Nutrition Doctor Relies upon Many Diagnostic Techniques

If, during your second visit—and maybe during your fourth, fifth, or tenth—you are still struggling with some symptoms, I may order a hair analysis to obtain a mineral profile.

It is convenient and requires very little hair, taken from the nape of the neck where it won't show. Seeking to understand a patient's mineral profile is different from seeking to understand a disease (or seeking a disease, for that matter). It is a way to get information that's *descriptive*. One patient may be lower in calcium and higher in manganese than another, but both may feel fine. Another patient's mineral values may be in the middle range, but if some minerals are out of balance with one another, then there could be room for improvement.

Hair analysis can tell me if you are low in zinc, chromium, manganese, and other trace minerals—or too high in such toxic ones as mercury, lead, cadmium, and copper. Further, it is just beginning to show promise as a diagnostic tool. Certain patterns seem to emerge in patients with arthritis, schizophrenia, diabetes, and other diseases. (See Chapter 30.)

Visit by visit, step by step, I gain insight into your health status and eating needs. And visit by visit I modify the diet and do what tests may be necessary to further identify (and treat) whatever problems remain.

Significantly, many of my patients eventually see a correlation between what they eat and their old symptoms.

Judith Brand, who first came in with arthritis, followed my diet very closely for several weeks. She stopped limping and went back to playing tennis—and as long as she stuck to her diet and took her vitamins, she felt great. Then one week she came in with a surprising flare-up of her joint pains (just when I thought we had seen the last of them, too), convinced that she had not gone off her regimen. I suggested that she review everything she'd had to eat or drink over the past few days to see if she could find any slip-ups.

Sure enough. When Judith came in the next week, she told me that when she checked her refrigerator closely, she discovered that her bottle of "diet" soda wasn't dietetic at all. Even this unwitting intake of sugar was sufficient to bring back her joint pains.

And, as Judith said to me, "To think that I used to eat that way every day of my life!"

Another young woman, Beth Marshall, who had been a chronic nighttime eater, was cured of nighttime eating within three days of starting her diet. To her amazement, she began to sleep through the night.

But on her fourth visit she reported to me that she'd been up again—eating. When I questioned her closely, she sheepishly admitted that she had eaten a piece of birthday cake. Then, she told me, she had gone on from there because "it hadn't seemed to make a big difference." In short, she was sneaking little bits of cake a few times a day.

But when she was back on her diet for three full days, she slept through the night once more. Her wakefulness was more convincing than my words in driving home the point that her self-indulgent behavior could (and did) make all the difference.

You Are Almost Ready to Get Started

I have stressed the importance of such preliminaries as an electro-cardiogram, a physical exam, and laboratory tests (including a glucose tolerance test) before embarking upon a new dietary regimen.

And I am suggesting that you go to your doctor for these tests. He would be remiss if he didn't ask you why you want them, and though he may do what you request, he may miss the significance of your test results. He may or may not think that nutrition will help. (More about *why not* in the next chapter.)

If he cooperates, both of you will probably gain insight into why the nutrition movement is becoming a revolution.

Whatever you do, though, be sure that you are fully aware of your medical condition when you begin to change your patterns—and do it (preferably) under the watchful eye of a health professional, one who can put your health situation and your nutritional needs in proper perspective.

Chapter 6

THE MEDICAL MENTALITY

Up to this point, I have implied that your doctor might be less than cooperative when you say you would like to try a nutritional approach to your health. And you may be wondering why I say this again and again, as though I know beforehand what he might say. Experience has taught me how doctors react to the prospect of nutrition, so in that sense, I *can* anticipate how he'll react. With few exceptions, our doctors are card-carrying members of a medical establishment. And they have a big stake in continuing that membership.

Why Our Doctors Toe the Line

Most doctors today belong to local and state medical societies, and about half of them belong to the American Medical Association (AMA). The goals of these medical organizations are no different from those of other self-interested associations. Members who stay in line are supported; those who go astray may be censured. The society must preserve solidarity among the ranks, maintain a unified front at all times. Thus, I urge you not to lose sight of the fact that an AMA statement seems to represent primarily the interests of its membership (the doctors) and not necessarily those of the public at large.

Fresh air and ideas from the outside are heretical, dangerous, and threatening. The more so since nobody has the time to examine new concepts carefully, and it is so much easier to reject them and their proponents out of hand.

Thus, when a physician gives his opinion he relies upon the strength of numbers. He may preface it with such phrases as "the consensus is that . . ." or "accepted medical practice dictates . . ." or "most doctors believe. . . ." When he uses these phrases he is both drawing strength from fellow doctors and toeing the party line. Neat, isn't it?

What happens when someone with a new idea comes along?

The Galileo Syndrome

Galileo asserted that the world was round (spherical) rather than flat (disc-shaped). He had evidence, he said. He had tests. He had proof. But did anyone believe him? Did they examine his mathematical proof with open minds? Hardly. (Well, they did look at his math, but because they assumed the world was flat, they refused to accept Galileo's data. Now, three and a half centuries later, we have seen the best evidence refuting the calorie theory thrown out, on the basis that it cannot be right because we all know that "a calorie is a calorie." The establishment somehow doesn't seem to accept the fact that it is possible to lose more weight on a low-carbohydrate diet than by fasting.)

When someone advances a new idea today—for example, that certain mental illnesses may be treated with massive doses of vitamins —the establishment reacts with a negative snort. "How can this be?" "It goes against all our teaching, all our practice!" "We can't believe this!" "It can't be true because we all know vitamins are to prevent deficiency!" And there the subject ends. Of course, the doctors who advanced the new ideas are censured and discredited. They lose their chance to discourse with the prevailing establishment.

They may be avoided by their establishment peers, bad-mouthed, or even expelled from their medical societies and associations. I know of many situations in which medicine has lost a valuable practitioner and contributor because the group in power has lifted a so-called dissident's license to practice. *And this only because he practiced differently, not badly.*

After all, the establishment must hold the line. A doctor whose ideas make him more effective than his peers is often viewed as a threat. Only the respectable, tried and true, "proven" cures and remedies may receive that sacred endorsement.

The standard of proof these days is the "double blind study," something the FDA requires of pharmaceutical companies when they attempt to prove that a drug is effective.[1] If, for example, a pharmaceutical company were trying to prove that aspirin cured warts, they would round up a great many "otherwise healthy volunteers" who were plagued by warts. They would try to match each group member to another person by age, sex, and other factors, and then designate the warty crowd as groups A and B, each member of group A having a counterpart in group B. This is known as a one-to-one correspondence.

Group A and group B would be told that they were getting "wart medicine" and that the groups' results would be compared at the end of the study to see which group did better.

If the group on aspirin showed significant loss of warts, then—in that particular study—the aspirin would be deemed effective. When more studies were done and the results repeated, aspirin would be regarded as a cure for warts.

Only one group would really get the aspirin. The other group would get an identical-looking placebo. To be sure the test was impartial, the doctors giving out the pills would not know which patient was getting what, since they would receive their precoded bottles of pills from a third party.

There is a variation of this protocol called the single blind, in which the patient doesn't know what he's getting but the doctor *does* know what he is giving. Contemporary medicine doesn't award this study protocol the same weight as the double blind.

Nutrition Medicine Does Not Lend Itself to the Double Blind

A doctor locked into a fixed treatment protocol would find it difficult to practice nutrition medicine effectively because a physician must be able to vary the dosage according to patient response.[2] So a double blind with all patients taking the same dosage would be virtually useless in a nutritional study, because every patient would require individualized dosage to get the same effect.

Unfortunately, the type of proof offered by nutrition specialists is not acceptable to the establishment, as a rule. Remember, most of today's medicine developed in studies that were not double blind. Rather, if an astute clinician observed that a number of similar cases responded to the same techniques, he would announce that he had found a regimen that worked. His research was always mediated by his own skills as a physician (impossible in the double blind). Dr. James Lind, in 1747, was able to prove that scurvy was caused by nutritional factors by feeding lemons to only two subjects out of twelve. Most of the medical knowledge inherited by all but the last two generations of physicians was acquired without the double blind protocol.

In the old-fashioned way of showing that something works, a doctor treats a number of cases of a given illness and tabulates the results. If I were doing a tabular study on arthritics' response to a new treatment, I would take a hundred or more consecutive cases and tabulate the results as "better," "worse," and "unchanged." My peers could then judge the effectiveness of my regimen by comparing it with the results they achieve using their own protocols. And if I reported that ninety-five out of a hundred patients got better or showed some improvement, I am sure that most of my colleagues would take notice. If their results on the regimens they now use are not as good, then they might feel it worthwhile to try what made my patients better. Unfortunately, it doesn't work that way.

Specifically, my records do indeed show that over 90 percent of hypertensive patients who followed my diet and vitamin regimen had either significant drops in their blood pressure or were able to reduce or completely discontinue their medication. Does this constitute proof that my techniques work? No, indeed it does not! The tabular studies are termed "anecdotal" by today's establishment, and are not considered sufficient for proof. Even if I were to review fifteen thousand patients and showed that the cure percentages held, my colleagues still could not accept my findings, simply because my study wasn't double blind.

Although pharmaceutical companies don't exactly like or welcome the testing the FDA requires, they will claim that their tests constitute proof, and use their results as selling tools in marketing their drugs to doctors. The doctor-to-be is exposed to this "here's proof—our latest double blind study" promotion from the first day of medical school.

Pharmaceutical companies do a lot more than promote their drugs. They give grants, provide scholarships, present awards, and distribute "reminders" and premiums—pens, calendars, tape-booklet learning programs, and the like. Some legislators have actively opposed such practices. Senator Edward Kennedy of Massachusetts has long campaigned against certain forms of drug marketing. He has come down hard on gifts to doctors and has worked to attempt to clean up the claims that may be made for various agents. But the pharmaceutical companies' aggressive market-related efforts have helped establish the double blind study as virtually the only acceptable proof that a drug or other agent is effective.

The double blind, appropriate as it is for testing potentially harmful drugs, is grossly inappropriate in assessing the medicine of tomorrow. For tomorrow's medicine, which I believe can be practiced today, involves identifying environmental and life-style factors that are harmful to our health. The next step, of course, is to overcome them.

Having read this book, you may go to your doctor convinced that nutrition is the answer, not drugs. But before you leave his office you may find a prescription in your hand. Did you ever stop to wonder why?

Because it is simpler to write a prescription. After all, the faster the doctor gets his patients in and out of his office, the more patients he can treat and the more disease he can stamp out. Or if he is in a clinic situation, the sooner he can go back to his critically ill patients, the happier he will be.

I'd wager that most doctors would feel naked without their prescription pads. Why? No doctor can escape the message of his medical training, which tells him that pharmaceuticals are the best form of treatment.

He has been taught that drugs clear up symptoms. Thus, to treat patient, match drug to symptom. There's relatively little concern about treating the whole person and balancing the system to eliminate *causes* of disease. Even though there is ample evidence for the nutritional cause of disease, doctors are still not taught that faulty nutrition may be at the root of many diseases and conditions. This is because a nutritional disease implies a nutritional correction. Not a pharmaceutical one. And by now the pharmaceutical industry is too deeply entrenched (both philosophically and economically) in our medical institutions.

So the doctors keep overprescribing drugs and underestimating nutrition.

When the Doctor Can't Write a Prescription

If your situation doesn't lend itself to drug therapy, you may have a particularly exasperating experience in store. Your treatment may consist of a truism such as, "Relax, it's your nerves," or "You'll just have to learn to live with it."

When a doctor doesn't know the answer, he may, in self-defense, use one or more of several tactics. If your doctor thinks something is noncontributory or unimportant, he may ignore your question. He'll just forget that it ever came up and will continue the discussion on the last topic he felt comfortable with. Or he may change the subject or turn the tables. For example, if your doctor feels uncomfortable when confronted with your complaint of chronic fatigue, he may bring up your job insecurity, your unhappy marital situation, or the fact that you've had trouble with your kids lately.

I seriously doubt that he sincerely believes these problems are the cause of fatigue, but it puts *you* on the hot seat, not him. A doctor is usually on safe ground when he asserts that a patient's life situation, whatever it may be, is a source of anxiety or frustration. Or he may counterattack on something entirely irrelevant—such as a high cholesterol reading. If the problem *you bring up* never seems to be dealt with, it may be because your doctor feels there is nothing he can do for it. He may feel just plain helpless and defenseless when you complain about something he's not sure he can effectively treat.

Another common ploy is to refer the case to another physician. Often, in fact, a referral to the right doctor is the greatest contribution to the patient a physician might make. But all too frequently it's merely a way to unload the patient he can't handle.

When a doctor has a pretty good idea of what is wrong, but feels that he lacks the experience or the self-confidence to deal with it, he may call upon his colleagues. It is politically sound, because he is showing support and approval of the physician to whom he refers, and it helps to create a reciprocal structure of obligation.

The problem with referrals, though, is that specialists tend to see only one narrow viewpoint. A referral does seem to obligate a specialist to do an exhaustive work-up in his field in order to rule out any possibilities the referring doctor may have missed. So the neurologist might order a brain scan to diagnose headache, or the gastroenterologist might order a GI series (X rays) for your chronic heartburn, just to be on the safe side. And if the referral is to a psychiatrist, is he likely to tell you, "No, your head's in fine shape"?

These tactics are understandable. And I sympathize. For the contemporary doctor is trained to deal in a stepwise logic. He tries to build a logical treatment structure for everything he sees. He is lost when he cannot identify a disease or a symptom. His training tells him to be logical, but it backfires when he has no clear-cut diagnosis.

Over-Reliance on Laboratory Data Leads to Under-Reliance on the Patient

The doctor's demand for scientific proof leads him to require laboratory confirmation of his suspicions. This may backfire when lab tests come back normal or when they indicate an abnormality in someone who has no symptoms. A doctor may refuse to treat a patient whose symptoms indicate a major dietary problem, but he will almost invariably attack an elevated cholesterol level.

Thus, all too often, a patient's words fall upon deaf ears. For some reason, many doctors simply assume that their patients are incapable of giving accurate information about how they feel. So the physician may rely almost solely upon the laboratory, and will then treat individual patients as though they were statistics.[3] When this happens, he will ignore those diet-related dizzy spells and aggressively treat only asymptomatic laboratory-found abnormalities.

I do not dispute that laboratory data is useful, and I do make heavy use of it myself. But many's the time that a patient's lab tests have been equivocal—for example, in terms of thyroid function. Although I could interpret the lab tests to mean that the patient's thyroid is within low normal limits, if the patient reports feeling sluggish, cold, and depressed, I look beyond the laboratory data. I may ask the patient to take his underarm temperature first thing in the morning, before getting out of bed, for a few days and report back to me. If the patient's temperatures are very low (below 97°) I then have evidence that the patient may indeed have a sluggish thyroid. No matter what the lab tests said. But if I didn't listen to the patient, I'd miss this clue and many others as well.

Why Your Doctor May Not Approve of the Nutritional Approach

In the first place, the nutritional approach may seem to be at odds with the pharmaceutical approach your doctor has been taught. Like me, he may feel that such drugs as digitalis and adrenaline have a place in medical practice—they can, after all, save lives. But he may not recognize that the real problem is the *long-term* use of many other types of drugs. Antidepressants, tranquilizers, antihypertensives, and, for that matter, any drug that could be avoided by using some alternate form of therapy are the issue. These drugs are prescribed for patients who then take them (and perhaps rely upon them) for years at a time.

But even beyond all his drug-oriented training, your doctor has probably heard the American Medical Association and "experts from leading universities" come down hard on nutrition.[4]

In fact, you will probably find that your doctor, if he is at all like the many physicians I know, indulges in a sort of medicine worship with an almost religious fervor. His faith in his own profession is unshakable. This comes out most illuminatingly when, in discussing an alternative technique he is not familiar with, he will ask this rhetorical question: "If that approach were so effective, don't you think we would all be using it?"

Your doctor may be reluctant to deviate from accepted, standard medical practice. Or he may not know enough about nutritional techniques to be aware that they are completely safe.[5] And it may not occur to him to use nutrition while gradually weaning a patient from his drugs.

Maybe You Can Try to Work with Your Doctor

A book such as this one certainly isn't intended as a substitute for medical care by the reader's own doctor. But it is a good way to let the reader in on some nutritional techniques that yield good results for my patients. If you tried some of them and were successful, it would be hard for your doctor to argue with someone who told him, "I tried it, and it works." I, for one, have never been able to argue with a patient's success.

Is a Calorie Just a Calorie?

Your doctor has probably heard that "a calorie is a calorie" and doesn't see why you, or anyone else, should avoid carbohydrates as long as you're getting as many (or as few) calories as you need.[6] He may not differentiate between refined and unrefined carbohydrates, using just that reasoning. Further, he may believe the authorities who say that a low-calorie diet is the lifetime answer to obesity. (In full understanding of the fact that over 90 percent of seriously overweight subjects on a standard low-calorie diet either fail to lose weight or gain it back, and that the majority of these dieters report emotional symptoms—usually depression.)[7]

Your doctor may have heard that "in this affluent society, we are all well nourished." He may consider middle-class synonymous with well-fed. He may not realize that *dysnutrition* is rampant among us all and that the malnutrition one may see in poverty areas isn't the only possible nutritional deficit.

Your doctor may have gone to school where his professors received grants from the food and drug industries. And may have been taught their "line."

In sum, he probably thinks that nutrients are safe but ineffective.

And he may think that dietary manipulation is pointless or risky. And that's where you may be able to set him straight.

Sometimes Doctors Are Not Even Willing to Give Nutrition a Try

In case you think that the medical opposition to nutrition is merely due to lack of interest, consider the militant reaction met by a psychiatric resident friend of mine when he attempted to institute nutritional diagnosis and treatment of mentally ill patients.

This young physician ordered a GTT on a schizophrenic patient because he had noted that the patient's behavior seemed to get worse when he ate more sugars. For this act, the board placed my friend on probation and told him firmly that "medicine is not practiced this way here," ordering him to stick to the accepted protocols of the hospital.

And when my friend ordered a low-carbohydrate diet for a grossly overweight patient, the order was overridden by his chief. Further, he reports that his hospital will not allow a patient to receive more than three grams of vitamin C per day and that individual B vitamins may not be ordered at all. A patient may receive only those B vitamins in the low-dosage multiple-vitamin combination approved by the hospital formulary committee.

The distressing thing about this doctor's experience is that he was trying to help his patients and that the techniques he wanted to try could in no way have hurt them. I find it surprising that the medical establishment in this hospital wasn't curious about what he might turn up. Maybe the results would have been startlingly good and everyone might have learned something. One wonders whether the medical hierarchy might have been unwilling to risk that the patient might get well, and thus weaken their antinutrition stance. After all, a low-carbohydrate diet and glucose tolerance tests certainly do not make patients sicker.

Another example of establishment attacks on nutrition is that of a leading antinutrition spokesman, Victor Herbert, M.D., who subjects other physicians to this logic: If vitamin C has antihistamine activity (which he admits it does), why not just take an antihistamine (i.e., a drug)? [8] He recommends a blocking agent (antihistamine) instead of an enabling agent (a vitamin). Now, does that make sense? The antihistamine has side effects such as drowsiness, dry mouth, and dizziness, to name but a few. Vitamin C certainly wouldn't cause these problems.

Just keep in mind that your doctor hears or reads statements like Dr. Herbert's on an almost daily basis. And nobody mentions that the vitamin C may have beneficial effects on gum tissue, capillaries, and even on resistance to cancer.[9]

Do you still wonder why your doctor might object? He is simply not trained or equipped to deal with the nutrition question. Let us hope that he will at least be open-minded and say, "Well, it can't hurt. Let's give it a try."

BOOK TWO

BOOK TWO

INTRODUCTION

I once asked an author how long it had taken him to write the book he had just published. He replied, "It took me all my life." I now realize what he meant, for I have had a similar experience in writing Book Two of *Dr. Atkins' Nutrition Breakthrough*.

The following chapters are products of my life's work as a physician and nutritional specialist. Incorporated in them are twenty-one years of experience in helping patients with everyday symptoms like headaches and the common cold and more complicated problems like depression and alcoholism. Behind me, and I hope in my future, are many pleasurable hours of guiding back to health patients with such degenerative diseases as diabetes, hypertension, and heart disease.

These patients continue to trust me with their health and their lives. I thank all of them. They have contributed greatly to my knowledge. Because of them—and, of course, the researchers who have turned the dream of treating illness with nature's own elements into a scientific reality—I have been able to develop a nutritional treatment regimen for a broad variety of physical and mental disorder. I know these regimens work because I have observed the progress of a significant number of my own patients who have successfully followed the nutritional recommendations set down here.

Book Two is a guide to good health. Included in it is information you can use to help yourself overcome the most common disorders physicians treat. All of these problems are caused or aggravated by dysnutrition—that metabolic imbalance due either to an overload of substances found in our over-refined diet or to deficiences of the vital nutrients we need to sustain good health. The goal for each individual is to conquer dysnutrition, and thus the illnesses which are caused by it.

Our health problems have been treated much too long with pharmaceuticals. There are safer methods, natural methods, detailed in the chapters to come. Implementing the information in this book to obtain the right selection of vitamins and minerals and the right blood sugar control diet, can both alleviate the symptoms of emotional problems, everyday illnesses, and degenerative diseases, and correct the very cause.

PART I
Improving Mental Health

Chapter 7

APPROACHES TO
EMOTIONAL PROBLEMS

The kind of medicine I now practice is generally referred to as orthomolecular medicine—or treating human illness by varying the concentration of substances *normally* present in the human body. This specialty—whether it is based upon large doses of vitamins or minerals, or upon a special diet—really has its roots in the field of psychiatry. The word "orthomolecular" was coined by Linus Pauling, who used it to point up the importance of making the biochemical environment just right.[1] When these treatment principles were expanded beyond psychiatry to include the entire health picture, the term "orthomolecular medicine" was adopted.

In 1951 Abram Hoffer and Humphry Osmond, on not much more than an educated hunch, first treated a schizophrenic patient with large doses of niacinamide and noted a dramatic response.[2]

We now know how fortunate it was that this patient responded—since not everyone with the same type of problem does. This lucky circumstance led to further trials involving nutrients as treatments for human illness. After a while, vitamins C and B_6 were added to the niacin regimen. More recently, the science has expanded with the understanding of the roles of vitamins B_{12},[3] folic acid, pantothenic acid, and of zinc, manganese, tryptophan,[4] and B_{15}.

At present, there are three basic approaches to psychiatric care: the traditional (verbal counseling), the psychopharmacological (use of drugs affecting brain metabolism), and the orthomolecular or nutritional. Although the three schools of thought are quite distinct, I suspect that the best psychiatrist would be one who is proficient in all three.

71

How the Three Approaches Interrelate

The drug-oriented psychiatrist may prescribe drugs that are geared specifically to eliminating the target symptom—such as anxiety. He and I do have something in common. We both recognize the importance of biochemical factors, and we each rely upon those tools we have learned to use. Drugs, however, may not get to the cause of the problem. And that's where the traditional talk therapist comes in. He would avoid drugs or limit their use to supporting the patient while he talks out his problems and uncovers the deeply buried neurotic difficulty. Most individuals would benefit from talking their problems out with the right therapist, but unless the biochemical factors contributing to the illness are identified and corrected, all the talking circumvents the fundamental problem.

The orthomolecular doctor, like the psychopharmacologist, treats the individual biochemically. However, he does it with enabling agents rather than blocking agents—with nature's tools, rather than man's. He recognizes that emotional symptoms are often the outward manifestations of a body that is out of balance. Thus, instead of focusing on a particular symptom, my nutrition-oriented colleagues and I *use the symptoms as clues to find out where and why there is a physiologic (not emotional) imbalance.*

The Role of Blood Sugar

For example, Jack L. Ward, M.D., a pioneer orthomolecular psychoanalyst, reported in the textbook *Endocrinology and Diabetes* that 891 psychiatric patients were tested for blood sugar disorders.[5] Four out of five of these patients displayed relative hypoglycemia according to his criteria. Dr. Ward concluded that there is a correlation between blood sugar disorders and mood difficulties. And although he does not claim that merely correcting the blood sugar abnormality will cure the psychiatric problem, he strongly suggests that a patient is more open to any kind of therapy once his blood sugar is stabilized. Briefly, he contends that any psychiatric patient should have a five-hour glucose tolerance test, because control of hypoglycemia plays a major role in almost every patient.

My Approach to Emotional Problems

I am not a psychiatrist. Yet I've been practicing psychiatry ever since I hung out my shingle. In fact, any doctor who treats patients *must* practice psychiatry, because every patient has emotions that affect his state of well-being either directly or indirectly.

Many times, patients come to me seeking nutritional treatment of problems which appear to be purely psychiatric.[6] Some of my most startling (and gratifying) successes have been achieved with patients who have obsessive-compulsive disturbances, anorexia nervosa, phobia (of which the fear of leaving the home, agoraphobia, is the most common), manic-depressive mood cycles, and the like.[7] Over the last thirty years, the nutritional treatment for schizophrenia, our most prevalent psychosis, has been developed by the orthomolecular psychiatrists to such an extent that the treatment protocol has been almost standardized.[8]

These conditions require the help of a trained orthomolecular physician, so it would not be appropriate to discuss them here. But many of us who apparently function normally are plagued with everyday emotional symptoms—depression, anxiety, addictions, inability to concentrate, confusion, loss of memory or self-esteem. These people can be helped immeasurably by nutritional techniques —often the same ones used in treating the more serious disorders— and I'd like to tell you how it can be done.

Chapter 8

INSOMNIA

I doubt that there's a doctor anywhere who has not heard, "I can't sleep. Can you give me a sleeping pill?"

The patient generally assumes that he or she has a right to a sleeping medication, that the doctor will see his or her *need* for it, and will prescribe one without question. This is the usual practice —but is it correct?

First and foremost, insomnia is usually a symptom of dysnutrition. In fact, the psychic or emotional stress, the environmental stress, and the everyday events that "cause" insomnia aren't really the causes at all.

These stresses would still be stresses, but you would take them in stride if your vitamin and mineral balance and your diet were right for you.

So when we talk about insomnia, we have to think about why your body is keeping you awake.

Recently, sleep problems have been the subject of a great deal of scientific, sleep lab investigation. Insomniacs, by definition, need a longer time after turning out the lights to get into the first stages of sleep. Sleep studies also show that insomniacs have disturbances of their deep sleep and their rapid eye motion (REM) dream phases, too. Worse still, many of the tossers and turners awaken in the morning (or are still awake) complaining of "no rest."

Several factors—such as a reaction to crisis or stress—may change sleep habits, and the sleep pattern never returns to normal. Most significantly, sleeping pills change sleep patterns, and may in fact worsen the very problem they are supposed to help.

You May Need Less Sleep Than You Think

Many of my patients who complain of insomnia don't have it at all. Somehow they have been indoctrinated into thinking that they *must* have a good eight hours' sleep every night, and they have not learned to be satisfied with anything less. Their "insomnia" may be their body's way of saying, "But I don't need all this sleep."

Sleep Requirement Is a Good Measurement of Health Status

I have noticed over the years that those who seem to enjoy the best of health require about six hours' sleep, or less. If you function well on four, five, or six hours' sleep but fear that you should get more, stop worrying. You are probably getting as much sleep as you require.

Sometimes sleep habits change quite dramatically when nutritional status improves.

Suzie Low, a patient who came to me for a skin problem, reported that she was going to bed one and a half hours later and awakening an hour earlier after only one week of following her new diet and vitamin-with-minerals plan. She was ecstatic. She felt more vital, more alert upon awakening, and she fell asleep more easily. And, significantly, she had not even thought she had any sleep problems before coming to me.

Among the most frequent complaints any doctor hears are "I'm too keyed up to get to sleep," and "I keep awakening throughout the night, and so I get up exhausted."

These patients' doctors will all too often prescribe sleeping medications, and many who come to me are using these drugs.

But I can (and do) help them without sleeping pills.

Here's How

One of the first things I do when a patient complains of difficulty in sleeping is to assess his dietary patterns—and medication, if any. I listen carefully and try to establish whether caffeine is contributing to the problem. Caffeine has a profound effect on some people, and many solve their sleep problems simply by not touching caffeine-containing drinks (coffee, tea, cola) after midafternoon. Others find that they must eliminate all caffeine-rich beverages and medications entirely.

Keep in mind, too, that though a nightcap may put you in the mood for sleep, and even may help you drop off, that little nip may have the opposite effect in the long run. You may soon awaken, because alcohol is a potent contributor to nighttime hypoglycemia, which in turn is the most common cause of nighttime awakening.

That Sleep Medication May Be a Non-Sleeping Pill

Sleeping pills may be addictive, causing physical dependency. Or they may just disrupt your normal rhythms, helping you sleep in the short run but not over the longer term. Each type of sleep medication comes complete with its own set of problems.

For example, those barbiturates that do induce sleep rapidly may not help you maintain it throughout the night. And those that help you sleep through the night may leave you with a hangover in the morning. Some have a long half-life and may not reach their full effectiveness for two or three nights. Dalmane (flurazepam), the most widely prescribed miracle sleep-inducer of all, has this property.

Older people in particular should be careful with sleep medications, for even flurazepam (which is probably one of the safest sleeping preparations on the market) has been reported to cause dizziness, drowsiness, lightheadedness, and staggering, among other things, in "average subjects." These effects would be more pronounced in the elderly, whose bodies clear the drugs more slowly.

Sleep Medications and Alcohol Don't Mix

If you like to take an occasional evening drink, remember that sleeping medications, in common with other psychoactive drugs, are particularly dangerous when taken with alcohol. Sleeping pills may interact with many other drugs as well, greatly multiplying the risks.

In short, sleeping medications simply are not anything to mess around with.

What About Stopping Sleeping Medications?

Anyone who has been taking sleeping medications for a prolonged period of time and wants to stop may need determination and bravery. Abrupt withdrawal from sleeping medications may, at first, make your problems worse.[1]

Usually, a patient who tries to withdraw from sleep potions experiences severe insomnia. There are two logical causes. The first is apprehension of the inability to fall asleep without the drug. The second is believed to be a "drug abstinence syndrome," which consists of jitteriness and nervousness. Further, once asleep, the patient may have disturbed sleep, fragmented and disrupted dreams, or even severe nightmares.

Research has, to some extent, explained why these phenomena occur. For example, if the habitually taken sleeping medication was one that suppressed rapid eye motion (REM) sleep, then there may be a rebound in the REM sleep phase, resulting in more frequent, more intense dreams. Nightmares may even be the result.

Sometimes withdrawal symptoms occur even when a patient is *not* attempting to withdraw from a drug. If he is taking a short-acting drug, he may experience withdrawal symptoms on a nightly basis when he sleeps beyond the drug's relatively brief duration of activity. At that point in the night when the drug's activity ends, the sleeping body reacts—unfavorably—to the state of sleeping without its aid.

In fact, sleep researchers recommend that anyone who takes one or more sleeping medications regularly should reduce dosage gradually to avoid withdrawal and rebound symptoms.

To sum up, sleep medications have the following drawbacks:

1. They may be habit-forming.
2. They may lose effectiveness after as little as two weeks of continuous use.
3. Patients who stay on the drugs may require larger doses as they become more tolerant to the medication.
4. The drugs may cause subtle metabolic interractions which have not yet been fully researched but which may be potentially hazardous over the long run.*

---

* Dr. Daniel F. Kripke of the Department of Psychiatry, University of California, San Diego, has serious concerns that some hypnotics (sleep medications) may be quite dangerous, saying that "use of hypnotics might be associated with 0.6% or more of total population mortality." He goes on to point out that medical examiner reports indicate that at least 1,400 deaths per year (and perhaps many times more) are associated with the use of certain sleep medications.[2] In fact, reviewing an American Cancer Society questionnaire given to 1 million people, Dr. Kripke discovered that those who admitted to taking sleeping pills "often" were 1.5 times as likely to have died, compared to controls who did not take them.[3]

The Insomnia–Blood Sugar Connection

Most doctors are not aware of this, but *most early awakening is caused by low blood sugar's various symptoms.*

For example, low blood sugar during the night can cause or contribute to palpitations, chest pains, nightmares, night sweats, headaches, dizziness, nonspecific anxiety (which may represent the nightmare you don't remember), and hunger. Most especially hunger.

I don't want to give you the impression that *all* early awakening is due to blood sugar fluctuations. One classic cause of early awakening is a full bladder. (In middle-aged or older males, this may signal bladder neck obstruction due to an enlarged prostate. In women it may point to cystitis, a bladder infection. It may, of course, be simply that you overloaded on fluids the previous day.)

The shortness of breath, abdominal pain, drenching sweat, or severe headache that awakens you may well be due to blood sugar instability. But they may be harbingers of a more serious condition. Depression, too, can cause early awakening, and if you suspect that could be your problem, turn to page 89.

If, however, you're sure that you're otherwise in good health, then it's likely that your nighttime awakening could be due to nutritional problems such as blood sugar instability or food allergy.

Adrenaline Release Contributes to Nocturnal Blood Sugar Instability

Because of poor eating habits, blood sugar often drops during the night, and this drop sets off several compensatory reactions—one of which is the release of adrenaline (the body chemical that makes you *feel* frightened) into the bloodstream. This release can be measured by analyzing a first-of-the-morning urine sample for adrenaline by-products (catecholamines), so that it is possible to find out in the morning how much adrenaline was released during the night.

Adrenaline release may cause your heart to pound. It may bring you bad dreams, anxiety symptoms, or night sweats. Thus, low blood sugar, by setting off the adrenal response, may be responsible for a feeling of foreboding when you awaken. Or, acting directly, it may cause hunger—and nightlong refrigerator raiding. Low blood sugar may even contribute to angina pains.

Since hypoglycemics, schizophrenics, and insomniacs have been shown to release excess adrenaline during the night, it seems logical that the single most effective measure for much early awakening is blood sugar control.

Proper Diet and Nutrients Can Ensure Productive Sleep

If blood sugar instability is a *cause* of sleep disorders, blood sugar control must be the first treatment of choice.

If you suffer from insomnia or any other sleep pattern that is giving you trouble, choose the blood-sugar-control diet most appropriate for you (see Chapter 28) and observe your sleep pattern closely for the next week. If you require the diet with the lowest carbohydrate level, then by all means use Ketostix to see if you have slept better on the days when your stix gave reactions in the purple ranges. (Ketostix, available in most pharmacies, are dipsticks for testing one's urine for the presence of ketone bodies. When used by metabolically normal persons, they indicate that the carbohydrate intake is sufficiently low to allow the stored body fat to act as a primary fuel source for the body. The Ketostix reaction is judged positive when the test sticks turn purple.) If your improved sleeping does indeed coincide with positive ketone readings, then you have confirmed a relationship between your sleep pattern and your blood sugar control—or your previous lack of it.

Once your diet is controlled, you should be sleeping better. But if you don't get as much improvement as you would like on a very low carbohydrate diet or on a diet that excludes simple sugars, you may well need nutritional supplements to get your sleep pattern back in shape.

Dr. Carl Pfeiffer, from whom I first learned about nutritional supplements that are helpful in sleep disorders, pointed out that nature has her own tranquilizers.[4] I admit that I was quite skeptical at first, but after a few of my patients tried his recommendations, I had to agree that there *are* supplements that help induce and maintain sleep.

The Sleep Vitamins

Inositol, one of the B vitamins, is my first recommendation because it has proven so reliable in helping my patients to sleep.[5] Most of them take from 1 to 3 grams an hour or two before anticipated bedtime.

Nutritional supplements work differently from pharmaceutical sleep-inducers in an interesting way. Many patients who take barbiturates to sleep find that they need increasing doses as they become habituated to the drugs. Not so with nutrients. In fact, many of my patients report that they can get by with less and less, eventually eliminating the supplements entirely.

I use more than inositol, however. If sleep problems persist, or if overstimulation occurs, then pantothenic acid (usually sold as calcium pantothenate) may do the job. Most of my patients start with 500 mg an hour or two before bedtime and may take as much as 2 grams.

L-tryptophan is the most well-researched nutrient in promoting sleep.[5] It is an amino acid (one of the building blocks from which proteins are made) not a vitamin. It is the precursor of the important neurotransmitter serotonin, which has been demonstrated to play a major role in the biochemical mechanism for sleep. Dr. Ernest Hartmann, director of the Sleep-Dream Laboratory of Boston State Hospital, pointed out that serotonin levels are directly proportional to tryptophan blood levels, and performed eleven different studies showing tryptophan to be extremely effective and virtually without side effects.[6]

I tell my patients to try about 1 gram of tryptophan the first night and increase the dosage gradually to 2 or 3 grams (if necessary) over a few nights, stopping when the desired result is achieved.

(There is a myth that protein foods help you sleep because they are a source of tryptophan. Although tryptophan is a part of all protein foods, it usually is present *in proportion* to the other amino acids—and tryptophan has been proven to have a therapeutic effect only when it is taken in tremendous *disproportion* to the other amino acids. This is because tryptophan competes with the other amino acids for a place on the transport system which carries the amino acids into the brain's cells.)

Niacinamide is a vitamin which enhances the action of tryptophan. In some patients it has antianxiety activity of its own, and may help to reduce some of the nervousness that keeps so many patients awake. I start with around 500 mg, but often build up the dosage to 2000 mg.

Calcium and magnesium have long been known as the sleep minerals.[7] I consider the raising of calcium levels especially important in improving sleep patterns, but I don't necessarily accomplish this in the obvious way, by giving calcium. I prescribe magnesium, because the two minerals stay in proportion, and when magnesium is taken the blood calcium levels go up. However, there is some advantage to taking them in balanced proportions of two parts calcium to one of magnesium. I often recommend that my patients start with about 1000 mg of calcium and 500 mg of magnesium per day. (For an example of a multinutrient formula, refer to the Sleep Formula in Vitamins at a Glance, page 320.)

Additionally, short-term studies indicate that there may be a temporary loss of these minerals on a high-protein diet, so they should be supplemented in any case.

By now, I hope that you have enough nutritional information to start tackling your sleep problem, and that a few days from now you will wake up feeling refreshed, revived, and ready for anything that comes your way.

Chapter 9

ANXIETY

Did you know that anxiety and tension are often symptoms of improper diet rather than responses to stress? That your emotional symptoms may be part of a metabolic problem and curable by simple dietary measures?

You would be surprised at how many patients walk into a doctor's office and say, "I need a tranquilizer," instead of stating their symptoms. We tend to equate the problem underlying the symptoms with the supposed remedy.

Under the circumstances, it's easy to see why Valium (diazepam) is the number one prescription drug in the United States and why it's been on the top-fifty list since 1966. More than 44.6 million Valium prescriptions were filled in 1977, and it is estimated that one American in four received a prescription for a tranquilizer or antianxiety medication in that year alone.[1]

If *your* problem is anxiety, you know you have company.

Nora Barnes, a patient who had been with me about six months, came in one day looking distraught. I knew she had a lot on her mind, so I asked her how her week had been.

"You just can't imagine," she blurted. "I suppose you're asking how I stuck to my diet, and I did well with that, but the rest of my life is out of control. Tommy fell off his bicycle and broke a front tooth. The oven almost blew up in my face. We had to rush my father-in-law to the hospital with chest pains. And Harold may be laid off at work. Everything's been like that all week. What I need is a tranquilizer!"

Nora had just done it. She translated her nervous, anxious, agitated feelings into a supposed cure. She obviously had no trouble in recognizing her anxiety and tension and in pinpointing the sources of it. But she was searching in the wrong direction for the remedy.

I sympathized with Nora. But my allopathic reflex—the ingrained reach for the prescription pad—didn't surface.

My approach to Nora, and to other patients with problems that cause anxiety, is in most respects much what you would expect from your family doctor. I listen carefully and advise as would any concerned friend. Sometimes my patients' actions speak louder than words: I see fidgeting, playing with strands of hair, cigarettes being lit and relit. And I have become accustomed to hearing people tell me they are testy, snappy, curt, or even preoccupied, before blurting out that something is worrying them dreadfully.

You are probably as much an expert on everyday, garden-variety anxiety as many of my patients, and most members of this society, must be. We all accept this comes-and-goes anxiety as an inevitable part of living here and now. But when the anxiety just won't go away, most of us begin to worry.

The Anxiety Attack

There is a more acute form of anxiety that comes on suddenly and is *really* uncomfortable—even terrifying.

Some people breathe too fast and take very shallow breaths (hyperventilate) and may even faint in response to a sudden anxiety-provoking situation. Others may notice increased heart rate, as a result of sudden adrenaline release, and wonder if their hearts are racing out of control (tachycardia). And still others may feel "skipped" beats and palpitations.

Distressing as these symptoms are, they are not mysterious. There is a solid biochemical explanation for what's going on.

Anxiety Is a Symptom of Hypoglycemia

Many of my hypoglycemic patients have acute anxiety attacks when stressful situations arise. Other patients are chronically anxious and cannot seem to control their apprehensions over things that should be taken for granted. And some of my patients are not even aware that they are anxious—but I can see and hear that they are.

Blood Sugar Levels Are Related to the Adrenaline Supply

Here is a typical anxiety reaction:

Your boss calls you on the phone and tells you he wants to see you at four this afternoon—and it's only nine in the morning now. He says he's received some "adverse reports from personnel" that he wants to discuss with you.

Or perhaps your spouse calls you and says, ominously, "There's something we're going to have to discuss when I get home." Instant anxiety for most of us, to be sure.

There are rare, enviable human beings who could take this type of call without worry. Such a person puts the whole matter out of his or her mind, works productively until four, and then strolls into the boss's office and finds out that the report is on someone else with the same last name. Or his spouse only wants to discuss vacation plans.

Most of us, however, don't take things like this so calmly. You wonder what could be the problem, and before you know it your heart is pumping like mad, your mouth is dry, your palms are clammy, and your stomach makes you wonder how it ever functioned at all.

The Anxiety Reaction

What happened is this: The medulla part of your adrenal glands responded to the emotional stress by pumping out adrenaline, which raised your blood sugar. (Adrenaline will increase your blood pressure and your heart rate, too.) But suppose you have had lifelong exposure to a typical "civilized" diet, with much more than your share of junk food. When this is the case (as it usually is), another mechanism must be considered. Namely, that after you have indulged in refined carbohydrates, your now hyper-responsive insulin mechanism responds by dropping your blood sugar to a point below that at which it started. The body must then call upon the same adrenaline mechanism to raise the blood sugar to normal. In this case, you could feel the very same symptoms that come with an anxiety attack without having to have the stress of an ominous occurrence to touch things off. As a matter of fact, A. J. Garber and his associates recently showed that hypoglycemia could cause adrenaline (and noradrenaline) levels to rise as much as tenfold within minutes.[2]

Similarly, when you consume a food to which you are allergic, the same blood sugar, insulin, and adrenaline changes may occur. The reasons for this are unclear, but the observations have been confirmed by several investigators—especially by Dr. William Philpott of Oklahoma City.[3]

Thus, if you are hypoglycemic, you may have anxiety attacks with no recent anxiety-provoking situation except the consumption of an improper diet.

The fact is that a hypoglycemic is at the mercy of a careening hormonal balance which can put him on an emotional roller coaster, causing moods to alternate between calm, testy, easygoing, and just plain impossible.

Although it is reasonably obvious that diet and nutrition play an important role in nervousness and anxiety, many orthodox physicians conveniently ignore this. When they hear the cue symptoms, their write-a-prescription reflexes fire and they issue orders for a drug to scotch the symptom.

The Traditional Treatment of Anxiety

Many years ago, the barbiturates were regarded as appropriate treatment for anxiety. (Of course, there was little else on the market at the time.) These drugs—of which phenobarbital is a classic example—were thought to be helpful in anxiety because they exerted a sedative effect. But we now know that sedation and removal of anxiety are by no means one and the same. Sedation involves making you sleepy; relief of anxiety should not.

And barbiturates have been found to be not much good for anxiety after all. (Imagine one quarter of an entire population drowsy but still anxious.) Barbiturates are addictive. They don't mix with alcohol, and they impair mental function and coordination as well.

Sometimes patients have a paradoxical response to barbiturates. In fact, this was so common during my house staff years that I was awakened almost nightly by calls to see patients who were agitated and disruptive because of the barbiturates which were, at that time, a standard bedtime order.

In the 1950s another drug, meprobamate (Equanil, Miltown), gained popularity. It had two major drawbacks. It was not consistently effective, and it could indeed make some patients dependent over the long term.

Sudden withdrawal after prolonged or excessive use had many adverse effects, and even though the drug is really fairly innocuous, there is a long list of adverse reactions that have been associated with its use.

So much was meprobamate prescribed that it became a part of our culture. Its heyday lasted until drugs like Librium (chlordiazepoxide) and Valium (diazepam), which belong to a class of drugs called the benzodiazepines, hit the market.

Librium was the first out, and did pretty well until Valium arrived. Valium took off like a kite in a high wind, and Librium followed with respectably upward-spiraling sales.

Valium, in fact, seemed to be perfect. It was "stronger" per milligram than Librium, and it seemed to control anxiety with remarkably few side effects. It was useful in premedicating surgical patients and in controlling skeletal muscle spasms. And in a pinch, a larger dose could be used to induce sleep.

Real perfection. Except for one thing.

Valium can cause dependency. And this fact is only just being recognized.[4]

Of course, all the benzodiazepines have always been known not to mix with alcohol. And even alone, they may cause drowsiness, fatigue, and muscle incoordination. Occasionally, confusion, constipation, depression, double vision, headache, and reduced blood pressure have been reported, and the physician's own manual on drugs also warns of nausea, slurred speech, hypotension, jaundice, urinary retention, vertigo, and insomnia. But these side effects are less of a real threat than is the more urgent problem of dependency.

Insidious Addiction

One of the worst facets of these drugs is the way their effect seems to creep up on those who take them. If you were to take a dose of Valium today, I doubt you would be craving it tomorrow. It is far more subtle than that. These drugs seem to be okay over the short term, and when so many patients report relief of symptoms at first, the natural tendency for both doctor and patient is to continue to use the drug. This is where the insidious effects begin.

The patient begins to feel better and doesn't want to be without the drug that made him feel less anxious. The doctor notes that the patient does, in fact, seem improved, so he may hesitate to recommend discontinuing the medication.

But when the prescription runs out, the real trouble may begin. The patient is probably not addicted after a short exposure. But chances are he will notice his lack of drugs after a day to a week, depending upon which benzodiazepine was prescribed and upon his individual susceptibility. All of a sudden, the newfound state of well-being evaporates, and the patient may feel worse than ever.

Many of my patients come to me after they have been on anxiety-reducing drugs for long periods. And helping them to kick the habit is often as challenging a task as I have.

That these drugs are not as safe as originally thought is only just beginning to be recognized on a broad scale. In fact, only in 1979 was the problem considered sufficiently serious to be brought to the attention of the United States Senate, to the point where the package insert has had to be relabeled to warn of the addiction potential.[5]

Proper Nutrition Can Control Anxiety

Since the levels of insulin and adrenaline are major biochemical correlates with anxiety symptoms and respond to blood sugar changes, *the controlling of the blood sugar is an important key to controlling anxiety.*[6]

I make sure my anxious patients stabilize their blood sugar levels (by adhering to the diets in this book) and then I go a step further. There are nutrients (vitamins, minerals, and amino acids) that have an antianxiety effect, and I recommend them, too. In fact, those nutrients that are helpful in insomnia are also useful in treating anxiety. I recommend that my patients take the sleep-inducing nutrients throughout the day, in *divided doses* with meals rather than all at bedtime.

My favorite nutrients in treating anxiety are inositol, niacinamide, pantothenic acid, calcium, magnesium, and tryptophan. (See the sleep formula on page 320.)

A Typical Case

Cindy Rawlins walked into my office complaining of "nameless dreads." She described her condition as being in "free-floating fear," with nervousness and seemingly unjustified apprehension. Cindy no longer said, "I'm anxious." She *knew* what her problem was. Simply put: "I need a tranquilizer." Like Nora Barnes, she had stopped thinking about the real problem and had focused upon what seemed to be the cure.

I told her that it wasn't an antianxiety drug she needed but better nutrition.

Cindy's glucose tolerance curve showed borderline hypoglycemia, and therefore I was quite confident that she would feel much better once her blood sugar was under control. I prescribed the diet lowest in carbohydrate, because Cindy was a little overweight—and she stuck to it unfailingly. She also took the basic vitamin formula (see page 319) supplemented with 1000 mg vitamin B$_6$, 1500 mg PABA, 3 mg folic acid, and, at bedtime, 1300 mg inositol. (With the exception of the inositol, the supplementary vitamins were not necessarily directed against the anxiety.)

By Cindy's third diet day, she was pleased to note that her nagging apprehensions had flown away. And by the seventh day, she felt self-confident for the first time in years. Her moderate overweight started to come off, and she was sleeping better, too.

As is evident, the right regimen cleared up Cindy's problems very rapidly. She really had not so much an emotional problem as a metabolic one.

Cindy's is not an isolated case. There may be millions like her, many of them now taking tranquilizers, who would find their anxiety symptoms relieved with two of nature's most reliable nutrition breakthroughs—the calmative nutrients and the blood-sugar-controlling diets. I have treated thousands of patients this way, and for most of them anxiety is a thing of the past.

Chapter 10

DEPRESSION

Depression can manifest itself in a myriad of symptoms. A depressed patient usually suffers from more than one of what has become known as "the constellation of depressive symptoms." Most clinically depressed patients suffer both from an inability to enjoy anything (anhedonia) and from some form of sleep disorder, whether too little or too much sleep. Some patients feel tired all the time and complain of vague aches and pains. Others develop specific pains or a mildly agitated feeling. Constipation, reduced sex drive, gastrointestinal complaints, avoidance of social functions, withdrawal, feelings of hopelessness, helplessness, and inadequacy are all symptoms, too. It's rare to see a depressed patient without some combination of these symptoms.

Depression May Feel Like a Physical Illness

One of the most interesting facets of clinical depression is that most depressed patients don't recognize that they are, in fact, depressed. This may lead to their embarking upon an endless medical search for both the cause of their symptoms and relief from them.

This search may be especially fruitless and confusing to both doctor and patient, because the physical symptoms are real and because symptomatic relief may provide some temporary help, though it will not get at the real cause. Even a very knowledgeable diagnostician may fail to identify depression as the primary problem after he has ruled out the more obvious physical maladies upon which the symptoms could be blamed.

Fay Smith was one of those "hopeless" patients who was sure she was going to die of her mitral valve prolapse (a usually benign heart condition; see page 209), or her fatigue, weakness, or chest pain. After years of seeing cardiologists who prescribed propanolol and other heart medicines, psychiatrists who prescribed tranquilizers, and this nutrition doctor who prescribed my standard vitamins and diet, she finally blurted out to me, "I'm so depressed."

I reacted immediately by increasing her intake of niacinamide, tryptophan, and pyridoxine to much higher levels, and within two days the entire syndrome began to clear. In a few pages I will explain how this happened.

Whatever its manifestations, from clinical depression to just feeling low, depression is a culture-wide illness of devastating proportions. It accounts for many visits to physicians' offices and many more days lost from work. It may be at the root of marital difficulties, of kids' failure to do well in school, and of on-the-job problems.

Treatment of Depression Has Changed with the Times

Generations ago, doctors had no choice but to wait out depression. In the 1930s, amphetamines ("pep pills") were touted as the answer to depression. Now we all know better.

Then along came electroconvulsive therapy (ECT), popularly known as shock treatment, for more severe cases. Although this frightening technique has been refined to the point where it may be beneficial in some cases, I would limit its use only to the most severe depressions and only as a last resort.

The 1950s psychopharmacology boom produced a class of drugs known as monoamine oxidase inhibitors, or MAOIs, including iso-carboxazid (Marplan), phenelzine sulfate (Nardil) and tranylcypromine sulfate (Parnate). These drugs seemed to be tremendously effective against depression, except that they displayed certain sometimes disastrous drawbacks.[1]

You Must Avoid Certain Foods When You Take MAOIs

In the first place, the drugs did not mix with tyramine, a breakdown product of the amino acid tyrosine. Tyramine is notable for its presence in "putrefied" foods such as aged cheese, beer, and wine, and in yeast, ripe bananas, avocados, pickled herring, and chicken livers. In addition, chocolate, excess caffeine, and a rather long list of foods and other drugs may also cause reactions.

Unfortunately, when a patient taking an MAOI ingested a food containing tyramine, significant elevations in blood pressure often occurred. Sometimes this would be accompanied by blinding headache and might be followed by a fatal intracerebral hemorrhage. Other side effects of MAOIs include dizziness upon getting up from a sitting or reclining position (orthostatic hypotension) which has caused some patients to fall, and resulted in disturbances in heart rate and rhythm in others. Also constipation, headache, overactivity, hyperreflexia, tremors and muscle twitching, mania and manialike states, jitteriness, confusion and memory problems, insomnia, peripheral edema, weakness, fatigue, dry mouth, blurred vision, anorexia, gastrointestinal disturbances, excessive sweating, and skin sensitivity reactions which show up as rashes. Less commonly occurring side effects include euphoria, blood cell changes, incontinence, sensitivity to light, sexual disturbances, and urinary retention, among others.

To my patients who are inclined to be overweight, weight gain was a particularly distressing side effect.

MAOIs are hardly agents with which to play games. Obviously, another drug was needed.

Enter the Age of the Tricyclic Antidepressant (TCA)

When they were first introduced, the pharmaceutical industry proclaimed tricyclic antidepressants safe and effective.* In point of fact, the tricyclics fulfilled the wildest dreams of the medical orthodoxy: a seemingly safe, seemingly effective pill to combat depression.

But how safe are tricyclics really? [2]

Reports of side effects and adverse reactions have included reduced blood pressure, hypertension, tachycardia, palpitations, arrhythmias,[3] confusion, disturbed concentration, disorientation. Dry mouth and blurred vision are quite common, as are increased pressure within the eye, constipation, urinary retention, and increase or decrease of sex drive.

Quite a list for a "safe and effective" new agent!

But despite these possible reactions, tricyclic antidepressants have been hailed as substantially safer than MAOIs. Taking them often

* Tricyclics include: doxepin (Adapin, Sinequan), nortriptyline (Aventyl, Pamelor), amitriptyline (Elavil, Endep), imipramine (Imivate, Tofranil, Presamine), desipramine (Norpramin, Pertofrane), and protriptyline (Vivactyl).

requires faith, since the side effects are usually felt within the first few days, while the benefits may take several weeks to accrue.

And again, my patients experience weight gain on these drugs.

Many have come to me for overweight that began when they started to take tricyclic antidepressants. And I have followed several patients who had been doing well on my diet until they were prescribed tricyclic antidepressants while under the care of another doctor. All of them gained an average of ten pounds in the first month—without any cheating on their diets. They all reported an absolutely frightening increase in their appetites and an insatiable craving for sweets and other carbohydrate-rich foods. This convinced me that tricyclics carry with them a very real risk of weight gain.

Originally it was believed that the weight gain experienced by patients taking tricyclics was due to a resurgence of appetite following the clearing of depression. But this has been disproven in part, and tricyclics are now known to cause weight gain unrelated to relief of depression. Rather, the weight gain seems to be the result of some metabolic side effect inherent in the drug's pharmacologic properties.

I have since helped patients to lose weight *and* shed their depression by taking them off TCAs and MAOIs while showing them how to accomplish the same thing nutritionally.

There are now on the market several combination drugs that include amitriptyline, some combining it with a "major tranquilizer," perphenazine (Etrafon, Triavil), and another with a "minor tranquilizer" or antianxiety agent, chlordiazepoxide (Limbitrol). The rationale for adding the tranquilizer is to help deal with the anxiety that so often accompanies depression. (By now you must know that if I think *one* drug is bad, then two must be worse!)

Essentially, these drugs have about the same side effects as the tricyclics alone, added to which are the potential side effects of the tranquilizer tagalongs.

This is not to deny the fact that tricyclic antidepressants do work for many individuals. They work because they block the action of norepinephrine, a neurotransmitter (i.e., a chemical involved in carrying biochemical signals to and from the brain). The drugs are slow to act and relatively slow to be excreted. Thus, if side effects develop, the symptoms may take some days to abate after the drug has been discontinued.

Many confuse the antianxiety agents (see page 85) with antidepressants. But they are different in that they affect different neurotransmitters. Neither class of drug as it stands today is an "upper," and neither works in all patients all of the time.

I have other ideas about treating depression.

If Drugs Are Out, What Is In?

The blood sugar control diet is the cornerstone of the therapy I recommend for my patients. Why? Because it works and because a majority of my depressed patients show unstable glucose tolerance curves.

One patient told me, "I feel as though I just got off an emotional seesaw," after being on a low-carbohydrate diet and vitamin-with-mineral regimen for just one week. And this patient was no stranger to psychiatry, either. She had been in supportive therapy, analysis, drug therapy, and the like. But her first real breakthrough came during her first week of carbohydrate restriction.

Nutrients Are Helpful, Too

During the years I have been treating depressed patients and following the nutritional literature, I have found that certain nutrients in particular are of benefit in treating depression. These include 1) vitamin B$_6$, 2) vitamin B$_3$ (niacin or niacinamide), 3) tryptophan, 4) zinc, 5) manganese, 6) vitamin B$_{12}$, 7) folic acid, 8) vitamin B$_{15}$, 9) pantothenic acid, and sometimes 10) thyroid. (Although thyroid is a hormone and not, strictly speaking, a nutrient, it is a substance normally found in the body and as such falls within the purview of orthomolecular medicine.)

With these nutritional aids, I have been able to devise a protocol for my depressed patients.

It starts with blood sugar control, along with the basic vitamin-and-mineral formula which you'll find on page 319.

I do a hair analysis to check for copper elevation and zinc/manganese deficiency. Dr. Carl Pfeiffer was the first to point out that the most common mineral imbalance among the clinically depressed was high levels of copper and low levels of zinc and manganese. Further, administration of zinc and manganese along with vitamin B$_6$ in significant doses leads to excretion of copper in the urine and thus lowers blood copper levels. This lower blood level will ultimately be reflected in the hair analysis.

With the copper/zinc problem in mind, I add chelated * zinc

* See glossary.

to the basic formula to bring the daily total to 150 mg per day (this is an extra 100 mg or so) and another 50 mg of manganese beyond the basic formula. Then, I give 500–1500 mg vitamin B$_6$ because it helps restore the zinc/copper balance.

I base the B$_6$ dosage on whether or not the patient remembers his dreams. For example, if a patient remembers only one or two dreams per week (even a fragment of a dream will do), I start with 1000 mg (1 gram) of B$_6$ in addition to what's in the basic formula. But if, on the other hand, there's less dream recall, I may start with 1500 mg. For those patients who remember more, I may start out with only the 200 mg in the basic formula and increase the dosage gradually if it seems necessary.

Pyridoxine (vitamin B$_6$) has been used quite successfully in treating the depression that is so common among women who are on The Pill. Half of them responded to B$_6$ with a dramatic lifting of the depression.[4]

Folic acid is another essential nutrient for treating depression. I usually give 6–10 mg, including what is in the basic formula. It is important to note, however, that some people are of a biochemical type characterized by a high level of histamine in the blood. (Histamine is the body chemical that is responsible for dilation and increased permeability of blood vessels, and plays a major role in allergic reactions.) The histamine level of such people *would be made worse by folic acid.* So you must evaluate your response carefully.

Usually, if the depression is a mild one, I send my patient home with the above regimen and when he comes in a week later I ask if there has been any improvement in mood.

Tryptophan for Depression

If, in my judgment, further treatment is necessary, I prescribe tryptophan and niacinamide in a ratio of approximately 2:1. I usually start with 1–2 grams and increase to 2–8 grams of tryptophan daily —in divided doses—with the greatest portion given at bedtime.

Dr. Guy Chouinard and his associates at McGill University in Montreal recognized that the life-span of tryptophan can be prolonged by administering niacinamide along with it. They devised a program in which depressed patients newly admitted to their hospital were started on small doses of tryptophan and niacinamide and built up to an ideal dosage of 4 grams of the former and 1 gram of the latter. (I prefer the 2:1 ratio to take advantage of the fact that niacinamide has an antidepressant effect of its own.) The study confirmed that the tryptophan/niacinamide combination at optimum dosage was at least as effective as imipramine, a tricyclic antidepressant, alone. The advantage of the niacinamide was that the amount of tryptophan could be reduced by one third.

Some patients respond dramatically to B_{15}, though I am not as yet quite certain what mechanism is operating here.

And some have responded to rutin (one of the full-spectrum constituents of the vitamin C complex) while many have had great results on injections of vitamin B_{12}, which I usually administer along with folic acid.

The B_{12} injections are very quick-acting, and my patients are able to report how they reacted on the very next visit. Some patients tell me that the shot made no difference at all, while others say the results were impressive.

When the injections do the trick, I add vitamins B_{12} and folic acid in tablet form to the basic formula and supplemental nutrients. Further, I try to ascertain when the effect of the shot wears off so as to give injections as often as necessary to avoid a letdown. Some patients need them as often as every day, and others no more than every month or two.

When B vitamins such as B_6 and niacinamide (B_3) are given, it is usually necessary to administer other members of the B complex to maintain balance. Thiamine (B_1), pantothenic acid, and vitamin C are all important and may have antidepressant effects of their own. (See Vitamins at a Glance, p. 322, for Anti-Depressant formula.)

Thyroid as an Anti-Depressant

Sometimes depression may be the manifestation of an otherwise "silent" sluggish thyroid. The answer, in addition to proper nutrition, may be the use of thyroid hormone, or perhaps kelp to provide iodine for thyroid function.

One patient of mine, Marjorie Knox, was a real problem case until we finally tried thyroid.

When Marjorie came to me, she complained of "doing everything at a snail's pace" and "being unable to get anything together." She had dropped out of architectural school because she didn't have the energy to keep going and complained that her mornings were the worst—typical in clinical depression. Although she did have a few good hours in the late afternoon, these just were not enough to make up for the rest of the day. Marjorie, who had lifelong acne, also had crying spells and lived on a cola and candy bar diet.

She had been to a chiropractor who had told her she had hypoglycemia, but the diet he gave her wasn't strict enough. So she then tried the Atkins Diet from one of my previous books.

Suicidal, depressed, and extremely cold-intolerant, Marjorie told me she wanted to "become a person again."

Marjorie's glucose tolerance test showed a fasting blood sugar of 104, with a rise to 177 at half an hour and a low of 88 in the fourth hour. The test was virtually normal, although she spilled sugar in her urine. Because she wasn't overweight, I put her on the Meat and Millet Diet and supplemented the basic vitamin formula with 100 mg of B_6, 150 mg B_{15}, 3 mg folic acid, and 1000 mg PABA. I also added 800 units of vitamin E.

I was a little disappointed when at the end of the first week Marjorie reported that she was no better.

So I added 1500 mg of vitamin B_1 and suggested a little patience.

There was no change in the second week, except that her skin had cleared up, and I then suggested that Marjorie take her basal temperature (in the armpit) first thing in the morning. I also had my nurse draw blood for a thyroid function test.

The next week she still felt no better, and the lab results were back. Marjorie's thyroid was borderline low only for one thyroid hormone and well within normal limits for the other.

Her basal body temperature had averaged about 96.3, which is low (in my experience, 97.8 is an average reading).

At this point, I reviewed Marjorie's chart very carefully and noted her extreme intolerance to cold. This was the final tip-off. Perhaps the cold intolerance and low basal temperature were the key to Marjorie's problem.

Sometimes the only way to be sure about the need for thyroid is by therapeutic trial—give it and evaluate the result. By the time the basal body temperature has risen .4 degrees, we can assume that a significant dose level has been achieved and can, at that point, evaluate its merit.

I wrote Marjorie a prescription for supplemental thyroid hormone as a therapeutic trial, just a small dose which could be increased gradually if necessary.

On her return visit the following week, a different person came into my office. Marjorie reported that about three days after starting the thyroid supplement she began to feel better. And after six days she had begun to feel that she could put the pieces of her life back together. Which she did. Marjorie has now returned to school, is studying architecture, and has not been plagued a bit by her old depressive symptoms.

In Marjorie's case, as in so many I have observed, I found again that medical practice is *supplemented* by good laboratory studies but must, in the final analysis, often rely upon the doctor's better intuitions.

High-School Teacher Plays Truant

Another depressed patient of mine, Harold True, came to me when he was thirty-two years old and feeling like an old man. He was a high-school drama teacher and simply could not find the energy to coach his classes.

He described himself as "incredibly depressed." He said, "I am a zombie. I'm unable to show up for work sometimes. Recently I told my class, 'You may see me, but I'm really absent!' "

He was having great difficulty just dragging his body out of bed in the morning. When he finally did manage to get up, he always felt fatigued and often experienced nausea and headache. After reporting this he made a feeble attempt at humor: "At least I know my nausea and headache aren't due to pregnancy. But the bad side is that what I've got has lasted more than six months."

Harold's first GTT (not done in my office) had been unremarkable, but that may be because he had only a three-hour GTT and a five- or six-hour test is usually required. He was told he had "borderline hypoglycemia" and was given the American Diabetic Association's diet, a plain balanced diet. And of course Harold didn't get any better. He had not given up there, though. He went to a second physician, a topflight professor at a major medical school and teaching hospital. When his nurse looked at Harold's GTT she told him, "I see you have hypoglycemia, but you won't get any help here. The doctor just doesn't believe in it."

Harold left that office with no help at hand.

The astonishing thing about Harold's encounters with the medical profession thus far was that no one had asked about his eating habits and no one had prescribed vitamins or a really modified diet.

When I received Harold's history, one of the first things evident was that Harold had virtually every hypoglycemic and depressive symptom in the book. He had nightmares too. In fact, the only dreams he was able to recall were nightmares, to the point where he dreaded going to sleep.

Since Harold's weight was only 147 and he is five feet nine inches tall, I put him on the Meat and Millet diet, in which he was allowed unlimited vegetables. He also received the usual vitamin formula, with 1500 mg of B_6, 6 mg folic acid, $3\frac{1}{3}$ grams tryptophan, and 1 gram of pantothenic acid to supplement it. On top of that he received an injection of folic acid, vitamin B_6, and vitamin B_{12}.

Harold's Return Visits

The second time I saw Harold, he looked a little better and said he felt only 80 percent as awful as before. He had all the same problems but a "little less so." He received another injection, and was advised to supplement his nutritional regimen with 60 mg of zinc and 1500 of niacinamide.

Two weeks later Harold was only "sixty percent as awful."

Thus, although I was elated by his 40 percent improvement in only three weeks, I added 300 mg of B_{15} to his regimen and another vitamin injection. Just two weeks later he reported, "Man, this is pretty terrific. I only feel twenty-five percent as awful as I did when I first walked in here." He commented that the B_{15} had "done a real number on my energy levels."

At this point, Harold's nightmares became much less frequent and he began to remember dreams.

A month later Harold came back and said, *"I feel normal. One hundred percent better!"* There were no signs of depression that I could see, and Harold reported once again looking forward to going to school and meeting the challenge of converting would-be thespians into accomplished young performers.

If I had a conjecture about the nutritional precursors of depression, I would identify them as the Modern Coke and Candy Bar Diet. I feel that I can say this with impunity because so many of my depressed patients seem to survive on just this lethal combination.

Cynthia's Depression

Although I treat many depressed patients, Cynthia Gill is remarkable for her history. At twenty-eight years old, she stood five feet eight and weighed in at a whopping 228 pounds. She had been on a major tranquilizer (sometimes used to treat depression, anxiety, and psychosis) for eleven years and told me she had been "constantly ill" for the past eleven months. When Cynthia was eleven, she had mononucleosis complicated by coma and encephalitis. During her recovery she gained fifty pounds, and by the time she was fourteen, she weighed 185. She had never been below that since. She also had anxiety attacks, lost hair by the handful, suffered from severe, blinding headaches, and felt run-down when she stayed away from milk and oranges.

Her father was an alcoholic, her mother diabetic, and this led me to think of a family history of carbohydrate intolerance.

Her thyroid was a bit low. She'd had four pregnancies, with three miscarriages and one surviving child—who weighed ten pounds thirteen ounces at birth. That made me think of Cynthia as prediabetic, at the very least.

Sure enough, her blood sugar was 142—in the diabetic range—and her hair analysis showed that she was low in zinc, high in copper. The usual ratio of zinc to cooper is 8:1; hers was 1.4:1.

It appeared to me that Cynthia had adequate cause for depression, and it wasn't something that could be cured by talking and listening.

Cynthia's regimen started with a no-carbohydrate diet, 3 mg folic acid, 1–2 grams pantothenic acid, 1 gram B_6, 3–4 grams inositol, and three kelp tablets, plus the basic vitamin/mineral formula.

During the first week she lost eight pounds, and over the first six weeks twenty-two pounds. Her diet seemed to help a bit, as did the vitamins and minerals, but she really didn't make much progress for a while.

Then I added chelated zinc to her diet and 2 grams of tryptophan. Carefully watching her serum (blood) zinc levels, we awaited results.

The improvement took place week by week, but the progress was not unbroken. As her condition improved she experimented with forbidden foods. Whenever she went off her diet her hair started falling out again. But over a period of time she learned to stay on her diet, took the folic acid, B_6, B_{12} shots, added B_{15} and PABA to her regimen. She didn't really shed the exhaustion and nightmares, however, until 1500 mg of niacinamide was added.

These three case histories demonstrate that there are many keys to the nutritional management of the depressed patient. Note that all our agents helped a little, but in each case it was a different natural substance that turned away the darkness.

I believe that nutritional medicine can relieve depression a full

85 percent of the time, yet there is probably no *single* nutrient that would perform much better than a good placebo, particularly if the test was designed by someone trying to prove nutrition therapy invalid.

These cases and hundreds of others from my files show that the real secret lies in understanding the teamwork of the nutrients and the biochemical individuality of response.

Chapter 11

ALCOHOLISM

The alcoholic is nothing more than a self-destructive, weak-willed individual who crawls into a bottle to shield himself from the realities he can't or won't face. He keeps on drinking even though he knows, like a smoker, that he *can* and *should* stop. Right?

Nothing could be farther off base.

The alcoholic has a metabolic problem akin to sugar addiction. He suffers from a *real craving* for alcohol that is the result of a biochemical imbalance.

Unfortunately, the medical profession tends to regard alcoholism as a psychiatric problem rather than a physiologic one, and treatment often centers on trying to persuade the drinker not to drink or on prescribing drugs that "reduce his underlying anxiety." The doctor might also prescribe other drugs which make the drinker violently ill if he swallows so much as a sip of alcohol.

But none of these treatments conquers the craving for alcohol. Thus it is almost impossible for the alcoholic to stop imbibing. If the craving were actually conquered when alcoholics dry out, would so many of them backslide?

Once we accept that alcoholism is a metabolic problem, we are halfway to the cure.

I am not underrating the difficulty of kicking the drinking habit. But I know that alcoholics can reduce their craving for alcohol by modifying their diets, and in this chapter I will tell you how.

What Is Alcoholism?

Too many people seem to think that a diagnosis of alcoholism must be made in order to get a heavy drinker to stop. This is an example of the thinking that often limits patient care: "First there must be a diagnosis; then, and only then, is there treatment."

I don't buy this. I would regard anyone's heavy drinking—whether alcoholic by one set of standards or not—as a nutritional problem, because alcohol per se is an antinutrient that robs the body of its store of B vitamins and minerals.

In fact, heavy drinking, even in a nonalcoholic, can impair liver function. And the liver is the main organ of metabolism in which so many of the body's biochemical functions take place.

I know that some people who are not alcoholic, by any definition, do drink heavily. But this is such a destructive nutritional practice that I believe all heavy drinkers should do as I advise alcoholics to do. Take stock. Heavy drinkers should drastically cut down on their intake, and alcoholics, of course, must stop.

If you are wondering whether you're a heavy drinker or an alcoholic, try this simple test: Choose your usual alcoholic drink and see if you can go for ninety days drinking no alcohol other than one standard-size shot of that drink every day, *no more and no less*. The alcoholic cannot do this. He can handle alcohol in only two ways: He can abstain completely, or he must overdrink.

Some people drink heavily as a part of their business life, and others lead social lives that include the cocktail hour and the "extended cocktail hour" as integral parts of the social process.

I call this last group the "country club drinkers," because they only drink socially, but never seem to be without a social occasion!

The Ramifications of Heavy Drinking

In addition to deficiencies of thiamine and the rest of the B complex vitamins, a heavy drinker may have deficits of vitamin C, zinc, magnesium, potassium, and manganese. It is in the alcoholic population that we find the true vitamin deficiency diseases such as beri-beri, the symptoms of which include emotional instability, shakiness, muscle tremors, and depression. Further, alcoholics may ultimately develop liver problems, eye problems, a tremor, and other neurologic difficulties.

What is not so well known is that the orthomolecular approach to alcoholism is highly successful. With usual supportive therapy and

Alcoholics Anonymous, 30 percent to 35 percent of alcoholics might be able to kick the habit. But if you give nutritional treatment in addition, you can expect 75 percent or 80 percent of alcoholics to be able to stay away from liquor.

The Alcoholic Has a Metabolic Problem

To an alcoholic, alcohol and sugar are almost interchangeable. And at many Alcoholics Anonymous meetings, coffee and sweets are served, as if this substitution would aid their membership in getting off alcohol. I am not criticizing AA, because the work they do is of unequaled value and they are the prototype for almost every self-help organization. Further, the transfer from alcohol to sugar addiction may, over the short term, be beneficial. But if the former alcoholic stays addicted to sugar, then I believe that there is a greater chance of his returning to the bottle than if he kicks *both* alcohol and sweets and keeps his blood sugar stable.

In fact, if you want to see someone who is doing well but still has most of the symptoms my hypoglycemic patients report in response to that questionnaire on page 48, all you have to do is talk to an alcoholic who takes sweets instead. An alcoholic who switches his addiction to sweets can be just as moody, unstable, and exhausted as when he was drinking.

What Improved Nutrition Can Do for the Alcoholic

Not only can an improved diet help the heavy drinker avoid or reverse the nutritional ravages wreaked by alcohol, it can also help him lose his craving for liquor and keep it lost—just as long as he stays away from the sugary foods that help trigger the insatiable craving.

If you are a heavy drinker (or if you are advising someone who is) a glucose tolerance test would be my first recommendation, for two reasons.

Just being willing to go for a GTT represents the first step in your motivation to improve your nutritional pattern and to stop drinking. Second, most heavy drinkers show some disturbance of their glucose metabolism and insulin response.

If you do have an abnormal glucose tolerance curve, this should provide a compelling reason for stopping the alcohol—you will know that you have a blood sugar problem and that it must be combated. Remember, a hypoglycemic glucose tolerance response is actually a first stage in the development of diabetes, which, in turn, is commonly associated with alcoholism. Many diabetics have alcoholics in their family trees, and many alcoholics have diabetic relatives and forebears.

Once you have your GTT results—and assuming they are abnormal—you will know that there are positive steps available to restore your nutritional and metabolic balance, and that in the process you will cut down on or eliminate the alcohol that is probably a good part of the problem.

Stopping the Craving

The high incidence of abnormal glucose tolerance curves and of diabetic relatives, as well as the ease to which heavy drinkers become addicted to sugar, all point to a cross-addiction. Since many of my sweets-addicted patients no longer crave sweets after a few days on a low-carbohydrate regimen, it seemed to me that the heavy drinker might benefit from the same regimen.

And it works.

The first thing I recommend to any heavy drinker in my office is that he immediately stabilize his blood sugar by going on a low-carbohydrate diet (see Atkins Diet, p. 270) if overweight, or a low-refined, low-simple carbohydrate diet (see Meat and Millet Diet, p. 275) if of normal weight.

This first step is vital to further controlling the craving and completely kicking the habit. And it is also vital to restoring the nutritional status of the heavy drinker—which is often unspeakably bad.

Mineral Analysis

No heavy drinker's work-up could be complete without a mineral analysis. Alcohol tends to deplete the body of certain minerals, and heavy drinkers often test low in several essential trace minerals. The advantage of this test, most conveniently done by examining a specimen of hair, is that the deficiency pattern of each individual can be identified and mineral supplementation tailor-made to each person. But there are certain deficiencies common to heavy drinkers.

If my alcoholic patient appears to have a low magnesium level, I may give 300–400 mg of magnesium, usually as a chelate.[1] (In this instance a chelate is a metal ion loosely bound to a protein molecule.) I sometimes find that I can get by with less magnesium by prescribing magnesium orotate, which seems to be more efficient.

Five hundred mg of magnesium orotate contains 30 mg of magnesium; I recommend this dosage be taken three to six times daily.

Zinc is another mineral in which the alcoholic is likely to be deficient—especially if he has cirrhosis of the liver. My alcoholic patients' hair analyses often show a manganese deficiency, so when an individual comes up short in manganese, I recommend 50 mg per day along with 150 mg of chelated zinc.

Another critical mineral is chromium, known as the "glucose tolerance factor" (GTF). GTF is important, too, because of the glucose intolerance so common in heavy drinkers. But chromium alone may not be enough to increase the body's supply of GTF, and it may be necessary (if the patient can tolerate the carbohydrates) to take brewers' yeast, which is a good source of the full factor. Currently I use a product which contains organic chromium concentrated from brewers' yeast.

Glutamine Is a Miracle Worker for Some

William Shive, an associate of Dr. Roger Williams, has demonstrated that L-glutamine, an amino acid, can stop craving in many (but not all) alcoholics.[2] A minimum dose of 1200 mg per day is appropriate, but I often prescribe as much as 2–4 grams if a patient complains of severe cravings. One caution, though: Glutamic acid doesn't work nearly as well as glutamine. Glutamine must be taken *as glutamine.*

Vitamin Supplements and the Heavy Drinker

Since alcohol is an antinutrient and prevents the absorption of folate (folic acid), thiamine, and vitamin B_6, it is of utmost importance to supplement these vitamins. Nonetheless, I believe that the entire B complex is important, though I do particularly stress folic acid and vitamin B_{12}, which I give as an injection at the first visit if a patient feels insecure about stopping his drinking. I also think that B_6 is particularly valuable because of its specific effect on the blood sugar as well as its key role in governing many reactions in the metabolism of protein.

Thus, in addition to the basic formula (see page 319), I might add a "B-50 formula" vitamin to augment the dosage of the vital B complex, and give weekly injections of what I call a "triple." The triple contains 1000 mcg (micrograms) of vitamin B_{12}, 50 mg of B_6, and 5 mg of folic acid. This formula seems to help most of my patients with cravings. Results are particularly good when my triple is given weekly along with the basic formula, L-glutamine, and minerals—along with an extra B-50 if it seems needed.

What's Happening at the Nutrition Frontier?

The nutrition breakthrough applied to alcoholism, not surprisingly, parallels what is happening in orthomolecular psychiatry. The successful clinical studies borrow techniques used in the treatment of schizophrenia. This does not imply that alcoholics are schizophrenics, but rather that the treatment of both conditions (and of many more) strives to correct the nutritional imbalances of each individual.

For example, Dr. Russell Smith of Whitmore Lake, Michigan, reported on the extremely successful treatment, relying principally on megadoses of niacinamide (vitamin B_3), of over five hundred alcoholics.[3]

And the late Dr. Nathan Brody of Laconia, New Hampshire, who treated thousands of alcoholics over a span of twenty-three years, used a megavitamin regimen emphasizing niacin, vitamin C, vitamin E, B_1, B_6, B_2, pantothenate, zinc, and manganese, and a blood-sugar-controlling diet.[4] He then followed the protocol of Dr. Carl Pfeiffer of the Brain Bio Center, Trenton, New Jersey, which is based on determining the histamine level of the blood.[5] The low-histamine patients are treated with niacin, folic acid, B_{12}, and pantothenate; the high-histamine patients receive calcium, methionine, and the folic acid antagonist diphenylhydantoin. All patients continue on zinc and manganese.

How to Stop Drinking

If you are truly addicted to alcohol, it can be rough to quit. The first step is to really want to stop. And it's absolutely necessary to successful treatment that no alcohol be taken in. The only really effective technique in stopping an addiction, or craving, is a prolonged period of abstinence to get the stuff completely out of your system. Thanks to AA, this concept is easily understood when applied to the alcoholic. (It is just as important when applied to the sugar addict or the person who is addicted to wheat, or chocolate, or coffee.)

A person must want to stop—and if he adheres to the blood sugar control regimen, he couldn't possibly consider taking in any alcohol.

So I tell patients the first week of their new diets that they must stop drinking *now*. If words help, I tell them, "Don't think of giving it up, know that you are *getting rid of it*." I ask my patients to imagine the worst conceivable case of DTs or of heroin withdrawal, and tell them to prepare themselves mentally for such an experience. I instruct them carefully on the Atkins Diet. Then I give them a triple, 2 or 3 grams of L-glutamine, extra niacin, B_6, B_{15}, and vitamin C, and tell them they may come in every day for another vitamin shot. So far, all have reported to me that the withdrawal experience was easier than anticipated.

The encouraging thing, though, is that I have found clinically that most of these patients on the low-carbohydrate diet and the nutrient supplements *do stop drinking and they don't go back to it*.

PART II
Treating Everyday Symptoms

INTRODUCTION

Nutritional breakthroughs have been taking place in psychiatry for three decades. To many orthomolecular psychiatrists, the treatment techniques are almost standardized; orthomolecular psychiatry has an orthodoxy of its own.

But there are breakthroughs which can be utilized by all of us—not the sick ones, but the healthy ones with everyday complaints. Headaches, menopausal symptoms, and fluid retention are just some examples of problems any of us might have. There are other symptoms—fatigue, dizzy spells, allergies, skin conditions, heartburn, bowel problems, sexual malfunctions, and the like—which could have served equally well as examples of the application of the nutritional principles that will help us to usher out the era of medications.

When we learn the nutritional techniques that are useful in some of these problems, then in consultation with a physician we can extend our newfound knowledge of what might constitute an ideal diet and vitamin-mineral regimen for each of us to develop a nutrition program suitable for problems other than those mentioned here.

Chapter 12

HEADACHE

Is there anyone out there who has never had a headache? I doubt it. Even the most hale and hearty sometimes succumb.

Most people pass off an occasional headache with annoyance and the knowledge that it will pass, but those who are afflicted with chronic or recurring headaches are in a different situation entirely.

There Is More Than One Type of Headache

Some people get headaches from noise, and others from fatigue or eyestrain. But others have headaches not quite so simply attributable to environmental factors.

For example, some of my patients get headaches at approximately the same time every day. I call these "time-locked" headaches.

Not all doctors are ready to acknowledge that most of these headaches are a common manifestation of hypoglycemia—analogous to the "daily low" experienced by some patients. The only problem in arriving at a correct diagnosis is that some patients don't realize that their headaches are time-locked, and it may take a week or more of daily record-keeping (itself a headache to some) to establish the scheduled nature of the problem.

Once this has been established, however, the cure is usually swift and simple. Control the blood sugar and you have controlled the hypoglycemic's time-locked headaches.

Unfortunately, not all hypoglycemia-related headaches are time-locked. Migraines may of course be time-related, and many *migraineurs* (the headache specialist's term for migraine sufferers) may be hypoglycemic, but the cure in the case of migraine may be more complex than the mere control of blood sugar.

Migraines: Multiple Symptoms, Multiple Probable Causes

Migraine is synonymous with miserable. Or worse. The migraine headache has often been referred to as the sick headache, and it is no wonder. Migraines often do make those who suffer them feel acutely ill.

The two kinds of migraine you hear the most about are the "classic" and the "common" types. Although the medical profession seems to consider the classic the most frequently seen type, it actually accounts for less than 20 percent of all migraine attacks.[1]

The classic migraine is characterized by a "prodrome," a set of symptoms that comes before the actual headache. This prodrome often includes visual disturbances. Some patients describe an aura where vision is dim and the surrounding edge is like a bright halo that shines or pulses; others may report diminution of vision or sparkling lights. This phase, which may include nausea, loss of appetite, cramping, vomiting, diarrhea, or simply a queasy feeling, usually lasts for fifteen to twenty minutes before the headache itself begins. But if these symptoms have not developed prior to the headache, they may come on after the head pain has set in.

A migraine may last as little as a couple of hours or as much as a couple of days. Most migraine patients find that they are very sensitive to light and noise and often prefer to go into a dark room, shut the door, and wait out the attack.

The common migraine is less sharply defined, and its prodrome is not as fixed as that of the classic one. Any combination of the symptoms above may occur, although vague and widely varied physiologic disturbances may precede the headache by several hours or days.

Migraines usually affect only one side of the head, but about one in three involves both sides. Some migraine sufferers notice inappropriate sluggishness, mental cloudiness, and irritability before, after, and/or during migraine attacks. Some of these symptoms may actually appear as much as a day or more before the actual headache process begins. Other patients lose consciousness or become disoriented, and some experience syncope (fainting) or confusion *during* attacks.[2]

The Non-Headache Migraine

Occasionally a migraine attack doesn't include headache at all. Doctors have described a syndrome called "migraine equivalents" which includes such symptoms as abdominal pain, nausea, vomiting, diarrhea, racing heart, dizziness, edema, and pain in the chest, thorax, or pelvis.[3]

After a migraine has stopped aching, the *migraineur* may feel exhausted or fatigued for a day or more.

Kids Get Migraines Too

The migraine is not a condition for the eighteen-and-over only. Although the majority of children with migraine do not have classic attacks, they do get headaches, described as throbbing, which occur most frequently with nausea, vomiting, irritability, and avoidance of light and noise. Up to one fourth of children with migraines seem to have a disturbance of consciousness, or stupor, many experience abdominal pain, and many become acutely confused.[4]

What Causes Migraine

Many women get migraine just before or during their menstrual periods, and many of them first experience migraines at the onset of menstruation in their early teens.

Women who take birth control pills are more likely to suffer from migraine,[5] either brought on or aggravated by The Pill, and John B. Brainard, M.D., feels there is strong evidence that highly salted foods bring on migraines too.[6]

Many have pointed to the connection between migraine and tyramine-containing foods (see list on page 90). Others point to alcohol, especially red wine. (My own particular headache trigger is the cheap wine that seems to be traditional at art gallery openings.) Chocolate, too, has been implicated because it is a source of phenylethylamine; and nitrite-containing foods such as hot dogs, ham (which is also heavily salted), bacon, and the like may be risky.

Coffee and tea cannot escape mention, either, as some patients react to them too.

There May Be More Factors Than We Have Yet Identified

Recently, there has been a great deal of research into the biochemical changes that occur during a migraine. The two most significant findings are a drop in the blood level of serotonin (a neurotransmitter) and a rise in free fatty acids.[7] This is noteworthy because some migraine sufferers relate their attacks to fasting, during which blood levels of free fatty acids rise. The headache occasionally seen at the beginning of a weight-loss diet may be due to this mechanism. Some patients relate their attacks to recent particularly fatty meals, others to emotional stress (when free fatty acids are released as a result of stress-related chemicals called catecholamines circulating in the blood), and still others to ingestion of alcohol within several hours.

It has been demonstrated that total free fatty acids are significantly elevated during migraine attacks, and some free fatty acids have been shown to release serotonin in test-tube studies.[8]

The Migraine Mechanism

Migraine headaches are vascular in nature. That is, they occur as a result of changes in the diameter of blood vessels in and around the head. This is why vasoactive foods—those that cause blood vessels to expand and contract—are implicated in bringing on a headache.

The initial phase of a migraine involves constriction of blood vessels, causing the visual symptoms. In the second phase, these vessels dilate, and the throbbing begins. So a migraine headache is a sequence: blood-vessel narrowing followed by widening.

The Cluster Headache Is Vascular Too

If a doctor tells you that you suffer from vascular headaches, he must be able to differentiate between cluster, migraine, and mixed syndrome. Cluster headaches differ from migraine in many respects. Whereas migraines affect four times as many women as men, cluster headaches occur in ten times as many men as women. A typical cluster headache lacks the prodrome so common to migraines. The headaches are usually on one side of the head only and begin with two to four minutes' unpleasant sensations in the temple or around the eye, sometimes accompanied by a little tearing of the eye, burning discomfort, or nasal stuffiness on the affected side only. Nausea and vomiting occur only occasionally.

Most cluster patients seem to get their headaches in their thirties, as opposed to the earlier age onset experienced by *migraineurs*. Typically, a patient awakens between 3:00 and 5:00 A.M. with sudden severe pain that drives him crazy for half an hour or so. Usually a cluster sufferer is able to go back to sleep.

Cluster headaches are so called because they tend to recur in rapid succession over a period of weeks or months and then go away for several months, only to recur again. Most patients have no warning; the headache begins suddenly and may abate as quickly as it came on. Some cluster patients are able to carry on with their business (unlike the *migraineur* who wants a dark room with no noise), and others become upset, often resorting to bizarre behavior to cope with the intensity of the pain. John R. Graham, M.D., reports that patients may be so "stirred and driven by pain" that they pace the floor actively and try to rid themselves of it, "sometimes in strange ways." During very bad attacks, he reports, "Patients in my group have jumped out of a moving car in traffic, locked themselves in closets or the bathroom so that their frantic endeavours won't embarrass their family, and yelled, screamed, wept, banged their fists or head against the wall, bitten the blankets, turned themselves upside down, and so on." [9]

It is painful even to imagine what it must be like to have these headaches come and go for years on end.

Cluster Patients Share Certain Characteristics

I was impressed by Dr. Lee Kudrow's reports that 90 percent of cluster patients in a three-hundred-patient group he studied were drinkers. Of that group, he adds, 60 percent had two or more drinks per day. (Most patients were wine or beer drinkers; perhaps this is related to the fact that wine and beer contain tyramine.) He also stated that in the majority of cluster-prone patients, a drink during a period when headaches occur regularly often induces an attack. Most patients stop drinking while their headaches are clustering. [10]

In addition, Dr. Donald J. Dalessio points out that most cluster patients are heavy smokers. [11]

Characteristically, the cluster patient is a hard-driven, perfectionist individual. It is believed by some that the headaches come on at night or on weekends because the patient has relaxed.

Cluster and migraine, however, are not the only headaches I see.

The Tension Headache

Some people develop muscle tension in response to environmental or occupational stress or poor posture which seems to lead to a headache. Typically, the pain starts in the middle of the day, increases steadily, and reaches its peak intensity by the day's end.

The headache usually starts with a dull, aching pain in the back of the neck. It then expands to the front of the head, the sides of it, and/or the area above the ears. Some patients may ache all over their bodies.

One kind of tension headache is related to physical stress, rather than emotional. You could call it a "Plumber's Headache," because it begins with the kind of muscle tension a weekend plumber would get if he spent a couple of hours on his back, underneath a sink, leaning upward. In fact, anyone doing physical labor that involves twisting, stretching, holding awkward positions, and working in cramped quarters may suffer from this result of muscular tension.

The Mixed Headache Syndrome

The patient with mixed headache syndrome classically shows no clear-cut pattern that would lead to an easy diagnosis. I think it could best be described as "a little of this, a little of that." The symptoms of a variety of headache syndromes are usually present, and traditional medicine often misses the boat by tackling each syndrome with a drug rather than by identifying the syndrome and getting at the underlying causes.

A Word of Caution

Although most headaches are *not* signs of conditions any more serious than migraine or cluster at worst, some may be warnings of serious pathology within the vascular system or the brain.

For example, some patients with severe hypertension have no warning at all until they get headaches. Some metabolic or endocrine imbalances may cause headache, as may some allergies (see Chapter 19).

Brain tumor, the most serious cause of headaches, is not very common. As you might expect, every frequent-headache sufferer probably wonders about that possibility until he or she is reassured by a physician that a headache syndrome unrelated to hypertension, tumors, and the like is at work.

If you have chronic headaches, you should *consult a physician* so that he may rule out more serious conditions before you go on to treat them nutritionally.

Though this book does offer an opportunity for self-treatment, it is not meant to be a guide to self-diagnosis, which can be exceedingly dangerous.

Widespread Disagreement on What Makes Headaches Tick—or Throb

Most traditional headache specialists are content to ignore the diet–headache connection. Dr. Ellen Grant, a neurologist at Charing Cross Hospital, London, set off a major controversy among headache experts.[12]

Dr. Grant studied fifty patients and achieved dramatic results by eliminating certain trigger substances from their diets. In her study, 87 percent of the patients had been on oral contraceptives, steroid drugs, tobacco, and/or ergotamine (supposedly a migraine abortive, which I will discuss at greater length later) for periods that ranged from three to twenty-three years.

All patients were advised to avoid cheese, citrus fruits, alcohol, chocolate, and other people's cigarette smoke, as well as hunger and "excessive stress." Women on oral contraceptives were advised to find alternative means of contraception. There was improvement in some patients, but since most continued to have headaches, Dr. Grant decided to investigate the food allergy picture.

She found a gold mine.

In an extremely high incidence of food allergy, a full 78 percent of patients reacted to wheat, 65 percent to oranges, 45 percent to eggs, 40 percent to tea, 40 percent to coffee, 37 percent each to milk and chocolate, 35 percent to beef, and 33 percent to corn, cane sugar, and yeast.

Headaches became much less frequent among patients who avoided up to ten common foods, and all the hypertensive patients in this group (25 percent of the entire group) lost their high blood pressure as a side benefit. Dr. Grant also commented that chemicals in the home environment may make allergy testing difficult for patients, because these chemicals (and others' cigarette smoke) may also act as migraine triggers.

Dr. Grant's final results were startling. Among patients who eliminated vasoactive foods (i.e., tyramine-containing foods; see p. 90), 13 percent were headache free, and when smoking was stopped a full 53 percent of patients ceased to have headaches. Finally, when allergy elimination was accomplished, 85 percent of patients had no more headaches.

Hypoglycemia May Be a Factor Too

Fasting, also linked to migraine, can be likened to the low blood sugar state of hypoglycemia. Migraine sufferers have been proven to have an unusually high incidence of abnormal glucose tolerance tests.

So even though the traditionalist may choose to ignore dietary factors such as low blood sugar and food allergy, there is ample evidence that these factors play a significant role in migraine headaches. Need I tell you how strongly I feel about controlling diet as a means of eliminating headache instead of taking drugs to ward them off or stop them once they have begun?

Traditional Treatment of Headache

To start with the simplest treatment, most patients either ignore their headaches or decide to treat them by taking a few aspirins or other simple analgesics. If the headaches continue, a trip to the doctor is likely.

In a doctor's office, most patients will give a history of their headaches and then answer the doctor's questions. By the time a patient has been through the mill and gotten to a headache specialist, he may be lucky enough to see one who considers allergies, food intake, and the like. But it seems to me that there are far too few such enlightened practitioners out there. Traditional treatment is likely to involve the proverbial "allopathic soup." In other words, a prescription for something potent.

I am afraid that even time-locked headaches are often unrecognized as being caused by low blood sugar. They are most likely to be passed off as "nerves," "tension," or "stress" and treated symptomatically with aspirin or anxiety-controlling drugs.

On the other hand, migraine and cluster headaches are more likely to be treated aggressively with potent medications, some of which may produce side effects indistinguishable from the very condition they are supposed to treat.

Drugs are prescribed for two purposes: the first is "prophylactic"—to prevent headaches. The second is "abortive"—to stop a headache in its tracks once it has begun.

Prophylactic and abortive treatment of both cluster and migraine headaches may rely upon ergotamine, a drug which Dr. Grant says precipitates migraines in some patients. Its side effects also include numbness and tingling of the fingers, muscle pains in the extremities, weakness in the legs, quickened or slowed heartbeat, nausea, vomiting, and localized edema and itching.

If this sounds suspiciously like the migraine prodrome, remember that ergotamine constricts blood vessels and that the migraine prodrome consists of symptoms that are a result of constricted blood vessels.

Patients on the drug should be weaned from it gradually, and its manufacturer advises that "no more than ten tablets per week" be taken. It is contraindicated in patients with coronary heart disease, peripheral vascular disease, hypertension, impaired kidney or liver function, and, not surprisingly, pregnancy (ergot preparations are used to bring on uterine contractions).

Methysergide maleate (Sansert) is also used to help prevent migraine and cluster headaches, and its use requires even greater caution. This drug is sufficiently dangerous that the package insert contains a "box warning" that cautions of connective-tissue changes and fibrotic thickening of cardiac valves which may occur after long-term use, as well as an extensive list of other problems.

Other drugs recommended for prevention of migraine include amitriptyline (a tricyclic antidepressant), clonidine and propanolol (the former does *not* have FDA approval for this indication, the latter does), isocarboxazid (Marplan) and phenelzine sulfate (Nardil—a monoamine oxidase inhibitor and a *very* dangerous drug, which was discussed in some detail in the chapter on depression), belladonna (a plant-derived alkaloid which can be quite toxic), and cyproheptadine (an antihistamine for which the FDA has not added migraine to its list of indications).

All do help some *migraineurs* to some extent, and none are without risk.

When a patient comes to my office who is regularly taking all or any of these drugs, I consider it my duty to wean him or her from them gradually.

Some patients receive narcotics for their severe headaches, and these patients may actually become addicted, or at least habituated. Fortunately, most doctors today do try to avoid prescribing this type of drug.

Ample Evidence Implicates Dietary Factors in Migraine

Although most formal discussion centers around migraine, dietary principles apply to any sort of vascular headache. Vascular headaches are unmistakable because of their throbbing and all respond to some of the same triggers (such as alcohol and tobacco). They can be avoided by bringing into play the same elimination techniques useful in migraine. In my own practice, I have treated many migraine patients, fewer cluster patients, and more nonspecific throbbing headaches than any other type.

At present I am working closely with several cluster headache sufferers and am seeing favorable results.

My first cluster patient was the most severe case I have ever seen. He had gone through such headache tortures with no relief from *any* simple medication that by the time he came to me he was almost irretrievably addicted to meperidine (Demerol). During the third hour of his glucose tolerance test, a typical cluster headache began. The lab results of the test showed that his third-hour blood sugar was an alarmingly low 20. Recalling the high incidence of drinking and smoking in cluster patients, I began to suspect that blood sugar abnormality might be a link in the chain of causation, perhaps missed by others because they may not be on the lookout for it.

Thus far, I have yet to see a cluster patient with a normal glucose tolerance test.

The techniques described below may be effective in most vascular headache situations.

Migraineurs Tend to Have Abnormal Glucose Tolerance Tests

Although it was obvious to me from my first contacts with migraine patients I treated that the overwhelming majority had abnormal glucose tolerance curves, it took others a while to catch on.

Although everybody conceded that low blood sugar was *occasionally* associated with migraine, nobody seemed to consider it a primary cause, nor did any group do routine glucose tolerance tests until recently.

I was particularly gratified to learn of the work of three physicians at the University of Missouri, Drs. James D. Dexter, John Roberts, and John A. Byer, who published what I consider to be the definitive study on the subject.[13] They studied seventy-four migraine patients whose attacks were time-locked to the midmorning or midafternoon fasting state. According to their five-hour glucose tolerance tests, six patients were diabetic and fifty-six were reactive hypoglycemics. Only 16 percent of the group had normal glucose tolerance curves.

All patients were placed on a low-sugar, six-meal regimen and improved greatly. The six diabetic patients showed an improvement of greater than 75 percent. Three were completely headache free.

Forty-three of the fifty-six reactive hypoglycemics were available for follow-up, and 63 percent of them showed greater than 75 percent improvement. Nobody got worse.

Although the authors conclude that "these data do not prove that a precipitating factor of migraine headaches is either the rate of fall of blood glucose or hypoglycemia," they do state that "there may be other metabolic factors which have been mentioned previously which precipitate migraines that are associated with low blood glucose." They go on to say that their study merely proves that a low-carbohydrate diet does indeed help migraine patients.

I hope that now those headache specialists who have refused to recognize any correlation between blood sugar and migraine will realize that blood sugar is a factor that must be reckoned with in all migraines.

And when I hear my headache patients tell me how much better they feel, I am confident that even if there are other metabolic factors, such as allergy and the like, controlling blood sugar is the first step on the road to controlling headaches.

A Classic Case of Headache

Most headaches are neither migraine nor cluster, but rather what I call garden-variety headaches. Some are associated with hypertension; many are attributed to a sinus condition; others to eyestrain, and so forth.

Rita Grable came to me complaining of ankle swelling, a tendency toward hypertension, overweight (she was five feet four and 187 pounds), and, incidentally, daily headaches caused by "sinuses." Her fasting blood sugar was 120 (high, to be sure), and during the glucose tolerance test her blood sugar level went up to 175, followed by a drop to 55 in the third hour. I put Rita on the Atkins Diet and the basic vitamin-and-mineral formula, and within a week she returned with less ankle swelling, fewer pounds, and the delighted observation that she had not had a headache for a few days.

For four full months Rita did not have a single headache, until one day she lost her head and absentmindedly (she said) ate a piece of cake. For the next two days she was plagued by her old "sinus headache."

Treatment for Most Headaches Adheres to Basic Principles

With the exception of tension headaches, I treat most headaches in a similar manner.

Tension headaches are in a class by themselves, because they may be related to anxiety and nervousness. In these cases, I recommend the same dietary and vitamin-and-mineral patterns as for anxiety—and my results are remarkable. It seems that once the blood sugar is controlled and the anxiety has been quelled, the headaches just evaporate.

Treatment for Headache from Migraine to Mixed Syndrome

We are entering an era where headache researchers are focusing more and more upon the biochemistry of headache.

Many biochemical factors have been implicated, and some of these give clues to what nutritional treatments may help. Others will probably yield more pieces of the puzzle in time.

For example, elimination of foods containing tyramine (see p. 90) is a valid nutritional approach. Histamine levels have also been implicated, especially in cluster headache, and this leads to part of my rationale for the use of vitamin C and niacin, both of which have antihistamine activity and are often recommended together. Monoamine oxidase, prostaglandins, and estrogens have been implicated, too. I feel particularly strongly that estrogens must be used with extreme caution in headache sufferers. In fact, I recommend that my headache patients on estrogen rethink either their dosage or their need for the preparation. In those patients to whom estrogen is essential (and there *are* some) I try to establish dosage at the lowest effective level. When the estrogen is *not* essential, I encourage its gradual elimination.

These factors, of course, are in addition to the now well-known connection between headache and blood sugar and insulin levels.

My approach may seem simplistic, but it has proven to be remarkably successful.

My first step, as always, is to be sure that the blood sugar is stable and that my patient is taking a vitamin-and-mineral supplement such as the one I recommend on page 319.

Next, in addition to the basic vitamin formula, I recommend vitamin C, because it is a biologic antioxidant in addition to having an antihistamine effect. Thus it can deactivate many toxins, and it is possible that its success may stem from its action on the very toxin that triggers an individual's headaches. I usually prescribe 2–4 grams of vitamin C to be taken at the first sign of the head pain.

Although vitamin C is not the answer to all headache, it is a simple, elegant little maneuver which seems to work in almost half of occasional headaches.

Secondly, both niacin and niacinamide will provide immediate relief in a significant number of sufferers. I prescribe 50 mg of niacin every few hours or 500 mg of niacinamide. The niacin is kept at a lower dosage because of its major side effect—flushing. This flush represents the dilation of the blood vessels, which probably is the basis of its effectiveness in headache.

Dr. Federigo Sicuteri, taking his lead from studies which showed that serotonin levels were lower in migraine patients, reasoned that administration of tryptophan, serotonin's nutritional precursor, should be effective.[14] He found that this was indeed the case. Approximately half of the migraine sufferers on whom he tried it reported improvement. His work was confirmed by P. Kangasniemi, M.D., in a study that involved eight patients (six female, two male) all of whom had suffered migraines for over ten years.[15] Four of the patients in this well-conducted double blind study experienced marked relief during tryptophan treatment, leading the authors to conclude that "tryptophan may be a worthwhile alternative for a . . . still incompletely characterized group of migraine patients."

I have been using tryptophan on my migraine patients since this article was published. Two grams per day is a maintenance level, and I prescribe double that dose if a headache cycle seems to be in the offing.

What You Do Not Ingest May Be As Important As What You Do

Although I regard vitamin and mineral supplements as tremendously important, I have come to believe that the restriction of carbohydrates and other dietary triggers may be at least as important.

A recent patient of mine who bears this out is Ollie Williams.

At the age of fifty-one he'd had cluster headaches for thirty years, mostly during three to four weeks each summer. He was overweight (200 pounds plus) and was diagnosed as diabetic in 1971. He had been taking many vitamins before coming to me, and he reported that he had moderate improvement of headache on vitamins.

Ollie's blood sugar was a whopping 170 in the fasting state and rose to 335 in the first hour. By the fifth hour it had dropped to 95—although 95 is not a low number, a drop of over 100 points is highly significant and indicates that low blood sugar symptoms may be expected.

Although diabetic and watchful about sugar, Ollie drank a great deal of apple and prune juices in addition to eating bread, rice, beans, and honey as well. His former doctor had prescribed imipramine (Tofranil) for him as a headache prophylactic (see tricyclic antidepressants in the chapter on depression), and I requested that he go off it to give nutrition a chance.

Ollie went on the Atkins Diet and took the basic vitamin-and-mineral formula along with extra B_6, inositol, folic acid, B_{15}, vitamin A, vitamin E, dolomite, alfalfa, and garlic. Three weeks later his blood sugar was down to 128. Thus he brought his diabetes under control.

During the first weeks the headaches went away, and they stayed away for two and a half months. Then on a follow-up visit he reported that he'd had a headache. When I suggested that there had been some sugar in his diet, he denied it flatly. So I requested a list of what he had eaten the day prior to the headache and noticed barbecued spare ribs. I suggested that Ollie go home and check the label on the barbecue sauce.

I got a sheepish phone call the next day. Most barbecue sauce, like ketchup and many other condiments, is laden with various forms of sugar—and the stuff in Ollie's kitchen was no exception.

I cannot overemphasize the role of nutritional triggers, and I believe that the best way to find out the cause of your headaches is this: If, after stabilizing your blood sugar and taking the basic vitamin-and-mineral formula plus vitamin C, tryptophan, and other measures I have suggested, your headaches have not improved greatly or departed completely, you must then consider a food allergy and look for it meticulously (see allergy chapter).

John B. Brainard, M.D., in his book *Control of Migraine*, identifies nitroglycerine, alcohol, monosodium glutamate, and tyramine as "chemical triggers." And he has also noticed that a sudden increase in salt intake may cause problems. Dr. Brainard found, too, that many of his patients (and he) reacted to nuts and pork.[16]

As I have mentioned, nicotine (tobacco) is a vasoconstrictor and may trigger vascular headaches. Even though I am not a chronic headache sufferer, I do get a headache when I walk into a smoke-filled room.

Dr. Brainard's list is compatible with my own no-junk-food, low-carbohydrate edict. If you suffer from migraines, you may want to review some of the ideas in his book.

How to Find Your Particular Headache Triggers

If you get headaches frequently (but don't have a permanent headache), you should start a notebook in which you record everything you eat. Mark down the date a headache occurs and look to the previous twenty-four hours for a recurrent pattern, bearing in mind that your headaches may have more than one trigger. Katharina Dalton did such a retrospective analysis on several thousand headache patients and found that within the twenty-four hours prior to the migraine, each had eaten one of a number of common foods that trigger headaches, such as citrus, chocolate, cheese, and alcohol.[17]

Although this doesn't prove cause and effect, it *is* a good place to start. And if your pattern repeats itself, you can test it in the following manner:

Leave out all suspicious items for a week. If you are like Dr. Grant's patients, then there is an 85 percent chance that your headaches will go away during that week. Then reintroduce your suspects one at a time, eating the same food twice in a single day to be sure. (Often we can get away with initial contact, but a second one may bring on the reaction.)

When you do get a headache, don't introduce a new food for at least four days. Then you can start your testing again. Once you have been through this list, you will have a pretty good idea of which foods you should avoid.

Chapter 13

MENOPAUSE

"I know that some illnesses are fatal and that others give excruciating pain, but for the life of me, I've never known suffering greater than what I feel with these hot flashes."

I sympathized, even though the closest I have ever been to a hot flash (or flush) was when I unsuspectingly took my first niacin tablet. At least the experience gave me a little insight into a complaint I so often hear.

Before Julie saw me, she had made the rounds. She'd had hot flushes for years, and nothing seemed to help. What was worse, they had begun even before she noticed any menstrual irregularities or other signs of menopause.

The first doctor Julie consulted prescribed estrogens. Putting aside her misgivings about the estrogen-and-cancer controversy, she took them willingly because she was so desperate for relief. Almost immediately she became bloated, and by the second month noticed that she was gaining weight. She also became dizzy, experienced weak, tired spells, and felt severely depressed.

In short, everything you could say about a patient with a blood sugar disturbance you could say about Julie when she took the estrogens. Clearly, estrogen supplements weren't the answer for her, as they are not for so many other women at her stage of life.

All Julie's Doctors Thought Alike

In her quest for relief, Julie consulted five other doctors, all of whom wanted to prescribe estrogen supplements. (Apparently, or-

127

thodox medicine had nothing else to offer.) Recalling her first trial, Julie politely refused them. She told me that when she turned them all down, she was thinking that the orthodox "cure" was surely worse than the disease.

Of course estrogens are not really a cure for menopause—which is not a disease. The menopause is something that will inevitably happen to every woman fortunate enough to live long enough. Some women are lucky and feel virtually no symptoms, others are uncomfortable briefly but get through relatively easily, and still others exist in a living hell throughout.

If you are menopausal or expect to be soon, you have surely heard about the flushing, tension, fatigue, and loss of libido that are the most common symptoms associated with it.

Menopause Symptoms Mimic Hypoglycemia Symptoms

Hypoglycemia and menopause share a myriad of symptoms, many of which are amenable to the same dietary treatment. In particular, the depression and the mood swings of both conditions respond to blood sugar control.

Those who have a difficult menopause may be having problems because they have low blood sugar in addition to "change of life." In fact, symptoms of low blood sugar may be accentuated in the menopausal patient just as they are in the patient with premenstrual tension.

The usual treatment seems disarmingly logical. Since the menopause corresponds to a lowering of estrogenic functions, simply replace the missing estrogen. A cult of enthusiastic proponents has made estrogen replacement a near panacea for women past the age of menopause. On this therapy, which usually consists of estrogen extracted from other species (horses) or of synthetic substances similar but not identical to our natural hormone, some women do marvelously well. But many others seem to do much worse.

Estrogen and Blood Sugar

The reason is that estrogens seem to aggravate dysinsulinism; [1] that is, they seem to accentuate diabetic and hypoglycemic tendencies.[2] Part of the evidence comes from women on oral antidiabetic medications plus estrogen who get a greater blood-sugar-lowering effect when both drugs are taken together.

One can tell in advance which women are more likely to react badly to estrogen supplements. One way is to look at the Harper Index Questionnaire score (see page 48). If the score is high, then problems are more likely to arise. Further, a glucose tolerance test is a good indicator. If the difference between the high and low readings is greater than 75 points, that's another red flag. Additionally, no insulin determination should be over 100 units. Lastly, if a woman tends to distribute her weight in the upper part of the torso, with hips and legs remaining slim, then she is probably not a good candidate for supplemental estrogens either.

Some physicians, of course, deny that estrogens play hob with the blood sugar, and it is easy to understand why. For they are viewing the *average* result of what happens to women who take estrogens, rather than individual cases. It works this way:

A clinical study is performed. Some women's blood sugar levels rise and others go down. But on the whole, they rise and drop about the same amount above or below the point at which they started. Thus, when the figures are averaged, the rises cancel out the drops, and the mean blood sugar elevation or decrease appears insignificant. This is a pitfall common to many analyses where there are two effects to be measured. It tells the researcher how the group behaves, but it is easy to jump to an inaccurate conclusion if the individual cases at each extreme are not evaluated. Many "negative results" concerning nutritional techniques are based upon this very fallacy.

Still, there are times when I concede that estrogen supplementation is justified. But when I recommend estrogen, I attempt to prescribe it in the smallest effective dose—which is, in fact, in line with the "good prescribing practice" endorsed by both manufacturers and researchers.

My Goals in Treating Symptoms of Menopause

When a patient complains to me of menopausal symptoms, I tell her that it would be wonderful to simply knock out the flushes and have done with it. But I do not believe that this is a realistic goal if hormone-free therapy is to be put into play.

My goal is to control the symptoms and to make them as manageable as possible. If a woman is experiencing vaginal dryness or loss of secretions, for instance, I may recommend either a lubricating cream or jelly (vitamin E cream is often effective) or an estrogen-containing one. Just remember that the estrogen from a cream may be absorbed and you may experience estrogen's side effects as a result. Rarely would I consider prescribing estrogens before I have seen what a nutritional program can do.

Nature's Allies in Coping with Menopause

First and foremost, I insist that my patients stabilize their blood sugar to counteract the effects of careening estrogen levels. This helps many patients' emotional symptoms and puts them on a much more even keel.

Naturally, it doesn't quite eliminate the flushes, and that's where the nutrients have proven of tremendous benefit.

The regimen I devised for Mary James is typical of what I recommend. Mary came to my office for treatment of her menopausal symptoms because she didn't want to take estrogens and her family doctor had offered no helpful alternatives.

After putting Mary on the Meat and Millet Diet (she was slim), and taking a hair sample for analysis, I recommended the basic vitamin formula (see page 319), plus 400 units of vitamin E, increasing the dosage slowly and assessing her progress. Mary's hot flushes stopped when she got up to 800 IU (international units) per day. In other patients, I continue to add vitamin E until I get up to 2000 IU or the flushes stop, whichever comes first. In most cases, even when the flushes do not go away, there is some improvement.

There are some patients, however, for whom vitamin E simply doesn't do the whole job. In such cases I rely on two ancient herbal remedies, ginseng and/or dong quai (available in some drugstores and health-food stores, but not always easy to find in the United States). Ginseng seems to be more associated with men's problems and dong quai with women's, but I have not found these natural substances to be that selective in my own practice. Sometimes one works better, sometimes the other.

Ginseng comes from a plant that has been used in the Orient for centuries for its medicinal properties. I have seen ginseng from Korea, Siberia, China, and the United States. Some brands from each of these countries are effective, others are not. I would recommend checking out ginseng before you purchase it by ordering the booklet "Ginseng" by Walter Ziglar (published by International Institute of Natural Health Sciences, Huntington Beach, California), who analyzed fifty-four different brands and tells you the results. I don't want to recommend one brand over another but prefer to let you be the judge of which one you will buy.

Other Nutrients Work Too

Another patient of mine had tried vitamin E, diet, ginseng, dong quai, and *still* didn't feel much better. Then I added lecithin to her regimen because of the favorable results I had had with other patients. That did the trick. Much to my delight, my patient came back the week after she had started on lecithin and proclaimed, "This is it. I feel fine!" Another patient responded dramatically to choline, a constituent of lecithin. Still another responded to superoxide dismutase (see page 175).

A typical hair analysis reveals that most menopausal women are low in zinc and manganese. So I add chelated zinc and manganese to the daily regimen along with 1 to 2 grams tryptophan and 500 to 1000 mg niacinamide. (See the chapter on depression for my rationale for using niacinamide with tryptophan, page 94.) Recent studies have shown that low estrogen levels lead to low levels of free tryptophan in the blood, and that low levels of free tryptophan are associated with depression.[3]

One patient with particularly recalcitrant symptoms came back about a week after starting her tryptophan and niacinamide to tell me, "I'm so relieved that life is no longer a living hell. My friends can't get over the change, and I've even told a few of them who take estrogens that there's *another* way to deal with menopause."

Dr. Carlton Fredericks pointed out that folic acid and PABA (which is part folic acid) have the effect of increasing the estrogen output.[4] This makes them useful in management of menopausal symptoms, but the effect can be a two-edged sword, as estrogen has a tendency to aggravate such conditions as cystic breasts. The nutrition doctor has to use his judgment to see which condition requires greater attention.

Other vitamins not to be overlooked in treatment of menopause are pantothenic acid and niacin, which are required for the manufacture of estrogen and other hormones as well.

What About Premenstrual Tension?

The premenopausal woman often has a difficult time just before her menstrual period comes each month. Many of the nutritional techniques I have just discussed can be beneficial here, but the greatest emphasis in managing premenstrual tension should be on the use of blood-sugar-stabilizing diets and vitamin B6, for reasons which may become apparent in the next chapter.

Chapter 14

UNEXPLAINED WATER RETENTION

Do the letters IE mean anything to you? Probably not. Yet as many as one quarter of all women suffer from the condition the letters represent: idiopathic edema, or unexplained fluid retention. (If you tend to retain fluid, be sure to check with your doctor to be sure you don't suffer from a heart or other serious condition before you assume your problem is idiopathic edema.)

IE, yet another manifestation of dysnutrition, has begun to get lots of attention from journalists and the medical profession. I have a rule of thumb that never seems to fail: Conditions that now occur with greater frequency are in some way related to the dysnutrition epidemic that parallels our modern eating habits. IE is one condition that seems to occur with increasing frequency—and I believe that the greater incidence of cases is real, rather than a result of improved diagnostic techniques or increased medical watchfulness. It seems to follow the same pattern as hypertension, atherosclerosis, and diabetes.

At present our traditional physicians are unable to do much for idiopathic edema, and perhaps this is because they still believe that it is indeed "idiopathic"—which means arising from unknown causes. But it is not. Idiopathic edema is caused by our "civilized" Western diet and can be controlled by a proper diet. But traditional physicians treat IE symptomatically and assault the patient with drugs. In this case, they are not pooh-poohing nutrition. Not at all. The problem here is that they have not even considered it!

Rhoda G. Had Made the Rounds

Rhoda G. came to me after she had been to five different doctors who had put her on five different diuretic regimens. All had restricted her sodium intake; none had asked her a single question about her diet. The diuretics these doctors prescribed did help her —but only temporarily. As soon as she stopped taking them, she swelled up all over again.

On her first visit she lamented, "Sometimes my friends wonder if I'm pregnant! And in the morning, my face is so puffy my eyes look like slits."

She felt as though she were on a seesaw. She never knew from one day to the next what her dress size would be, and her breasts were so tender that she dreaded putting on a bra.

Further, the diuretics were not without unpleasant side effects. She often felt irritable and at other times weak. But it was her distressing leg cramps that pointed to the diuretics as the cause of these difficulties. (Diuretics cause the loss of potassium and other minerals essential to the proper functioning of our muscles. Muscle weakness and cramps are an extremely common side effect.)

Rhoda Could Count on Being Swollen Much of the Time

Like so many of my female patients, Rhoda felt frustrated by her relentlessly recurrent swelling. She often had difficulty bending her fingers (from swelling due to fluid retention) when she awakened, and she hated to see her puffy face look back at her from the mirror first thing in the morning.

By evening the swelling in her face had usually gone down— literally. Though her face would look more normal, her ankles would usually be swollen and her legs would be tremendously uncomfortable. What's more, if she took off her shoes in the evening, she knew she could never get them back on without elevating her legs. Although she seemed to retain water all day long, at night the tables were turned. Rhoda was up all night urinating.

Before her periods, Rhoda's problem got so severe that she had to use her alternate wardrobe, one full size larger.[1]

(Interestingly, IE is more common in overweight women and can be alleviated by weight loss. It also tends to disappear after menopause.)

IE May Be Related to a Disturbed Carbohydrate Metabolism

The reason I believe that idiopathic edema is nutritional is that most of my IE patients have an abnormal glucose tolerance curve.

It's a rare IE patient who has a normal one. Dr. J. Mostow demonstrated this twenty years ago when he showed that sixteen of twenty-one women with IE had hypoglycemic GTT results.[2] In Rhoda's case, her blood sugar rose to 161 in the second hour and dropped to 49 in the fourth. And she was concerned because her symptoms included irritability, crabbiness, and severe mood swings in addition to the edema. I bring in Rhoda's other symptoms here because the medical profession considers them to be part and parcel of the IE syndrome. But they are symptoms of hypoglycemia as well.

So IE may not be idiopathic after all. Perhaps the most convincing argument that idiopathic edema is a nutritional problem is that most patients' symptoms clear up on a blood sugar control diet, just as do those of the hypoglycemic. But in the case of the patient with IE, there is one major bonus—the water retention clears up along with the mood and energy problems.

How I Treated Rhoda

Since Rhoda was moderately overweight, I put her on the Atkins Diet and on the basic multiple vitamin formula (see page 319).

When she came back the following week, she was a few pounds lighter—some of it loss of fat, much of it from water loss.* She was, understandably, more cheerful. But she still complained of some bloating.

She put me to the test: "Would you," she asked, "please give me a prescription for a diuretic to finish the job?"

I was astonished by her request. But I realized that Rhoda, although she had not been successful with diuretics, did not understand what was wrong with them.

The Problem with Diuretics

A diuretic is a potent drug and a kidney poison that blocks the kidneys' ability to reabsorb sodium (along with other electrolytes and trace minerals) which in turn reduces the fluid volume of the body. This reduction in fluid volume occurs because when sodium and other electrolytes are lost, increased excretion of water results. Pharmacology often shares with physics the rule "For every action, there is an equal and opposite reaction." In this case, when the

---

* This diuretic effect of a low-carbohydrate diet has been thoroughly documented. It can be utilized in more serious conditions, such as congestive heart failure.

diuretic is withdrawn, the kidneys try to *conserve* sodium—the opposite reaction—which results in increased fluid volume. Thus, diuretic use may bring about an exaggerated tendency to retain fluid after a course of medication has been discontinued. Most doctors recognize that this rebound effect may result in water retention more severe after treatment than before.

In fact, two doctors from London, writing in the prestigious journal *Lancet,* were so impressed with the frequency with which diuretics seemed to *cause* IE that they postulated that IE is not idiopathic, but rather a condition caused by indiscriminate diuretic usage.[3] In the flurry of letters provoked by their accusation, it was established that, although not all IE is caused by diuretics, a great proportion of it can be blamed on these drugs.

A second type of pharmaceutical diuretic, spironalactone (Aldactone), acts quite differently. It blocks the action of the body's water-retaining hormone, aldosterone; it is an anti-hormone. Too often it produces undesirable side effects, such as breast swelling and tenderness, based on its interaction with other hormones. I personally limit its use to those cases where aldosterone levels are clearly elevated.

Certain Vitamins May Do a Better Job Than Diuretics

After I had finished telling Rhoda why I objected to diuretics, I explained that specific vitamin supplements could well be the answer to her remaining water problem.

There are a limited number of vitamins with diuretic effects, and vitamin B_6 is the one that works most consistently. I like to supplement a good vitamin-and-mineral formula with 500–1500 mg vitamin B_6 per day. The best technique for determining B_6 dosage is to increase it gradually until one can remember dreams several times a week.

Vitamin C has also been shown to have a diuretic effect, and it seems to enhance the action of B_6 as a diuretic.[4] The dosage of C is variable and may range from 1½ to 12 grams per day.

Rhoda asked me if it were at all possible that these vitamin dosages could be too large, and whether she could experience any unpleasant side effects. Certainly the amounts of each vitamin *looked* large—and I thought her question was justifiable. So I reassured her that these levels of vitamin B_6 have never been shown to be dangerous and that the worst effect of too much vitamin C could be slightly loose stools.

There May Be an Answer in Herbs Too

Although Rhoda didn't need more diuretic effect, there was another measure I could have recommended, had she needed it. There are herbal diuretics (available in health-food stores) which contain several herbs with diuretic properties. Don't get caught in the snare of thinking that because herbs are natural they have none of the toxic potential of drugs. Keep in mind that many of today's drugs are in fact the natural and synthetic chemicals derived from herbs. So, although I am more inclined to recommend herbs than pharmaceuticals, I administer both types of remedy only with the greatest of caution.

Non-Dietary Aids

In addition to vitamins and diet, elevation of the feet and support hose may help. Since some patients find that their swelling increases when stressful situations arise, it may help to learn to cope more constructively with stress. The most striking non-nutritional help comes from regular exercise such as bicycling, swimming, jogging, or whatever you choose to improve your vascular tone.

Rhoda Became Half a Rhoda

Rhoda has been free of edema for the past year. In fact, just the other day she told me how "dried out" and comfortable she now feels. No more breast tenderness, no more swollen feet at the end of the day. She is slim now and pleased with her appearance and the way her clothes fit, and she feels as though she has shed more than a lot of water and some fat. She has shed a psychologically disabling condition.

When idiopathic edema is associated with overweight, as it usually is, the treatment for both is the same. The most effective diet is one that not only eliminates refined carbohydrates but also produces ketosis—that is, *the same diet that's right for most overweight patients.*

The very criticism of the diet decrying the fact that it induces fluid loss is also the most convincing argument showing how valuable this technique can be in conditions such as idiopathic edema, where *control* of body fluid volume is essential.

PART III
Resisting Disease

Chapter 15

THE IMMUNE SYSTEM

Have you ever wondered why, in the midst of an epidemic, there are always some who do not get sick? Or conversely, in beautifully clear weather, why a few individuals are unable to shake their recurrent colds, bronchitis, or sore throats? This individual quality of resistance to illness is dependent on a complex network of infection-fighting blood cells, antibodies, and many other biochemical processes in our bodies, all collectively known as the immune system.

When I was a medical student it took only a few days to learn all that was known at that time about this defense system within our bodies. In the last few years there has been a veritable explosion of information dealing with every facet of our immune system. The issue I raise concerns the possibility that nutrition can enhance its effectiveness. As was true with early nutrition studies, the emphasis to date has been on *deficiencies*. What is now needed is to explore the nutritional augmentation of the immune system in the normal person, that is, the person who has no deficiencies. We are now at the dramatic point where this information is being gathered. When it is fully developed, it will constitute one of the greatest breakthroughs in nutrition.

Actually, there are many ways in which nutrition can strengthen the immune system. Our immune response comprises several different types of activity. One type depends on our *white blood cells,* which remove external particles, including viruses, bacteria, plant and animal material. Another type of activity depends on circulating proteins, known as *humoral antibodies* or immunoglobulins, which react and pair with specific foreign substances (antigens), neutralizing them. In addition, other important protective proteins (such as properdin, complement, interferon) are classified as *nonspecific factors* which help to maintain the level of immune response. Finally, the *skin and mucous membranes* contribute to our good health by protecting us against the entry of bacterial and viral invaders.

What Nutrients Affect Our White Blood Cells?

Most of us are aware that our white blood cells are the infection-fighting cells which destroy and consume invading organisms. We know that pus is the remains of these white cells (neutrophils and phagocytes), and we know that we usually have a bacterial infection when our "white count is elevated."

We do not as yet know many details about the nutritional factors supporting these white cells, but we do know that studies in deprived areas throughout the world show that malnutrition, particularly deficits of protein and iron, definitely impairs this function.[1] Further, Dr. Brian Leibovitz and Dr. Benjamin V. Siegel, in reviewing the scientific literature, were able to demonstrate many ways in which vitamin C is necessary for the ideal functioning of these neutrophils.[2]

A better-studied area of our immunity involves another group of white blood cells. These are the lymphocytes that originate in the thymus and are called T-lymphocytes. They are responsible for delayed hypersensitivity, usually seen as a skin reaction which appears in susceptible individuals some time after contact with an allergen has been removed.

Although these T-lymphocytes are not effective against bacteria, they are primarily responsible for our immunity to viruses, protozoa, and fungi. A considerable body of research shows that folic acid, B_{12}, choline, methionine, and presumably B_{15}, a group of nutrients collectively known as "methyl donors," are all effective in enhancing the T-lymphocyte function, which is also known as cell-mediated immunity.[3] Vitamin B_6 has been shown to be important, at least to the extent that a deficiency of B_6 markedly suppresses cell-mediated immunity in experimental animals.[4] Recent work also points to the possibly significant role played by the mineral zinc.[5]

Dr. David Horrobin, director of the Clinical Research Institute of Montreal, advances with considerable evidence the hypothesis that one of our prostaglandins, PGE_1 (see page 230), may play a major role in the function of the T-lymphocytes.[6] Nutritionally, this hypothesis fits in well with the observed facts, for the synthesis of PGE_1 depends on vitamin C, B_6, and zinc, as well as the extremely important category of nutrients—essential fatty acids.

How Does Nutrition Affect Our Antibody System?

Antibodies are small spherical proteins that circulate in the blood serum. Each has it own specific task, reacting to and neutralizing one particular type of foreign substance. Most of our common allergy responses and many of our food allergies demonstrate this antibody system.

Our antibodies are made by another type of lymphocytes called B-lymphocytes (B standing for bone marrow, where they originate). According to Dr. Samuel Dreizen, animal studies have shown the antibody-forming response to be inhibited by deficiencies of pyridoxine, folic acid, pantothenic acid, thiamine, riboflavin, niacin, tryptophan, protein, and vitamins A and C.[7] Clinically, the nutritionist finds that large doses of Vitamin B_6, C, and pantothenic acid are most effective in treating patients with an antibody-based allergy response.

Nutrition and Other Immunity Factors

Researchers are just beginning to study nutritional effects on the other protective elements known as nonspecific factors. So far, generalized malnutrition has been shown to impair most of these factors. Specifically, the properdin level may depend on pantothenic acid and possibly magnesium; lysozyme appears to depend on vitamin A; and according to Dr. Benjamin Siegal, the activity of interferon, heralded as both a virus- and cancer-fighting protein molecule, can be enhanced by vitamin C.[8]

In all this discussion of antibodies and white blood cells we tend to overlook that our most effective shield against infection may well be at the "portal of entry"—our skin and mucous membranes. Specific deficiencies of vitamin A, niacin, riboflavin, pyridoxin, folic acid and B_{12}, vitamin C, protein, and iron have all been shown in one clinical study or another to affect unfavorably the integrity and function of the skin and mucous membranes.[9]

In a like manner, our ability to heal wounds can protect us. I am currently working with a colleague, a plastic surgeon, in studying a vitamin and mineral combination that enhances wound healing and reduces surgical complications. The program consists of placing preoperative patients on a high-protein, low-refined-carbohydrate diet and providing, for at least one week before the operation, 100,000 units of vitamin A, 5 to 8 grams of vitamin C, 2 to 3 grams of bioflavonoids, 800 to 1600 mg of pantothenic acid, and 150 mg of chelated zinc. This program is maintained for one week after the operation as well, with the addition of 800 units of vitamin E. (Vitamin E helps in wound healing but, because of its ability to prevent platelet clumping, might have the effect of prolonging surgical bleeding or oozing. I therefore recommend withholding its use until after surgery, and after all bleeding has stopped.) Our preliminary findings indicate a major improvement in the surgical response of patients so treated. (See Vitamins at a Glance.)

Current research in all these areas is beginning to indicate that our immune systems may prove to be the key to winning some of the most serious medical struggles—such as the battle against cancer—as well as some of our most annoying ones, such as the still unavailing fight to find a cure for the common cold.

Chapter 16

COLDS AND VIRUSES

A common scene in any family practitioner's office is this: A patient comes into the office with a respiratory infection and complains, "I have a temperature of a hundred and three, I'm coughing my head off, and I feel too sick to go to work. Please give me a shot of penicillin."

The patient wants to get rid of his distressing acute symptoms, and he has been programmed by our culture to rely upon his doctor's intervention when he gets sick.

The doctor, however, is a bit more sophisticated than the patient. He knows that antibiotics are useful in bacterial infections but ineffective in common viral ones. And he also knows that most respiratory infections (unless proven otherwise) are viral.

Unfortunately, the doctor is under pressure to show that he is willing to do something for the patient, which usually translates into writing a prescription. Thus he may rationalize that although a viral infection is beyond the reach of antibiotics, the patient could conceivably fall prey to a "secondary bacterial invader." So the doctor will issue the requested prescription; and the patient will have it filled, take the medication, and get well.

The doctor knows that most viruses are self-limiting and usually go away by themselves. But the patient often equates his getting better with the antibiotic he has taken and concludes that it "knocked out my virus."

The next time the patient gets a respiratory infection, he may say to his doctor, "Penicillin always knocks out my bronchitis. Will you renew my prescription?"

Obviously, not all infectious diseases go away by themselves. And antibiotics are indicated in bacterial infections. But today, all too often the antibiotic is used indiscriminately.

This is particularly unfortunate for several reasons.

What's Wrong with Antibiotics?

First, bacteria often develop resistance to an antibiotic after it has been around for a while, necessitating a whole new generation of "magic bullets" to fight old infectious bugs.

And there are specific problems. Penicillin may cause a severe, life-threatening allergic reaction in some patients. Or it may cause a rather itchy rash, which may crop up long after you've forgotten why you took the penicillin in the first place.

Other antibiotics may knock out the *helpful* intestinal bacteria and cause diarrhea due to an overgrowth of monilia (the "yeast infection"). Antibiotics also tend to cause weight gain, and deplete the body of vitamins C and K. Nausea, skin problems, and sun sensitivity are other occasional symptoms. Tetracycline shouldn't be taken by pregnant women or children under the age of eight because tooth development or coloration may be impaired.

Take Two Aspirin and Call Me in the Morning

When the doctor, for whatever reason, does not prescribe an antibiotic, he probably recommends aspirin. Perfectly innocuous, right? Wrong.

A study conducted by doctors at Cleveland's University Hospital has shown that aspirin compromises the infection-fighting ability of the white blood cells.[1]

The Low-Carbohydrate Diet Helps Build Resistance

The low-carbohydrate diet has a long and distinguished history. One of the first benefits attributed to it dates back to the early 1930s when F. Hoelzel described improved resistance to infection among patients on a low-carbohydrate regimen.[2] At about the same time R. M. Nesbit pioneered the use of the ketogenic diet in treating urinary infections.[3] (The diet's effectiveness was probably due to the fact that a ketogenic diet acidifies the urine and that bacteria do not thrive as well in urine of greater than normal acidity.)

One can even use the low-carbohydrate diet in some types of

intestinal flu, especially those associated with diarrhea. Here, it works another way. The low-carbohydrate diet slows down the activity of the large intestine and can put a sudden end to a bout of diarrhea.

Vitamin C and the Common Cold

When a patient tells me he took several grams of vitamin C for his cold and "got better," I'd love to believe that his recovery was because of the vitamin C. But I discipline myself not to jump to conclusions. I remember that colds may go away as quickly as they come and that the recovery might be a coincidence. And I remind myself that though vitamin C may have *helped* push the cold away, it is unlikely to have performed a two-hour miracle.

There are studies that prove vitamin C works in the common cold, and there are an equal number that show it does not.

Linus Pauling, for example, reports a 35 percent drop in illness per person (based on the number of "sick days" compared to the controls) among people who took vitamin C for colds.[4] But the American Medical Association's official position is that there is no justification for the generalized use of vitamin C in the common cold.[5] What is particularly intriguing about these two oft-repeated conclusions is that *they were both drawn from the same data.*

But rather than talk about a lot of studies and review conflicting results, I would prefer to tell you how I combat the common cold in my own practice.

Vitamin C and Vitamin A

Although 1½ grams of vitamin C every two hours when a cold seems imminent may help to lessen the severity or even chase the cold away *if the vitamin C is taken in the first twenty-four hours,* I find that vitamin C alone is not nearly as effective as vitamins C and A together.

When I think I might be coming down with a cold, I take 1½ grams of vitamin C every two hours. But I also take 100,000 units of vitamin A per day for five days, then half that for another five days. After this ten-day period, dosage should settle down to the usual 10,000 IU per day—unless the ideal dose for you happens to be more than that.

You may rightly wonder what effect these vitamins might have on you. Too much vitamin C might give you loose stools, and if you've reached your individual threshold and your stools become loose, just lower your dosage or switch to calcium ascorbate, which can cut way down on this complication.

You may have heard that too much vitamin A can be toxic. This is very true. But large doses of vitamin A, in the range I have described, when taken for a few days have never been proven toxic and can, as borne out by my patients' results, be a real help in dealing with the common cold.

I am especially concerned that vitamin A has such a widespread reputation for toxicity, because I feel that it has become the scapegoat vitamin. Whenever an opponent of the nutrition movement wants to prove a point, he cites the potential toxicity of vitamins A and D to support his ultimate conclusion that we should get off those dangerous vitamins and take our medications.

Worse still, vitamin A's therapeutic qualities have been underrated or ignored in the exaggeration of its potential dangers.

In my own personal experience, there have been those evenings when I felt so sick that I thought, "Tomorrow's going to be the first office day I will have missed in fifteen years." I then hasten to take vitamins A and C until the following morning, when although I may not be feeling one hundred percent, I am invariably well enough to put in a full day at the office. Sniffling a little, perhaps, but certainly not sick.

Is Vitamin C Effective Against More Serious Illnesses?

Much vitamin research is going on in Japan. One group of researchers has been able to prove that diphtheria toxins are inhibited by vitamin C.[6] Another has shown vitamin C to be effective against hepatitis, measles virus, viral pneumonia, herpes zoster, facial herpes (the bug that causes "cold sores"), certain types of meningitis, and other disease-causing organisms.[7] A group in the United States has shown that laboratory animals and humans may produce more infection-fighting white cells when there are adequate levels of vitamin C to help things along.[8] It is amazing how many of the different mechanisms our bodies use to ward off infection have been proven to be favorably affected by vitamin C. It may well be that the only reason vitamin C has not been proven effective against more different viruses is that it has not been adequately tested.

The one real drawback I can attribute to vitamin C is that some people may experience a "rebound effect" and develop a dependency. For example, some of my patients who take very large daily doses develop sniffles when they stop taking it. The sniffles clear up when they reinstitute the vitamin. I can't call this a cure for the cold; it's simply putting back the vitamin C upon which the patient has become dependent.

If you are taking large amounts of vitamin C and want to cut down on your dosage, you should consider what I tell my patients: Taper your dose slowly.

Another criticism leveled at vitamin C is that it may keep people who rely upon it from seeing their doctors and perhaps from obtaining antibiotic prescriptions (where appropriate) for fighting their infections. This age-old criticism can be leveled at any alternate therapy—that it keeps the patient away from "proper" medical care.

I know of only one reason not to supplement antibiotic therapy with vitamins A and C; that is, if diarrhea develops. (Of course, both vitamin C and antibiotics may cause this reaction.)

The ABCs of Cold and Virus Fighting

I have covered vitamins A and C, but what about B?

The B complex is important for every function your body undertakes. But in colds and viruses, pantothenic acid (a member of the B complex group) may well be invaluable because of its stress-fighting capabilities. (For further discussion, see the chapter on arthritis.) I usually recommend that my cold-ridden patients take from 400 mg to 1500 mg of pantothenic acid per day, along with vitamins A and C.

Just remember that when taking a B complex vitamin in large amounts, you must increase your intake of the rest of the B complex to some extent. Proper use of the B complex does not allow for megadoses of one B complex factor without appropriately increasing dosage of the others. (For an in-depth discussion of how to use vitamins, see Chapter 29.)

Like most of the B complex, pantothenic acid is generally free of side effects. It may cause an occasional bit of drowsiness, which is likely to be less severe than the drowsiness sometimes caused by the antihistamines you buy over the counter or by prescription.

Are Any Minerals of Help in Colds?

There is considerable evidence that of all the minerals, zinc plays the most important infection-fighting role. There is a major shift of zinc in our bodies whenever we come down with an infection. And Dr. Bruce Korant of Wilmington, Delaware, demonstrated that zinc has antiviral activity in tissue culture.[9]

I use chelated zinc, 150 mg daily, as part of the regimen whenever one of my patients complains of a respiratory infection. And zinc is a part of the virus-fighting vitamin-and-mineral formula I have devised for my office patients. (See Vitamins at a Glance, page 319.)

The common cold may seem to be an unimportant illness, but the nutrition breakthroughs that help you shrug colds off so easily are of great significance. They represent ways in which we can strengthen our immune system. And, as suggested in the next chapter, our immune system may play the greatest lifesaving role of all.

Chapter 17

CANCER

Doctors through the years have considered the immune system useful for fighting infectious organisms and in wound healing. Only recently have they begun to recognize that this very immune system can be useful for fighting off illnesses which have never been considered "catching." The one exciting the most interest is cancer.

The match-up of what we know about our own immunity with what we know about cancer holds hope of providing answers we have all been seeking. The question raised is a tantalizing one: If the body's immune system helps to control cancer, then is it not possible that the true breakthrough against cancer may be found in the strengthening of our immunity factors?

Although I have not treated cancer since my residency training at the cancer hospital affiliated with Columbia University, I have seen enough of it among patients in my practice and among family and friends to have a healthy respect for its horrible impact.

I believe that cancer is a subject that must be dealt with in this book. Not because I feel I have a "cure"—I do not—but because cancer is the most frightening example of the vast gulf that divides the orthodox medical community and the nutrition movement.

Nonorthodox cancer treatments—ways of improving the cancer victim's odds—abound. But no matter how promising these past and present treatments have been, they have suffered the same fate. Ruthless suppression.

It is as though the political and regulatory powers in charge of our health care system were involved in a no-holds-barred campaign to make certain that cancer remains an everyday reality in our culture. Thus, chemotherapy, radiation, and surgery—the establishment's favorite cancer-fighting tools—are the only treatments that have not been dubbed "ineffective" or even "quackery."

The War on Cancer

The term "war on cancer" is more than just rhetoric. Cancers are treated as many physicians treat other diseases: There is an invader that must be attacked, removed, or in some way killed. Don't worry about how sick the treatment makes the person with cancer. Kill the cancer, and forget about the rest.

This reasoning borders on the irrational. For chemotherapies and radiation cause so many diverse systemic effects that patients sometimes die of the side effects rather than of the tumors themselves. Chemotherapeutic agents, by their very nature, are cellular poisons. How can they do their recipient much good?

The Nutritionist's View

Although cancers should not be in the body, they are not *foreign* objects. They are made of tissue, and they are grown by the body itself.

Thus, it is possible that cancer represents a condition in which the host's defenses are weakened, a condition in which the balance of power between the host's resistance and the disease process is tipped in favor of the disease. It is not logical to weaken a patient further with radiation, chemotherapy, and surgery.

Rather, cancer treatment should begin by augmenting the victim's resistance so that he can ward off the inroads of the runaway cancer cells. Most of this strengthening comes under the heading of immunology. And this type of treatment has been almost uniformly suppressed.

There have been so many potential breakthroughs against cancer. And again and again, the discoverers' careers have been ruined because of establishment politics. Whole bodies of knowledge have been buried because the establishment has been afraid of the more natural cancer therapies. Years of research have gone down the drain, and the scientists' will to do further work must perforce deteriorate with such frustration.

A *Partial Who's Who in Nontoxic Therapy*

The list of promising, yet suppressed, cancer treatments is very long. It extends well beyond the current recipient of orthodoxy's disfavor—laetrile. In the 1920s, Dr. William Koch was reporting cancer cures with glyoxylide, a substance designed to stimulate cell oxidation, but he and his treatment were mercilessly suppressed.[1] The same fate befell Dr. Max Gerson, whose cleansing diet seemed to improve the overall health of cancer victims;[2] Dr. Robert E. Lincoln, whose bacteriophages, viruses that kill bacteria, cured cancer through improving the patient's balance of power;[3] and Dr. Andrew Ivy, whose krebiozen was really an immunological agent, or vaccine. A book chronicling the persecution of Dr. Ivy, *A Matter of Life or Death* by Herbert Bailey, is must reading.[4] The indignation it aroused in me provided much of the motivation for my position.

Currently, the same struggle against harassment, resistance, suppression, nonrecognition, lack of funds, even exile, is being waged by Dr. Joseph Gold, whose hydrazine sulfate improves the metabolic balance between healthy and cancer cells;[5] Dr. Lawrence Burton, who is able to rebalance the body's immune system, using protein fractions taken from the subject himself;[6] Dr. Stanislaw Burzynski, whose "antineoplaston" peptides guide the cancer cells toward normal growth;[7] Dr. Virginia Livingston, who finds the bacteria *Progenitor cryptocides* in the blood of all cancer victims and treats patients successfully by improving their immune response;[8] Dr. Harold Manner, who absolutely proved in animals the effectiveness of the current metabolic therapy with vitamins, laetrile, and enzymes;[9] and Dr. Josef Issels, whose program of immuno-augmentation seems to include most of the techniques mentioned.[10]

What all these researchers have in common, aside from some very promising results, is that they stressed that *the patient's system must be strengthened to be able to resist the cancer*. In other words, cancer treatment—to them—means building health rather than destroying it with radiation and chemotherapeutic poisons. And this positive approach carries with it the assumption that as the body becomes stronger it will fight the tumor. This does not always mean that the tumor will shrink, or go away.

Instead, it is assumed that the body could live with a tumor, just so long as it didn't grow or spread. If I found that I had a cancerous growth, I would be very happy if it stayed in my body but simply did not grow or invade my lymphatic system. That would give me a lot more peace of mind than being involved in a war in which both the tumor and my general health were destroyed.

I Wish I'd Said This

Robert Bradford and Michael Culbert, editors of *The Metabolic Management of Cancer*, provide such useful insight on the subject that I want you to read it in their words.

> The root philosophical causes of the controversy over the metabolic management of cancer, the non-political reasons why it is under such attack by standard or "orthodox" medicine, are these:
>
> First, an allopathy-dominated medical establishment does not understand metabolic therapy (holistic medicine).
>
> Second, "orthodoxy" considers cancer to be a number of "tumor diseases," with multiple causes and varying treatments —perhaps 100 separate diseases with many more manifestations. The *sine qua non* of modern oncology is, by its very name (*onkos* meaning "lump") the tumor itself—whether the tumor grows, remains stable, or diminishes. We refer to this obsession as the *false criterion of the index of tumefaction.*
>
> Metabolic physicians hold that cancer is a chronic, systemic, metabolic disease characterized by the uncontrolled proliferation of trophoblast, or trophoblast-like cells and brought about by a dietary deficiency and weakened immune system, with numerous outside factors helping "organize"—but not *causing*— the condition. . . . Metabolic physicians . . . agree cancer is, characteristically, a metabolic dysfunction, not "lump and bump disease."
>
> This consideration is an almost cosmological deviation from standard or "orthodox" oncology and Western medicine for, first and foremost, it teaches us that tumefactions are *symptoms* of the disease state, not the disease state itself. Hence, treating the symptoms—however vital this may be in life-threatening situations—[is] by no means a treatment of the disease. The diminution of a tumor does not mean the cure of cancer; indeed, under standard immune system-depressing modalities, the diminution of the tumor may simply be an ancillary development to the slow killing of the host through the weakening of the immune system.
>
> Up to now, the entire energy of oncology has gone into the

development of ways and means to remove, reduce, poison, or burn out tumors. The aim of the metabolic management of cancer is NOT the removal, reduction, poisoning or burning out of tumors, but the blocking of their spread (metastasis) and the shoring up of the health of the whole person to resist the metabolic dysfunction and overcome it. Tumor reduction may or may not play a major role in this effort, but is—other than in life-threatening situations—incidental to the overall treatment.

Cancer tumors, depending on their gradation, are composed of anywhere from 50 to 90 percent natural or *somatic* tissue. In fact, the bigger the tumor, the more composed it is of natural tissue. The capacity of poisons and radiation to reduce a tumor is actually an indication of how negatively they are affecting the whole body.[11]

Can the Establishment Really Be Trying to Suppress Cancer Cures?

It sounds unbelievable that cancer cures could be suppressed, doesn't it? When most people first hear about it, they react just as I did—because the very idea of suppressing a cancer cure is unthinkable. But it takes place with absolute regularity, no ifs, ands, or buts about it.

I remember talking to a West Coast nutritionist known for his innovative therapies. I asked him, "Do you have anything that will work against cancer?" He thought for a moment and said, "Yes, I think I do. *But please, don't tell anyone.* I don't want to lose my privilege of practicing nutrition medicine. I'd rather not make it known that I've got a technique that could help some cancer victims."

Now this man understood nutrition. But he also understood the realities of health care politics.

What If You Have Cancer?

The problem of what to do if you have cancer is not an easy one. It almost seems that you cannot accept both orthodox treatment and nutritional management at the same time, and that you have to choose one or the other risk and go with it. Chemotherapy, for example, seems antagonistic to management that seeks to build up your body's natural resistance.

(There are several programs of cancer treatment which do seek to integrate chemotherapy and the nutritional-immunological approach. Two that have been described in print are those of Dr. Hans Nieper and Dr. Mario A. Soto De Leon.) [12]

An example of this dilemma in cancer management may be seen in the now-controversial area of the use of vitamin C. Dr. Ewan Cameron, at the Vale of Leven Hospital in Scotland, and Nobel Prize-winner Linus Pauling treated one hundred terminal cancer patients with vitamin C and compared them with one thousand control patients treated identically except without the vitamin C. [13]

The average survival time of the vitamin-C–treated patients was 210 days, and for the controls only 50 days. Ten percent of the vitamin C patients survived more than three years.

Their observations were corroborated by two Japanese doctors at Fukuoka Torikai Hospital who found a greater than sevenfold prolongation of life in 55 patients classified as terminal. [14]

In contrast, a study at the Mayo Clinic found vitamin C to be ineffective. [15] The difference between the studies, as Dr. Pauling so astutely pointed out, was that only a handful of the patients in the Scottish or the Japanese groups had been exposed to chemotherapy or radiation, while virtually all of those in the Mayo Clinic study had prior chemotherapy or radiation. Dr. Pauling offers this as convincing evidence that *vitamin C will work only if our immune system stays intact.*

Those in the establishment feel very strongly that any not generally recognized treatment is quackery. And though a cancer victim may be dying, the orthodox oncologist (cancer specialist) is usually loath to allow his patient to try anything unorthodox that might turn the tide. In fact, this unwillingness to try unconventional alternatives usually overshadows any humanitarian feelings on the part of the doctor.

There are, of course, exceptions. But most of the time, the scenario runs something like this:

A patient says to his or her physician, "Look, I'm in pain. I'm not getting any better, and you're doing the best you can. I'd really like to get some laetrile—or maybe some vitamin/enzyme therapy that I've recently learned about. Could it hurt?"

And the response is usually something like this: "If you try any of that claptrap, I'll walk off the case."

That is hardly a compassionate attitude on the part of a physician who is helping us over our most difficult, most final illness.

So the question, "What form of treatment?" still remains.

Perhaps this is because orthodoxy somehow finds itself fighting for its own belief system, based on its wage-war approach, and has become more interested in perpetuating the belief system than in perpetuating the life of the cancer victim. Patients who have tried cures from the other camp are often viewed as traitors to the medical profession and to the major cancer hospital system. The net result is the rather predictable suppression of seemingly effective nontoxic treatments and powerful attempts at discrediting their discoverers.

It seems that the early successes of unorthodox approaches point up the fact that the cancer establishment has, year after year, been spending millions of our well-intentioned charitable donations and tax revenues pursuing paths that are not going to cure cancer. Their world has viewed the appropriate, accepted treatment of cancer as being surgery/radiation/chemotherapy for so long—and business, industry, and the medical profession have such a stake in this treatment—that anything at odds with the traditional triad threatens to undermine the system.

What Then Does the Cancer Victim Do?

If you, as a cancer victim, wage war on cancer the establishment way, you are weakening your body's ability to knock out the tumor. And you are going against the "build up the victim" mode of treatment. If you concentrate on the latter treatment, then you risk losing all the facilities, trappings, and attention that go with the medical establishment, such as access to funds, hospitals, insurance coverage, and other forms of medical and nursing care.

So if you go nutritional, it will be a very lonely road. But if you go orthodox, it's a debilitating, often toxic one.

In short, either path is a rough one at present.

An Example of the Problem

A recent conversation I had with one of my patients, a young woman in her early forties, points this up.

She called to say, "I know you'll be able to help me. What can you suggest nutritionally to help offset the effects of chemotherapy?"

"Why have you submitted to chemotherapy?" I asked. I knew she had just had a mastectomy for breast cancer, and that she was a firm believer in nutrition, so I hardly expected chemotherapy to be a *fait accompli* for her.

"I didn't feel I had any choice. They said that without it I'll have two or three years to live, but with it I'll have a better than ninety percent cure expectancy, and they think they can keep me from losing all my hair."

"Are they willing to put those promises in writing?" I asked, pointing out that I knew of no form of chemotherapy that upped one's chances from zero to 90 percent. Most published results on long-term effects of chemotherapy indicate either no advantage, or a very slight one, in long-term life expectancy.[16]

This is the way I saw her dilemma. If the chemotherapy worked and she had no recurrence, she would make out all right, but if it failed, she would have lost her chance to succeed with all the alternative programs. Chemotherapy potent enough to risk hair loss knocks out the immune system, and *all the alternative treatments depend on having the immune response at its best*.

The Problem of Proof

Behind the dilemma facing the individual is a knottier one—that of proving whether the treatments work. It is a problem universal to all natural therapies: How do you prove that what you are doing is effective?

Proof, the kind the establishment accepts, needs money. Only if the researcher has the luxury of government and foundation grants can he study the course of the illness on the patients he treats, along with an equal number of controls who don't get the treatment. (The immorality of observing a group of controls dying of cancer is something I hope I will never have.)

I would like to have been able to tell my patient: "If you take massive doses of vitamin C, vitamin A emulsion, laetrile, protein-digesting enzymes, and autogenous vaccines,[17] you will have an X percent greater chance of survival." But since only a few hardy pioneers, themselves ostracized from the medical community and its funds, have done the work for the purpose of saving life, not establishing proof, there is no basis for any such statement to be made.

One reason so many of us and our loved ones still die of cancer is that the government is failing in its responsibility to its citizens to test these promising, life-extending, unorthodox potential breakthroughs the way it tests the mutilating therapies.

Nutrition and the Immune System

My main thesis has been that the best weapon for prevention, control, and perhaps cure of cancer is to have an intact or, preferably, strengthened immune system. The pioneering efforts I have referred to are examples of that; so are many of the vaccines, such as BCG * or Maruyama vaccine; so is the induction of a high body temperature (hyperthermia).

But as I stated in Chapter 15, nutrition plays a major role in strengthening the immune system. In this way, as Dr. Richard Passwater indicates in his book *Cancer and Its Nutritional Therapies*,[19] nutrition will prove to be helpful in managing the cancer patient and, more importantly, in the prevention of the disease.

Among the vitamins with ample research attesting to their effectiveness are vitamins A, C, E, and B_{17} (laetrile), and the minerals zinc and selenium.[20] Most of these (A, C, E, and selenium) are biologic antioxidants and are thus capable of protecting us against the many carcinogens in our environment. Most (zinc, C, A, and possibly E) also have been shown to enhance our immune systems. The most comprehensive documentation of these points is available in Dr. Passwater's book.

Vitamin A and Cancer

Despite an impressive roster of studies indicating a favorable effect upon tumors (or, more accurately, upon those who have tumors), vitamin A usage poses a dilemma.[21] Somewhere around the 100,000-unit level for chronic usage, the risk of toxicity prevails, and higher doses seem to be necessary to increase cell-mediated immunity. The problem can be partially avoided by giving vitamin A in a form that bypasses the liver, where excesses become toxic. This bypass can be achieved by vitamin A emulsion and by synthetic A derivatives (retinoids).†

* Doctors at M. D. Anderson Hospital in Houston, Texas, have shown BCG vaccine to be helpful in malignant melanoma treatment. Sixteen out of nineteen patients so treated had their lives prolonged and were still alive after forty weeks had elapsed.[18]

† Austrian researchers showed that 150,000–300,000 units of 13-cis-retinoic acid, or 1.5 million units of vitamin A emulsion significantly increased all the parameters measuring T-lymphocyte immunity in a group of lung cancer patients.[22]

The Role of Selenium

Impressive evidence is now accumulating about the possible anti-cancer benefit of the trace mineral selenium.[23] Selenium has been seen to increase the effectiveness of vitamin E and tends to protect the body against a variety of types of cancer. It has been found effective in reversing some experimental mouse cancers, and in humans the incidence of cancer seems to correlate inversely with the selenium level of the diet. That is, the lower the amount of selenium in the diet, the greater the risk of cancer. Along with vitamin E, selenium enhances the immune response and acts as an antioxidant, helping to remove peroxides from the blood. These peroxides (and other free radicals) have the effect of damaging cell membranes and thus increase the risk of tumor development. About 50 to 150 micrograms per day of selenium is the preferred dietary level.

What About Laetrile?

Laetrile (B_{17}) is obviously not a cancer cure, but most of the documented evidence indicates that it does have a favorable effect on the cancer victim, particularly in improving the patient's well-being—regaining lost weight, decrease in pain, improving ambulation.[24] Occasionally a "cure"—what is generally termed a spontaneous remission—takes place.

Further, I believe the animal studies performed impeccably by the late Dr. Kanematsu Sugiura of Sloan-Kettering and by Dr. Harold Manner of Loyola University to be extremely valid demonstrations of the favorable effect of laetrile on spontaneously developed tumors in mice.[25]

Because of this work, plus the numerous clinical studies presented by the many physicians who use laetrile, my indignation is aroused beyond anything I have yet experienced when antagonists to the nutrition movement like Dr. Victor Herbert go to such great lengths to convince the medical profession that B_{17} is not only ineffective but a dangerous poison.[26] As if chemotherapy is not! The sad part is that these irresponsible voices have succeeded in convincing some 98 percent of the medical profession that they are right.

Laetrile Is Not Controversial

I believe that if you carefully study the actual published data (safety, adverse reports, animal research, and clinical reports) you will agree that *laetrile is a mild palliative which has to be used in conjunction with other nutrients, enzymes, and immune-system stimulants to be effective.* Those who feel it has no place are simply unaware of all the facts, or they are those individuals designated by the orthodoxy to protect its own interests, regardless of scientific truth or human suffering.

Since I Don't Treat Cancer Patients

I am not going to write extensively about the treatment of cancer, since I have had very little experience with it. The only way I have saved the lives of cancer victims is by referring them to other doctors who have the expertise in the rather comprehensive treatment protocol called nutrition metabolic therapy. But I think a few words about the *prevention* of cancer are in order.

First of all, do not be taken in by all the publicity about fats in our diet causing cancer of the colon. It is based on circumstantial evidence—which could just as easily indict sugar—and perhaps some financial self-interest (Dr. Ernst Wynder, leading promoter of this concept, heads the American Health Foundation. When that group was formed, its board of directors was amply populated with leaders of the corn oil industry.[27]) What has been shown is that polyunsaturated fats contribute to an increase in cancer incidence.[28] This is one reason vitamin E can be so valuable.

Secondly, Nathan Pritikin claims that fats cause an increase in breast cancer, while Dr. Carlton Fredericks states the opposite.[29] Whenever these two disagree, as they so often do, I would put my credence in Fredericks.

The Newer Cancer Tests

The greatest dilemma is faced by those who have had a cancer diagnosed and treated surgically, with all the diseased tissue presumably removed. The problem they face is called "secondary prevention." A certain percentage of these patients unfortunately will later suffer a spread of the very tumor that was taken out. The theory is that some of the cancer cells remain in the body to form a focus for a growth in a new location, or locations—known as metastasis. The key to managing this problem lies in knowing whether, and when, the cancer cells have actually begun to spread.

Until recently, medicine had relatively little to offer in these situations, except certain blood tests that indicated when tumors had moved into liver and bone. And the treatments that were available, radiation or chemotherapy, rarely changed the outcome of the illness. In the past few years, a number of blood tests have been developed, all of which measure the condition of the immune system.

One test, called the immuno-status differential, is nothing more than a computerized analysis of all the white cells found in a smear of the peripheral blood (easily taken from the earlobe by pinprick).[30] This analysis gives the doctor an index of how well the immune system is working, and what changes have come about in it. This information has a surprisingly high correlation with the progression of the disease, which seems to take place when the immunity factors are decreased. It gives the doctor a way to follow the internal progress of the patient and to judge whether the treatment, be it immunological, nutritional, radiation, or chemotherapy, has been successful.

In a like manner, Dr. Lawrence Burton has devised a test which measures antibodies present in the cancer patient's blood serum. It indicates whether the patient is resisting the illness or succumbing to it. Great accuracy has been claimed for this method.

A third test determines the amount of fibrin in the bloodstream, and promises to add another checkpoint to the battery of available tests.

The advantage of these blood tests is that the doctor can now hope to judge the progress of the cancer patient *before* any detectable spread of tumor can be directly determined by other means. The doctor who opts to use the nutritional or immuno-supportive treatment may see these laboratory findings return to normal without ever finding a detectable spreading of the tumor. The same may also be true if a toxic therapy is used, but I wonder about exposing a patient to the risks of such treatment without proof that the tumor has indeed recurred.

Nutrients for Prevention

I would use the same general approach to vitamins and minerals that I use in other conditions, except that if the patient were a high cancer risk (as might be detected, for example, through some of the above blood tests), I might use 40,000 to 50,000 units of vitamin A, 6 to 8 grams of vitamin C, 100 mcg of selenium, 100 mg of chelated zinc, and I would try to find some laetrile. (The legal availability of laetrile varies from state to state. Obviously I cannot recommend it in those states where it is not legal; but I strongly recommend it in those where it is.) Failing that, I might try to supplement with a source of nitrilosides (the group of nutrients of which laetrile is a member) such as bitter almonds or apricot kernels.

Is There a Solution?

If there is a solution, it is to go to the specialist who says, "I would make any sacrifice to see that the cancer is cured." Unfortunately, these individuals tend not to rise in the political structure. The major cancer hospital, with its expensive cobalt machines, is not a likely place to find such a doctor.

If the scientists and researchers who believe any sacrifice worthwhile were in charge, then they would look at vitamins A and C, hydrazine sulfate, antineoplastons, laetrile, enzymes, immune-system stimulants, and other proposed cures and conclude: "Maybe there's a lead here. The claim is encouraging, and maybe the substance could guide us to the breakthrough we've been seeking." Instead, those in charge seem dedicated to keeping out the very people who look to untraditional, but maybe effective, cures.

Putting Cancer and Nutrition in Perspective

If the medical establishment recognized nutrition as a better way of dealing with cancer, I think it would become obvious that nutrition should be able to counter most other diseases. And what then? The entire pharmaceutical industry would come crashing down. Nobody would be willing to trust drugs anymore, and everyone would rely upon nutritional techniques in most illnesses.

The leadership of the drug industry, the American Cancer Society, the AMA, and other medical groups would be threatened with extinction; there would be lobbyists and politicians displaced and out of work. In short, there would be widespread disorder and havoc in the medi-business community.

If you have cancer, the choice is of course yours. But before you make any choices, weigh all your options carefully.

PART IV
Correcting Degenerative Disease

INTRODUCTION

Most research in clinical nutrition has been directed against our chronic, degenerative diseases. Thus it should come as no surprise that there is now a wide array of nutrients effective against these life-shortening conditions.

In analyzing what nutritional techniques could do for our major chronic illnesses—heart disease, diabetes, hypertension, arthritis—I find possibilities that are truly overwhelming. Consider that each nutritional benefit adds cumulatively to the total, and you will begin to see how they are capable of changing the clinical impact of these, and many other, conditions.

Progressive illnesses, which we had previously been content to slow down, now bear real hope of being reversed. It is this cumulative effect of the new diet, the mineral balancing, the use of vitamins as safe pharmaceuticals, that together form a regimen capable of turning back the clock. Not a single breakthrough, but the total regimen, constitutes the exciting frontier provided by nutritional medicine.

Let me show you why I believe these aggressive, yet nontoxic, therapies deserve the title—Nutrition Breakthroughs.

Chapter 18

ARTHRITIS

Recently I appeared on a talk show in Cincinnati, discussing the usefulness of nutritional therapies in the management of arthritis. Even before the end of the show the studio phone was ringing. A spokesman from the Arthritis Foundation accused me of offering arthritics false hope because I had stated that arthritic symptoms may be altered by nutrition and proper diet.

But I don't believe that arthritis is hopeless, and I don't think arthritics should either. The Arthritis Foundation's phone call is merely a reflection of its link with the medical establishment and the pharmaceutical industry and their mutual opposition to the nutrition movement. The Arthritis Foundation's reaction is not surprising. It wants to maintain control of the medical profession's thinking about arthritis, much as the American Cancer Society and the American Heart Association maintain control over their respective domains.

But I cannot see why the medical establishment, especially that segment devoted to patient care, is so closed-minded, so influenced by power groups, and so resistant to trying new treatments.

Two Extremes of Thought

There is probably more divergent opinion regarding the role of nutrition in arthritis than in any other condition. Establishment doctors rarely even consider it, whereas virtually every nutrition doctor will tell you of several ways in which nutrition has proven effective for his patients.

As of mid-1979, the Arthritis Foundation reported that arthritis afflicts some 31.6 million Americans—one person out of seven. Of these, 22.5 million have either osteoarthritis (16 million) or rheumatoid arthritis (6.5 million), and the remaining 9.1 million American arthritics suffer from gout and all the other arthritic conditions.[1] Like most of the conditions discussed in this book, the worldwide incidence parallels the degree of Westernization of the culture being studied.

Osteoarthritis Is Not Inflammatory

Osteoarthritis is a degenerative disease and is associated with getting older. It's the "wear and tear" arthritis that is usually characterized by degeneration of the joint cartilage. Most people, if they live long enough, will develop this problem to one degree or another as the moist surfaces at the ends of the bones that form the joint tend to become rough. As the cartilage and other tissues around the joint break down, the joint becomes less comfortable and more difficult to move; there is little or no inflammation.

Osteoarthritis usually progresses from stiffness and soreness due to overuse (it may first strike women right around menopause) to constant discomfort as the surfaces of the joint become more damaged. One of the most logical "cures" is to rest the affected joint when it kicks up. Of course, poor posture, obesity, injury, and mechanical strain may be factors too.

Rheumatoid Arthritis Is Crippling

Rheumatoid arthritis is three times more prevalent in women than it is in men. It usually begins earlier than osteoarthritis (between the ages of thirty-five and fifty), but it can strike at any age from early infancy onward. Rheumatoid arthritis is the most crippling of all the arthritic conditions and appears to do most of its damage to the joints. Unfortunately, it also damages the body's connective tissues that support the bones and internal organs. In advanced cases, the lungs, skin, blood vessels, muscles, spleen, heart, and even the eyes may be affected.

Rheumatoid arthritis is characterized by swelling and inflammatory changes in the synovial membrane lining the joints. Inflamed tissue over the joint's surfaces causes pain, and scarring from repeated bouts of inflammation and remission is a source of joint damage.

Rheumatoid arthritis is the arthritic condition associated with severe deformity, and each recurring attack seems to be more debilitating and to cause further damage, until the final phase when the joints become permanently enlarged with only a little range of motion.

There Are Vast Possibilities for Therapy in Arthritis

Arthritis is *not* hopeless. But it is not a condition with a single simple cure either. There seem to be as many therapies as patients, and some patients may respond better to one regimen or diet than to another. The key to controlling arthritis is to pursue a variety of nutritional methods until you find what works best in your case.

Despite protestations from the Arthritis Foundation, such nutritional experts as Abram Hoffer, Allan Cott, Frederick R. Klenner, and Roger Williams all selected arthritis as one of two illnesses that are most likely to respond to nutritional therapy (the other condition was heart disease).

If you talk to a dozen nutrition authorities, you'll hear at least a dozen ideas for the control of arthritis symptoms. This is simply because there are so many nutrients and regimens which have a favorable effect on the course of the condition.

It is of course hard, if not almost impossible, to evaluate quite scientifically what *actually* happens, because patients on almost every regimen have remissions and exacerbations. But when you see long-term control of symptoms on a nutritional regimen, then you must assume you are doing something right.

Nutrition seems to have more to offer than any other form of treatment. When I see patients treated by orthodox therapies progressively lose function and mobility over a period of years, I realize that those therapies have little to offer over the long term.

Drug Treatment of Arthritis and Where It Falls Short

One maxim that comes to mind when I think of the drug treatment of arthritis is "The more potent the drug, the more potent the side effects." This makes considerable sense, since most so-called side effects are actually undesirable direct effects.

The least potent drug commonly used in the treatment of arthritis is aspirin. It has long been the first line of defense, because it is effective in relieving stiffness, pain, and inflammation and because it was believed to be so safe. (It is quite true that an occasional aspirin *is* quite safe. It's just that arthritis is a relentless condition that dictates steady usage.)

Unfortunately, aspirin in large doses over a long period of time may cause gastrointestinal bleeding. In fact, in his extremely important book *Hazards of Medication*, Eric W. Martin points out that 70 percent of patients who repeatedly take aspirin suffer "occult" (hidden) loss of blood, both from local stomach irritation and from aspirin's ability to prolong the normal bleeding time by reducing platelet clumping.[2] Other side effects include ringing in the ears after a few days' dosage, asthma attacks, and indigestion or acid stomach.*

Aspirin's Greatness: It's Not As Bad As . . .

One good thing I can say about aspirin in arthritis is that it's not as bad as cortisone. When cortisone (a synthetic adrenal cortex hormone) became available in quantity in the 1940s, a lot of doctors jumped on the bandwagon and prescribed it for their arthritic patients because it seemed to make them feel so much better.

Cortisone is a very, very potent drug. It does provide relief from pain, stiffness, and the symptoms of arthritis. It seemed like a miracle—except for one thing. *Its side effects were at least as potent as its therapeutic effects.* Euphoria was a pleasant effect, but not so pleasant were fluid and salt retention (which lead to weight gain), increased blood pressure, moonfaced appearance, diabetes, de-

---

* Dr. Jacqueline Verrett, in her book *Eating May Be Hazardous to Your Health*, reports:

> At the insistence of the FDA he [an experimenter] is using aspirin as a control substance to determine whether or not the animals are susceptible to birth defects. And the reason he is using aspirin, in the words of one FDA official, is that the drug is such a "potent and reliable teratogen" [a substance that produces birth defects and fetal deaths over and over], as Dr. [Bernard] Oser has confirmed. His experiments show that the offspring of animals given aspirin during pregnancy are born with serious abnormalities—such as spina bifida, in which the spine is incomplete (a human born with this defect usually does not survive long), and oxencephaly, in which the brain is exposed. The doses are high—between 150 and 300 mg per kilogram of body weight daily—but some humans do take large doses of aspirin. Also, when the doses were lowered, fetal deaths went down but abnormalities went up.
>
>   . . . Yet the FDA is so sure aspirin is a cause of birth defects that it uses the drug as a yardstick against which to measure the teratogenic power of food additives, and then it doesn't tell anyone but just quietly files away the information as it keeps coming in.[3]

creased resistance to the spread of infection (often fatal), osteoporosis (thinning of the bones) with spontaneous fractures, severe
psychiatric disorders, degeneration of nerves and other neurologic
difficulties, cataracts, acne, excessive hair growth (particularly in
women), disturbance in the metabolism and utilization of protein
and fats, and heart and kidney failure as a result of the retention
of salt and water in tissues.

These effects made it obvious to all that cortisone was not a
miracle cure.

So, because cortisone was even worse, everybody looked back to
aspirin, which the medical profession is increasingly recognizing as
"not so safe as believed."

With cortisone out of the picture and aspirin not effective enough
in well-tolerated doses for many cases, our resourceful pharmaceutical industry came up with a new class of drug to supersede
aspirin.

The Newest Group of Drugs

The prototype of this class was indomethacin (Indocin), followed
by ibuprofen (Motrin), tolmetin sodium (Tolectin) and several
others—all touted as "non-steroid anti-inflammatory agents."

All three drugs have been associated with severe gastric disturbances and "potent reactions" to their anti-inflammatory, pain-
killing effects. But, since the medical profession considers them
"moderate" in safety, let me review the side effects only of indomethacin, the one that has been around the longest.

Your first warning may come from the official package circular,
which cautions, "It is not a simple analgesic. Because of the possibility of adverse effects, some of which may be serious, the drug
should not be used casually." These adverse effects include: single
or multiple ulcerations, including perforation and hemorrhage of
the esophagus, stomach, duodenum, or small intestine. Death has
been known to occur. Gastrointestinal bleeding with ulcer formation, perforation of pre-existing lower-bowel lesions such as diverticu-
ula and cancerous spots, increased gastrointestinal pain in patients
with other types of GI problems. Nausea, vomiting, loss of appetite,
abdominal pain, stomach pain, and diarrhea have been reported.
Serious changes in the blood chemistry and composition may occur,
among them bone marrow depression and various anemias. Other
reactions include acute respiratory distress, rapid fall in blood pressure (resembling shock), asthma, skin rashes and hives in hyper-

sensitive individuals. Some patients experience hearing disturbances and ringing in the ears. Psychotic episodes have been reported, as have depression, confusion, and depersonalization. Coma, convulsions, peripheral neuropathy, drowsiness, light-headedness, fainting (syncope), and headache may all occur, too. Blood pressure may rise, blood may appear in the urine, or the patient may retain water—and some patients have experienced loss of hair or an alarming skin condition called erythema nodosum.

I offer this list not to caution you against this specific drug, which in fact is not notoriously dangerous, but as a rather typical example of the myriad of risks that anyone may be exposed to when he consents to take a typical prescription drug. In this case, it is one frequently prescribed, quite casually, in response to some statement like: "I have this nagging pain in my shoulders and aspirin doesn't seem to give me much relief."

With such a long list of side effects, what makes this type of drug safer than cortisone? Simply the fact that some patients may manage to escape the side effects, whereas in the case of cortisone, *anyone who takes enough of it for long enough is likely to get into trouble.*

Still another class of drugs which has posed the problem of excessive toxicity is that represented by phenylbutazone (butazoladin), which has also been implicated in ulceration of the gastrointestinal tract, perforations, and occult blood loss. Use of this drug has always been limited by its severe gastric effects. In my own practice, water retention and weight gain have made it an extremely unpopular drug among my overweight patients. It may also cause changes in the blood composition and bone marrow depression. Nonfatal hepatitis, skin rashes, allergic reactions, kidney problems, cardiac problems, eye symptoms (including optic neuritis, retinal hemorrhage, and retinal detachment), kidney pathology and disturbances in kidney function, hearing loss, agitation, lethargy, and mental/emotional symptoms are all possible.

And this is why nutrition has such clear-cut advantages; it rarely causes adverse effects and often brings about beneficial ones.

Nutrition Is the Best Alternative to Drugs

Nutrition is just plain better.

Unfortunately, even the orthodox arthritis specialist (rheumatologist) may not be aware of this superiority, because he reads what the Arthritis Foundation wants him to see. The doctor who reads avidly, however, will find ample evidence that nutrition can and does help many patients.

Although a great many studies point to nutrition techniques as holding great promise, most of the studies are really preliminary and have yet to be nailed down as a proper clinical trial should be. Despite the potential offered by these preliminary studies, establishment apathy has resulted, so far, in a lack of follow-through along these hopeful avenues of research.

The Scientific Community Provides a Rationale

A recent advance was based on a "pharmacologic" rationale. It began this way. Since arthritics improve when given cortisone, why not give the nutrient upon which the synthesis of adrenal cortex hormones depends? A wealth of animal studies have demonstrated convincingly that the B vitamin pantothenic acid is an essential link in the chain of steroid hormone production.

Thus, several groups of researchers studied the effect of pantothenic acid upon arthritis. It had already been shown that arthritis sufferers have lower blood levels of pantothenic acid than non-sufferers.[4]

The stage was set for clinical trials, and Dr. Eustace Barton-Wright of London's Greenwich and District Hospitals administered 100 mg of pantothenic acid to forty patients with osteoarthritis and to twenty with rheumatoid arthritis.[5] This technique gave favorable results only after the sulfur-containing amino acid, cysteine, was added to the regimen.

Ascorbic Acid to the Rescue

Vitamin C, too, has been considered. It is especially useful if a patient has taken cortisone (or other steroids) or aspirin, which are notorious for lowering the vitamin C levels.[6] Further, the joint fluid is thinner when blood levels of vitamin C are higher.

To show how effective—and how safe—vitamin C can be, let's look at a meticulous experiment performed by Drs. E. S. and M. G. Wilkins of Simon Fraser University near Vancouver. Using tissue cultures, the Wilkinses compared the effects of vitamin C and that old standby aspirin. Aspirin did inhibit the growth of the rheumatoid cells (they grew at a rate of 54 percent of normal), but the *normal* joint cells were even more suppressed (only 21 percent of normal growth). Vitamin C, however, was totally lethal to *all* the rheumatoid cells, in the same concentration that allowed 93 percent of the normal cells to survive.[7] Their work provides a lesson in the advantages of vitamins (enablers) over drugs (blockers).

Further, vitamin C may be useful because of its chelating effect, in that it may help an arthritic get rid of toxic heavy minerals that seem to play a role in the arthritic condition. Dr. Fred Klenner, the vitamin C expert, has stated that "a person who will take 10–20 grams of ascorbic acid a day along with other nutrients might well never develop arthritis." [8]

I rarely give vitamin C without its companion nutrients, the bioflavonoids. This is because C and the bioflavonoids occur together in nature and apparently work together in the body to maintain the health of connective tissues.

In fact, in the days before nutritional treatments became such unpopular subjects, Dr. Peter J. Warter of Trenton, New Jersey, found that a mixture of vitamin C and the bioflavonoid hesperidin was effective in managing forty-two patients with rheumatoid arthritis and seventeen with osteoarthritis.[9]

Dr. Ellis and B6

Dr. John M. Ellis has written extensively on the use of vitamin B6 in arthritis, especially in a syndrome involving mainly the hands and fingers.[10] The condition Ellis described also included weakness in flexing the fingers, leg cramps, and severe shoulder symptoms. In fact, he had great success with his patients when he gave only 50 mg per day. I think the results are more spectacular when the dosage is much higher.

Just two days after I prescribed 1 gram of pyridoxine to Nancy Merrill, who has as typical a case of the condition Ellis described as I have ever seen, she told me that "I've just lifted my hands over my head for the first time in years! And I feel better than I've felt since I got out of my teens."

Dr. Ellis points out, however, that rheumatoid arthritis usually does not respond to vitamin B6.

Dr. Kaufman and Niacinamide

One of the first vitamins to receive mention in the treatment of arthritis was niacinamide. This dates back to the 1940s, when Dr. William Kaufman, then practicing in Connecticut, thought niacinamide was worth writing a book about.[11] I do not yet understand how it works, but it seems to help the arthritic, perhaps because the rheumatoid arthritic excretes far more tryptophan than non-arthritics do, thus decreasing the amount of niacin available. B_6 and B_3 correct this abnormality.[12] Another possibility is that niacin mobilizes arachidonic acid (a fatty acid) and stimulates the formation in the body tissues of substances called prostaglandins, some of which combat inflammation.[13] I usually make it a point to include B_3 (500 mg, three or four times daily) in the vitamin program I devise for my arthritic patients.

Vitamin E gets into the picture here, too. Two Israeli doctors administered 600 IU of vitamin E to twenty-nine arthritics, and more than half reported marked relief of pain, compared to only one of the placebo-control patients.[14] Thus, vitamin E appears to have a place on the list of vitamins shown to be valuable to some patients in treatment of arthritis.

My personal favorite, PABA, yet another member of the B complex group, also seems to be an anti-stiffness factor that's effective in many fibrotic conditions. (It was shown to be effective in such connective tissue disorders as scleroderma, dermatomyositis, and Peyronie's disease.)[15] I mention it here because it has given my patients such good results in combating stiffness.

What Are the Latest Theories?

To learn why so many nutrients are effective in arthritis, we should review some of the most recent theories of what causes the arthritic process.

Some of the same biochemical changes that affect the arterial wall in atherosclerosis (see page 226) are also evident in arthritic joints. Free radicals, which are highly reactive, unstable molecules with unattached electrons, and which by their chemical nature are obliged to react immediately with one of the body's normal chemicals, have been shown to initiate damage to the joint membrane in acute rheumatoid arthritis.[16]

The Value of Anti-Oxidants

As is true in heart disease, perhaps the most damaging free radicals are peroxides. These unstable chemicals are the results of a sort of molecular supersaturation with free oxygen. Their tendency is to oxidize any molecule they contact. Much of the benefit derived from the nutritional antioxidants vitamin E, vitamin C, and the mineral selenium can be attributed to their ability to prevent peroxidation damage.

We can carry the principle of antioxidation one step further by using the same enzyme maintained in our bodies' own cells to protect them against peroxidation. Superoxide dismutase (SOD) is an enzyme residing within our cells for the purpose of inactivating the peroxide radicals. Much basic biochemical research has made peroxide "suspect number one" as the chemical that initiates the rheumatoid process.

Since SOD has become clinically available, I have been using it on my arthritic patients, and it seems to work. (Although I always wonder whether any enzymes will maintain their biologic effectiveness when taken by mouth and having to pass through the highly acid stomach contents.) But it requires a lot—usually more than a dozen pills taken throughout the day are needed to get any results.

The most intriguing lead, nutritionally, may well be that there are several superoxide dismutases, some which require copper and zinc to be active and others which require either manganese or iron. All of these minerals (with the possible exception of iron) have been reported effective in treating arthritis. Of these, the most promising is copper.

The Copper Story

Dr. John R. L. Sorenson of the University of Arkansas and Dr. Werner Hangarter of Kiel, West Germany, reviewed the use of copper complex in the treatment of rheumatoid and other forms of arthritis in about 1,500 patients, and found them to be "useful antiarthritic drugs, but much less toxic, and with no irritation of the intestinal tract." [17] *

All these bits of scientific data have contributed to the regimens I use in treating arthritic patients.

---

* There are many observations to support their views: First, there are marked changes in the blood copper level, proportionate to the severity of the rheumatoid activity. Secondly, copper is necessary to the function of several important enzymes, superoxide dismutase, a major anti-arthritic enzyme, and lysyl oxidase, an enzyme involved in the repair of inflammation. Sorenson recommends copper aspirinate, which brings about a favorable ratio between anti-inflammatory and pro-inflammatory prostaglandins.

How I Treat Arthritis

As in any other degenerative condition, my first step in treating arthritis is to recommend the basic carbohydrate-control diet appropriate for your weight. Thus, if you are arthritic and overweight, I would recommend the lowest carbohydrate-level diet of all. And if you are underweight, the Meat and Millet Diet. If of normal weight, then you should be on a comfortable diet that incorporates moderate amounts of the complex unrefined carbohydrates (see p. 275). In other words, use the Meat and Millet regimen without overdoing its carbohydrate choices.

The first vitamin supplement I would add is the basic vitamin-and-mineral formula (see page 319). It is of vital importance to all tissue healing and to maintenance of the body's tissues in general.

After the basic diet has been followed for a good week, and the multivitamin formula is being religiously swallowed, I add specific supplements to the regimen.

I recommend that patients with rheumatoid arthritis take about a gram of pantothenic acid a day (for its steroidlike effect) and that patients with osteoarthritis take a similar quantity of B_6.

Those of my patients who have already been treated with steroids may well be in need of more vitamin C and bioflavonoids, so I prescribe 4 to 8 grams of vitamin C and 2 to 4 grams of bioflavonoids.

Although there are 200 IU of vitamin E in the basic formula, I recommend an additional 400 IU or more per day.

Hair Analysis May Be of Great Value

Because I like to discover how each nutrient works in a specific individual rather than use all nutritional treatments possible, I would probably send a patient home for a week or two on the above regimen. But before I did so, I would order a hair mineral analysis as a further diagnostic test.

While awaiting the results, I most often supplement my patients' regimens with manganese for the following reasons: The overwhelming majority of my patients are low in it, and it helps maintain the proper balance between zinc and copper.* At the same time, for some reason it helps many arthritics feel better.

---

* Dr. Charles Rudolph, Jr., found fifty-two rheumatoid arthritis patients' hair samples to be lowest in manganese, followed by copper and iron.[18]

Other researchers, including Dr. Benjamin Frank, have pinpointed manganese as being the most consistently valuable mineral an arthritic can receive.[19]

When the hair analysis results do come back I still have an uncomplicated picture, because all I have added is manganese, which is usually low. Thus, I can supplement those minerals which seem to be in short supply or try to rid the body of any toxic minerals which may be overabundant.

More Vitamins

If the nutrients I'm giving—for example, vitamin B_6 or pantothenic acid—seem to be yielding positive results, I often increase the dosage to see if greater dosages might provide even greater benefit. Conversely, if the reaction seems negative, I might reduce the dosage.

If my patient is not making the kind of progress I would like to see, I might add a gram of niacinamide (vitamin B_3) to the daily regimen. And if such a patient is not taking pantothenic acid, I would be inclined to add that too.

One Step at a Time

In general, I add nutrients one at a time to see which prove to be most beneficial.

My overall goal, of course, is to wind up with maximum results from as few supplements as possible over the long term.

Mineral Supplements

When I supplement the minerals, I prefer chelates, because these complexes seem to be better utilized in the body.

Thus, if a hair analysis shows that my patient's copper is low, I add chelated copper. In the future, when copper salts such as copper aspirinate are available, they should, according to Dr. Sorenson's research, prove more effective. Although at first glance this aspirin compound looks to be a drug, its action is probably attributed to a better delivery of copper to the tissues. This type of copper salt has also been reported to be effective against ulcers, as well as seizure disorders.[20]

If the arthritis is of the rheumatoid variety, I would be inclined to start a therapeutic trial (that means, give it and see if it helps) with copper anyway. So much of the latest research suggests that copper plays a vital role in the health of the joints. (Perhaps one day we will find out why the copper bracelet your arthritic aunt wore was not really quackery after all.)

As yet, it is too early to know why some arthritic patients have high hair copper levels and others have low ones. In rheumatoid arthritis, copper is usually elevated in both the serum and the joint fluid. But does that mean it is causing arthritis or arriving on the scene to help out? On the other hand, zinc and iron may be elevated in the joint fluid and *lower* in the serum.[21] As yet we don't know what all this means for the arthritic patient. In managing the patient with degenerative arthritis, I will go by the hair analysis and try to balance copper and zinc. At this stage, it is almost impossible to give guidelines as to how much to take, beyond stating that copper and zinc seem to be very important in arthritis and that they should remain in proportion in your system.

Naturally, if a patient's zinc level is low, I prescribe chelated zinc, zinc orotate, or zinc aspartate. And, if zinc and copper are *both* low, I supplement them in appropriate proportions. Still, however, there is considerable guesswork here, since hair levels do not necessarily correlate with blood levels (see pages 294 ff.). And we do not yet know which are the more significant.

More Than Vitamins and Minerals

Early in the course of treating my arthritic patients, I consider other biological substances. My favorite is the substance our own joints and tissues rely upon—superoxide dismutase (SOD). It is much more expensive than vitamins and minerals, its absorption through the stomach is questionable, and it is used up in minutes. But it *is* what your inflamed joints *need* where the action is. So I devote a week to a therapeutic trial of SOD, making no other changes in diet or other agents. I start with six of the 50 mcg enteric-coated tablets and build up to eight, twelve, and sixteen per day until I get an effect—or don't. More often than not, the patient reports improvement.

The list of food factors effective in arthritis is a long one. High on the list is bromelain, the pineapple enzyme, and papain, the papaya enzyme. Alfalfa is a major benefactor to many arthritics, as is an extract of New Zealand mussels (available in most health-food stores).

Don't Forget Cod-Liver Oil

Popular nutrition writer/lecturer Dale Alexander has dedicated his life to teaching us the virtues of cod-liver oil as a joint lubricant and vitamin source for arthritics.* I suspect it also works by improving the types of prostaglandins we develop (see page 229). I often recommend one or two tablespoons of cod-liver oil at bedtime, taken with milk. (If you are milk sensitive, make sure you do not mix it with more than one ounce of milk.)

I Haven't Finished Yet

When stiffness is the problem, the vitamin that I think of is PABA. Two grams or more goes a long way toward relieving stiffness and loss of joint mobility. (The potassium salt of PABA has been used in doses up to 24 grams in other connective tissue disorders.)

If my patient has *still* not improved to the extent I would like, I may on the next visit administer a test dose of vitamin B_{12}— 1000 mcg, injected along with 5 mg of folic acid.[23] I have seen these two vitamins give dramatic relief to a small but significant number of arthritic patients. If the injection works, I then add 750 mcg of B_{12} and 6 mg of folic acid in tablet form to the daily regimen.

It may sound to you as though the treatment of arthritis can go on forever. And in a way it does. The condition surely *does* persist, and it often takes quite a while to find out what combination of supplements does the best job of relieving symptoms. And worst of all, the problem may not be in the supplements—it may be in the diet.

Food Allergy May Play a Role

As though finding the right combination of nutrients were not problem enough, food allergy may well be a major trigger in arthritis flare-ups.

Thus, if the simple use of vitamins doesn't seem to do the job, I often ask my patients to keep a list of the foods they eat, and attempt to correlate any flare-up with specific foods in the diet.

* Alexander's work was corroborated clinically by Dr. Charles Brusch and Edwin Johnson in the July 1959 issue of the *Journal of the National Medical Association*.[22] They tested ninety-eight patients with spectacular success. It has never been reported on since then.

It's not simple, though, for sometimes a food causes a delayed rather than an immediate reaction. So the list system is hit-or-miss, educated guesswork at best.

However, when a possible trigger is identified, it is worth eliminating to see what happens. I have my patient stay away from it for at least two weeks, and then eat the suspect food at least twice in a twenty-four-hour period. The first thing we look for is this: Did the arthritis clear up or improve during the two-week "vacation"? If so, then the second question is: Did the arthritis get worse after the food was again eaten?

Two examples of food allergy in arthritis are fairly well known to medical scholars. Dr. R. Shatin of Perth, Australia, wrote several papers describing patients whose symptoms vanished when the wheat gluten was eliminated from their diets.[24] He prescribed the same gluten-free diet that has proven so useful in schizophrenia and several large-intestine syndromes.

And Rutgers horticulturist Dr. Norman Childers pointed out that the nightshade food family, which contains such diverse vegetables as tomatoes, peppers, paprika, and white potatoes, is responsible for many arthritic flare-ups.[25] I have many patients who attribute their success to the elimination of the nightshade family.

Of course, any given patient may have more than one trigger food (and most do), so sometimes it is necessary to refer a patient for extensive—and sometimes expensive—food allergy testing. (See Chapter 27.)

Fasting—the Ultimate Diet

If by this time nothing whatsoever has worked, then it is time to reevaluate the food allergy situation—to the point of fasting.

This is because a no-food regimen means that nothing you are sensitive to is being eaten. Most patients' symptoms seem to improve after a few days' fast, usually between the third and the fifth days, but a fast of this duration should not be undertaken without your doctor's approval. Then food should be reinstituted slowly —no more than one new food per day—while you carefully watch for arthritic symptoms and food reactions.

Even in Relief, There May Be a Dilemma

Sometimes a patient presents a physician with a really tough choice. For example, Anne Epperly did well with respect to her many varied symptoms, except that her arthritis did not improve. So she decided to embark upon a cherry-juice fast she had read about, and to her delight, her arthritis symptoms cleared up promptly. Unfortunately, however, her new eating pattern was very high in carbohydrates—and her old carbohydrate-related depression and fatigue symptoms, which had been controlled by her low-carbohydrate regimen, came back.

Now I was faced with a therapeutic dilemma: to continue with the arthritis-relieving cherry juice, or to go back to the depression-and-fatigue-fighting low-carbohydrate diet?

Eventually, working together, we found a regimen that worked for her arthritis *and* her blood sugar. We kept the blood sugar control diet and relied on a more intense vitamin regimen.

So you can see that finding the perfect diet for any individual—especially one with a metabolic problem or a degenerative disease—is not all that easy. The treatment of arthritis can be complex and time-consuming. However, if the doctor and patient persist, some measure of relief can eventually be achieved. For example, of the last thirty patients who consulted me for osteo- or rheumatoid arthritis, the following results were tabulated: much improved, 19 patients; moderately improved, 8 patients; no improvement, 3 patients. In all cases, drug therapy was either reduced or eliminated.

Chapter 19

DIABETES

People think of adult-onset diabetes as a condition that strikes in the middle years. But although that is when the end-stage symptoms become evident, adult-onset diabetes may well begin with a child's very first lollipop.

It is not something that strikes, either. It is self-imposed.

I am not *blaming* the diabetic for his or her disease. He could not have known that he was causing his own diabetes, just doing what everybody else does. He may even have been eating a "good" diet and following his doctor's advice implicitly.

Yet he developed diabetes just the same.

How Diabetes Gets Started

Let me tell you about Alice, who is really a composite of my diabetic patients. Her hypothetical case will, I think, show you just how adult-onset diabetes develops.

Even as a toddler, Alice knew how to get what she wanted—sweets. All she had to do was refuse all those things she didn't like.

She had plenty of allies too. For instance, the minute Alice's grandma saw her, she popped candy into her mouth. Even Alice's doctor rewarded her with lollipops for being good.

Though Alice's dentist tried to convince her parents that sugar foods would rot her teeth, and they in turn cut down on desserts and tried to eliminate the candy, Alice was wily. She got around the candy ban by cajoling and trading with her school friends.

Of course candy and soda were not the whole problem. Those school lunches, the handiwork of the school dietician who made sure that each meal consisted of something from each of the basic four food groups, were something to contend with—metabolically, that is. The dietician wanted to be sure that Alice and her schoolmates ate everything she put on their plates. So a typical meal consisted of sweet 'n' sour stew, candied carrots, raisin bread, chocolate milk, and sugar-froth lime-green chiffon delight. Sound familiar? Sure it does! We *all* got the likes of this in our grade school cafeterias.

By high school, everyone was hanging out at the soda fountain, and later on at the pizza parlor. Alice went along, and if what she ate there was not the problem, then what she washed it down with surely was.

After high school came the startling discoveries of beer and booze. Alice didn't neglect coffee either—it was so perfect for ungluing the eyes in the morning and ideal for combating that hangover.

Finally, however, Alice noticed that things were not going quite right. Her friends thought she might be a little "strung out," and she had frequent unexplained bouts of "nerves," dizziness, and inability to concentrate. She also had unfightable and completely undeniable fatigue.

This is when Alice had her first serious encounter with a doctor. And a serious encounter it was, for though nothing positive was accomplished, Alice left his office with tranquilizers for the anxiety attacks and a little friendly advice that included, "Take it easy, get enough sleep, eat three square meals a day, and stop worrying."

Alice's problems were compounded by The Pill, which caused some bloating, headaches, and a nebulous depression. And when she began to gain weight (more than two dress sizes), her doctor assured her that it couldn't be The Pill's fault. Both Alice and her doctor agreed that the weight gain was doubtless the result of her newfound craving for sweets.

These new symptoms necessitated another trip to the doctor, who responded to the new complaints with a diuretic to make life bearable again. But those diuretics did their share in contributing to Alice's gradually growing propensity toward diabetes.

By this time in her life, Alice's overweight became a *real* problem. Especially since she was less active and no longer participated in a mandatory physical education program as she had in high school.

From High School to Work

Alice took a job before she finally met the man she married. Now she skipped breakfast at home and grabbed a bite at the office when the coffee cart with the ever-present doughnuts came around. And when she changed jobs she was "lucky" enough to work near the vending machine canteen which held that endless selection of the world's "finest, most nutritious foods."

Lunchtime was a disaster area again, with a quick trip to the local fillerburger outlet for a meat-flavored, food technologist's dream on a nonperishable, easy-shipping, quick-toasting bun—accompanied by an exotic concoction of ketchup and french fries. Naturally Alice washed all this stuff down with her favorite cola drink (no brand names, please) or a milkless, sugar-laden thickshake.

And finally those extra pounds added up to a glaring embarrassment. Along with the overweight, Alice had recurring bouts of exhaustion and a "case of nerves." She began to think she must be working too hard. Alice's problems should not have come as a surprise to her; after all, she had a *terrible* diet, never exercised, and filled herself with booze and sweets when relaxing. No wonder she felt worse by the day.

By this time Alice was earnestly trying to get rid of all these symptoms. She was snappish with her fiancé, and began to wonder whether he'd have second thoughts about the wedding. So back she went to the doctor—for more advice on getting into shape.

The doctor attributed her emotional symptoms to anxiety over her approaching marriage, pronounced her fit (if a bit flabby), and gave her his wisest counsel: "Walk instead of ride, and push yourself away from the table." That uttered, he handed Alice a prescription for more diuretics, a different brand of tranquilizer, and some diet pills.

Nutrition to the Rescue?

Unfortunately, Alice lost only a few pounds—and these came right back when she went off the diet pills which had made her intolerably jumpy. And she didn't feel any better for her efforts, either. Worse still, she did nothing more for her problem, because she was so disappointed with the "help" she got that she felt her situation was hopeless.

All the while, of course, she was eating less, but she was not eating less of those things responsible for putting her on the diabetes-bound roller coaster.

Then one day a girl friend of Alice's dragged her to vegetarian nutritionist's lecture. Alice listened, decided she had nothing to lose, and gave the nutritionist's program a try.

She gave up sweets in favor of lots of fruits and juices—still full of sugar. She ate the usual assortment of starchy and green vegetables and the ubiquitous yogurt. Unfortunately, Alice favored the chocolate frozen kind on a stick! And now, on this new health kick, Alice felt "at least ten percent better." (Sugar-filled though this diet was, it was better than her previously overprocessed, highly synthetic regimen chock-full of the miracles of modern technology.)

For a while, problems eased up. But as time went on, Alice's lifestyle (marriage, job promotions, and finally kids) made it harder and harder to stick to a vegetarian regimen. After all, dinner parties meant rolls, desserts, and after-dinner mints, not to mention a drink or two of the alcoholic variety. And there were church suppers where you couldn't offend Lissie-May by not just *tasting* her new gelatin mold.

Alice Finally Decided She Needed Help

Alice grew tired of going to her doctor and hearing the same old thing. She began to think her problem might be more than the effect of a sedentary life-style and "nerves."

And she was right. Her doctor had completely forgotten about the metabolic consequences of hyperinsulinism and how they could be devastating well before Alice's middle years.

If her doctor had inquired into her eating habits, he might not have suggested that Alice change them anyway.

Alice went back to the same doctor a number of times, and he couldn't seem to find anything really wrong. But the list of complaints began to resemble the questionnaire I use to develop a sense of a patient's hypoglycemia symptoms, and Alice simply felt as though she wasn't functioning. So she began to pay attention to various health-related magazine articles and finally switched doctors, begging for the glucose tolerance test that would doubtless explain the reason for all her symptoms.

As it so often is, it was refused. After asking around for a good long while, she found a doctor who agreed to perform one. Eureka! The test was done, and the results were hypoglycemia—and hyperinsulinism, too. At last Alice thought she had a handle on the problem.

But did she get help? Not yet.

For the doctor who did the GTT told her to eat a candy bar whenever she felt the symptoms coming on. Following this advice, naturally Alice got still worse.

The Final Phases

Alice dragged herself around, year after year, hoping she would find a solution to the problems, gaining a few pounds here and there, and feeling a little worse all the time.

Finally she became chronically thirsty, urinated constantly, and miracle of miracles, that extra weight mysteriously began to drop off.

So she changed doctors again—and this time the new doctor's routine tests indicated that "diabetes has struck."

Sure it struck. But the little ripples of onset had been going ever since Grandma handed out those sour balls, gumdrops, and peppermint creams.

Diabetes and Insulin Levels

Alice's diabetes finally became overt when symptoms of insulin deficiency arose. But latest research indicates that she must have gone through several decades of high insulin levels (caused by the junk foods, junk beverages, booze, and coffee) that assaulted her system day after day from awakening to bedtime.[1] And the diet pills, diuretics, tranquilizers, The Pill, and other drugs all contributed to that end, too.

But how, after all these years of *high* insulin levels, could symptoms of insulin deficiency occur? Are not high insulin levels at the root of adult onset of diabetes?

A Diabetic Is Not Simply a Diabetic Anymore

Until quite recently, a diabetic was a diabetic, because the only criteria for diagnosis were blood and urine glucose levels. But when Drs. Rosalyn Yalow and Solomon Berson developed a practical, inexpensive means of determining blood insulin levels, the whole diagnostic picture of diabetes took on a new, sharper definition.

Their research established that there are really *two* groups of diabetics: high-insulin and low-insulin types.[2]

The difference between the two groups is that the high-insulin diabetic tends to be obese and is less likely to suffer from the vascular, kidney, nervous system, and eye complications so likely to strike the low-insulin diabetic.

This could, of course, be due to the possibility that the high-insulin diabetic is merely suffering from an earlier stage of the disease.

What all this says to me is that the high-insulin hypoglycemic and the high-insulin early diabetic are links in the chain that ultimately ends in the low-insulin diabetic syndrome, in which the pancreas is exhausted and can no longer produce the amounts of insulin needed.

That is why many researchers think of hyperinsulinism, or high insulin levels, as the initial metabolic departure from normal in the development of diabetes.

The pattern progresses like this:

During your teens and early twenties, you may have had low blood sugar with some elevations of insulin. Then, perhaps in the next decade, the low blood sugar readings would persist, but the pattern would show that an elevation of sugar levels would begin to appear, usually in the first hour after taking glucose. Finally, in your forties, the high sugar readings would persist longer—as though some elusive anti-insulin factor were present, tying up your insulin and making it ineffective. At this point, your blood sugar would drop suddenly, and you would feel symptoms. Eventually, maybe in your fifties, the insulin response simply gave up, and your blood sugar stopped dropping after the rise. Thus, your blood sugar would be elevated in the morning, and you just might find glucose in your urine.

At this rather late stage, the unsuspecting physician makes his diagnosis via routine testing. The knowing physician, on the other hand, could have made his diagnosis a good twenty-five years before that.

It's about time the medical profession (and everybody else) recognized these intermediate stages in the development of diabetes and the necessity of performing glucose tolerance tests, with insulin levels, at reasonable intervals.

Just think how many obese, middle-aged, tired, anxious, irritable, depressed individuals might detect their diabetes when it could still be reversed easily.

So when anyone asks you, "What are the *first* symptoms of diabetes?" you could answer them by reciting the long list of symptoms that are attributed to low blood sugar. Excessive thirst and urination along with unexplained weight loss don't happen until decades later.

The Best Treatment for Diabetes Is Prevention

From Alice's example, you can begin to see why diabetes has become epidemic, and is getting more prevalent all the time. It is caused by our overconsumption of junk food and beverages and is enhanced by the blood-sugar-altering drugs that are too thoughtlessly prescribed. Lack of exercise contributes, too.

All these factors have increased alarmingly throughout the twentieth century. Although, to be sure, diabetes was seen before the twentieth century, adult-onset diabetes must now, logically, be in its heyday.

Prevention involves a healthy diet, restoration of the missing nutrients, more than adequate exercise, and avoidance of the many drugs that increase our insulin levels. Once these measures are instituted (and maintained) during any of the high-insulin stages of diabetes (or pre-diabetes), the process is halted or reversed, and overt diabetes rarely, if ever, occurs.

The Orthodox Approach

Although orthodox treatment may differ slightly from doctor to doctor, the same general outline seems to apply. It does not seem realistic to me, but I think you should see it in its entirety and judge for yourself whether it makes as much sense as my prevention approach.

1. The orthodox physician cannot treat diabetes until it is obviously there. So he waits for it to develop and *then* thinks about making dietary changes. Diabetes specialists are now talking about raising the criteria for abnormal blood sugar levels during a glucose tolerance test. A reading of 130 at the second hour has been considered abnormal, but it is being suggested now that the "abnormal cutoff point" be raised to 150. This means that many patients who are now considered borderline diabetics and who should watch their diets will be classified as normal and go unmonitored.

2. An orthodox physician recognizes only the most severe hypoglycemia and does not consider *any* hypoglycemia a forerunner of diabetes. Thus, the American Diabetes Association, the Endocrine Society, and the AMA have warned physicians that hypoglycemia

is being "overdiagnosed." [3] Unfortunately, this means that a physician who heeds their warning will not identify and give dietary advice to those patients who are strong candidates for diabetes.

3. When a patient *is* finally diagnosed as diabetic, the first treatment should be dietary. I do not deny that a lot of traditional doctors do put their patients on diets. The problem is that the diet most physicians direct their patients to follow is virtually identical to that on which the diabetes developed in the first place. It is high in carbohydrates without putting limitations on simple sugars. In fact, the newest recommendations call for a diet that is even higher in carbohydrates than the inadequate traditional one, and there is still no distinction drawn between simple and complex carbohydrate sources.

This cloud, however, does have the proverbial silver lining. Some diabetologists are beginning to recommend that there be a set ratio of complex to simple carbohydrates, stressing the complex ones. This, at least, is a step in the right direction.

4. The traditional line holds that an overweight diabetic should lose weight. I am all for this, of course. But the diet recommended —the balanced, low-calorie one—is sufficiently difficult to follow that a high percentage of diabetics will not succeed in shedding the extra pounds. This is in marked contrast to 95 percent of overweight diabetics who take off pounds on a low-carbohydrate regimen.

5. When diet alone does not control diabetes, the traditionalist turns to insulin or insulin-stimulating drugs. (I have no gripes about insulin, used properly, and I'll get to that later.) The non-insulin drugs in current usage, the sulfonylureas, were first recommended in the 1950s and were tremendously popular until the University Group Diabetes Program (UGDP) study indicated that patients taking them did not live as long as those with similar diabetic problems who took insulin. [4]

Many diabetologists, of course, disputed the validity of the UGDP study by pointing to many flaws in the research design per se.

The problem with sulfonylureas is that they will not work on insulin-deficient diabetics. What seems worse to me, however, is that the sulfonylureas *stimulate the release of insulin* in a patient who is already releasing too much insulin. As I mentioned earlier, these patients seem to have some resistance to their own insulin, so it hardly seems logical to get them to secrete even more. The drugs aggravate the diabetes more than they help it.

In treating over four thousand diabetics I have not once seen fit to prescribe one of these medications.

There is another class of oral antidiabetic that I have, on rare occasions, used. It is phenformin, which works *against* insulin. The FDA, in its own inimitable way, deemed phenformin to be dangerous and took it off the market.

And this takes me back to the subject of insulin. Because when diet doesn't do the job, that is what's left.

Insulin and Insulin

There are two types of insulin, and both are injectable. One is short-acting and is referred to as "regular" insulin, and the other is longer-acting and includes NPH, PZI, and lente insulins.

Both are effective in controlling blood sugar levels, but the longer-acting type leaves a patient with *constant* blood levels of insulin. These constant levels are probably higher than the blood levels the patient would have if the patient's own pancreas were releasing insulin after meals and then letting the blood level drop.

Regular insulin, on the other hand, is shorter-acting. It has to be taken more frequently, but it comes closer to mimicking the way the pancreas would function if it were behaving normally. This is described by doctors as a more physiologic action.

A patient on regular insulin really has to be a bit more motivated than one on the long-acting, but there is a benefit in the discipline. Dr. Peter Forsham, among other researchers, is convinced that frequent doses of fast-acting insulins come closer to achieving natural, physiologic blood insulin levels. And he believes that not only is the control of diabetes better when short-acting insulin is used, he is also confident that "properly insulinized patients have an appreciably lower incidence of small vessel disease that may contribute to large vessel pathogenesis." [5] In other words, he believes that diabetics on short-acting insulin have a lower incidence of cardiovascular complications.

Another reason I favor regular insulin is that my patients seem to be able to get by with less than is required of the long-acting type. And insulin has a set of diabetic complications all its own, so it follows that the less of it a diabetic has to use, the better. Insulin has been implicated as a possible cause of cardiovascular complications. This does not in any way mean that insulin isn't necessary and lifesaving, but it does indicate that too much of it may be troublesome.

First, when it is produced in excess (as in the high-insulin diabetic) it is not efficient in dealing with blood sugar, so we have to add more. Professor Robert W. Stout of Belfast University has demonstrated that the cells that are instrumental in the formation of atherosclerotic plaque (see Chapter 22) grow under the influence of insulin.[6] He was able to prove that experimental animals injected with insulin developed atherosclerosis. And if their aortas were injected with insulin, the atherosclerosis would develop at the exact site of the injection.

Second, in high-insulin diabetics and in overweight members of the general population, there is more heart disease than in people whose insulin levels are normal.

That is one of my objections to long-acting insulin—it is present in the blood stream even when not needed. And I do not believe that excess insulin stimulation at the cellular level is in any way desirable. This excessive insulin load has transformed our diabetic population from one that died of diabetic coma in the old, pre-insulin days to one that dies of cardiovascular complications.

Diet and Nutrition

I wish there were earthshaking breakthroughs in the treatment of diabetes. But there aren't. There is, however, a promising finding that may well make a great difference to both diabetics and hypoglycemics. It is the discovery of a *glucose tolerance factor* (GTF) that is a complex of trivalent chromium, glycine, nicotinic acid, and the amino acids glutamic acid and cystine, among others.

Just as cobalt is an essential mineral in vitamin B_{12}, chromium is an integral part of GTF, which is essential to the metabolism of carbohydrates. GTF should really be considered a vitamin because, like the B complex vitamins, it is active in carbohydrate metabolism, is essential to the human organism, and has a mineral fraction.

Dr. Richard Doisy of Syracuse University made some synthetic GTF and showed that with it the blood glucose level of laboratory animals could be brought down, but only about half as much as when the animals were given brewers' yeast, which contains natural GTF.[7] So it looks as though we have a little way to go in analyzing GTF to find out exactly what's in it, and in duplicating it in the laboratory.

Once this has been accomplished, there may be one more helpful agent in the management of diabetes and blood sugar disorders.

How I Treat Diabetes

First and foremost, I stress carbohydrate restriction and stabilizing blood sugar levels. My goal is to keep blood glucose down and prevent it from spilling over into the urine.

Although we don't yet know all the answers to treating diabetes, I get spectacular results in reducing or eliminating insulin by instituting a low-carbohydrate regimen.

Unfortunately, the control is not always for a lifetime, for some diabetics seem to "adjust" to the new regimen after a while and spill sugar again—meaning that they need insulin again. I counsel every patient whose diabetes is controlled by diet to keep careful tabs on his urine sugar. Of course, every diabetic should be under the supervision of a physician.

Since blood sugar control by diet is far preferable to blood sugar control by insulin, any vacation from insulin and its potential side effects may well help to prolong a diabetic's life-span.

I have recently done a study of forty-four consecutive diabetics in my office practice. I included only those who were not previously in treatment, so most of them would have to be classified as mildly diabetic. Before they started on my regimen their mean blood sugar level was 160; after they had been on the diet with vitamins and minerals, their mean blood sugars were down to the borderline reading of 111.

Improvement Went Beyond Blood Sugar Levels

Not only did blood sugar levels dip into the "normal" range, cholesterol levels in general went down 20 points (from 245 to 225) and the triglyceride levels plummeted so consistently that the mean went from 171 to 94. Best of all, this group's fasting insulin levels went from 41 to 24 (the normal range extends up to 25 units). Needless to say, all who were overweight lost weight, and in another group of forty diabetics who were on oral medications, most were able to stop taking them. Ninety percent of the insulin-taking patients were able to reduce their dosages, usually to less than half their starting levels.

All the overweight diabetics started on the ketogenic diet, monitoring their progress with Ketostix. The nonoverweight (the normal or under-normal weight group) went on the Meat and Millet Diet, completely eliminating simple and refined carbohydrates.

The Diabetic and the Pritikin Diet

You may note that this sort of success with diabetes is also claimed by backers of just the opposite diet. A good example is the Pritikin diet. Although Nathan Pritikin attributes his diet's success to its low fat content, most authorities would agree that his diet is effective because of the high ratio of complex to simple carbohydrates.[8]

Unfortunately, Mr. Pritikin's diet is also low in protein, low enough to induce a deficiency in some patients. It cannot match a ketogenic diet for controlling hunger. If the diet is followed implicitly, I am sure the blood sugar will improve, but diets with sharply lowered carbohydrate intakes far outstrip these high-carbohydrate diets in the matter of lowering the blood sugar.

I have found that if the ratio of complex to simple carbohydrates is kept high, protein and fat sources can be added to the diet without sacrificing good results.

The diet with a high ratio of complex to simple carbohydrates is obviously the diabetics' diet of the future, although the American Diabetes Association has not yet officially espoused it. Phyllis Crapo, working with the Stanford University group, demonstrated that each source of carbohydrate can produce a different amount of insulin. The range of insulin secreted varied from 45 units of insulin one hour after a dose of sugar, through 27 units after a dose of potato starch, to only 12 units after a dose of rice starch.[9] What is needed are more studies on every carbohydrate. The ideal diet for diabetes could be based upon those foods that provoke the least insulin response.

Vitamin Therapy Can Make a Difference

Although diet alone can do quite a bit, it is really not enough. I feel that a program of vitamin-and-mineral therapy can add a therapeutic advantage.

I have found no vitamins and minerals so effective in the management of diabetes that, in and of themselves, they will correct the blood sugar abnormality. There are several nutrients for which this claim has been made, but I have been disappointed with their effects when I have tried them in my practice. The single exception is vitamin B_6, which has been shown to help the diabetes of pregnancy—gestational diabetes. Vitamin B_6 was administered to a group of pregnant women with impaired glucose tolerance, which had arisen only since the pregnancy began. All of the women had been shown by vitamin analysis to have a relative deficiency of vitamin B6, and when this vitamin was replaced they all showed improved glucose tolerance. This, in turn, enabled them to get through their pregnancies with fewer complications to mother and fetus.[10]

Dr. William Philpott provides some rationale for the use of B6.[11] He maintains that diabetes is really the result of a series of allergy-addiction responses to foods commonly found in our diets, and that the hallmark of this allergic state is elevated blood sugar, which, his studies show, occurs after the trigger foods are eaten. He has found that vitamin B6 can prevent this blood sugar elevation. Philpott also claims to achieve the same effect with vitamin C.

Dr. K. E. Sarji, at the annual meeting of the American Diabetes Association in 1978, reported that she had observed that diabetics have significantly lower levels of ascorbic acid (vitamin C) in their platelets, compared to control subjects. She went on to say that this might be associated with the increased clumping of the platelets so commonly observed in diabetics.[12] And we know that this platelet clumping is associated with atherosclerosis, or hardening of the arteries. Thus it is possible that taking additional vitamin C might help the diabetic go one step farther toward avoiding the vascular complications of diabetes.

Vitamins and minerals do exert a favorable effect on the well-being of diabetic patients in general, and for this reason I recommend them routinely.

The Russians, in less well documented research, suggest that "vitamin" B15 also has a favorable effect on a diabetic's blood sugar levels.[13]

My own recommendation emphasizes the B complex vitamins because they are so important in carbohydrate metabolism, relying heavily upon vitamin B6 (500 to 1000 mg per day in addition to what is already in my basic formula). I also recommend at least 1500 mg of vitamin C in addition to the basic regimen, for a daily total of at least 3000 grams.

Inositol, too, is important, because it may help the diabetic avoid some of the neurologic problems that tend to go along with years of diabetes. I prescribe 2 to 6 grams per day for those patients who have difficulty with neuropathy, or who have lost their knee or ankle reflexes. Doctors in St. James Hospital in Leeds reported good results with a smaller dosage.[14]

I believe that vitamin E may be a useful adjunct in treating diabetics who have vascular complications. Drs. Evan and Wilbur Shute of Canada have pointed out that vitamin E is particularly useful in accelerating healing among diabetics with compromised vascular systems.[15] I make sure that most diabetics in my practice get approximately 800 IU of vitamin E in addition to the basic formula—and even more than that if vascular disease is a prominent feature of their illness.

Minerals—a Most Important Nutritional Aid

Diabetes is one condition in which minerals are more important than vitamins. Chromium, zinc, manganese, and magnesium deficiencies all seem to play a role in the development of diabetes. To me, these are the Big Four of essential trace minerals, not only because they play so many key roles in metabolic pathways, but also because they are so frequently deficient in our overly refined Western diet. Dr. Charles Rudolph, Jr., studied the mineral analysis patterns taken from hair specimens of eighty diabetics and found these four minerals to be significantly lower than normal.[16]

Because of all the recent work with GTF, chromium, and brewers' yeast, I recommend brewers' yeast to those patients of mine who can tolerate the extra carbohydrate it contains. For those patients who cannot, I recommend either chelated chromium or, preferably, a GTF chromium, which is derived from yeast grown on a chromium-rich culture medium. Many patients react to this product with an upsurge of stamina and well-being.

There have been hundreds of scientific papers attesting to the importance of magnesium in heart disease. Magnesium protects us against the same type of heart disease that is the number one complication of diabetes. And why not? It activates six of the nine enzymes known to be involved in the metabolism of sugar (glycolysis).

Dr. P. McNair states that there is some evidence that diabetics who develop retinal problems have low magnesium levels.[17] This work has been corroborated by Drs. Mater and Levin at St. George's Hospital Medical School in London.[18]

Zinc, too, has been shown to be effective in atherosclerosis, especially the peripheral vascular kind (see Chapter 23).[19] There also appears to be a relationship between zinc and carbohydrate metabolism. Zinc is involved in the granulation and storage of insulin. Diabetics lose more zinc in the urine than do normal subjects.[20]

The evidence that manganese deficiencies lead to impaired glucose tolerance has thus far been confirmed only in laboratory animals.[21]

How I Use the Minerals

First I do a hair analysis to ascertain the specific mineral pattern of the individual I am treating. While awaiting the results, I start with extra GTF chromium.

In addition to chromium, I often recommend manganese and magnesium—up to 50 mg of manganese and 400 mg of magnesium per day—and I usually suggest an extra 100 to 150 mg of zinc per day. In short, I like to recommend the basic formula plus extra B complex, concentrating on B_6 and brewers' yeast along with minerals.

Fiber in the Diet

There are numerous reports about such fibers as guar gum, pectin, and wheat bran and the favorable effect they have upon the diabetic's laboratory values.[22] Frankly, I am not sure whether the fiber itself has an effect or whether most of the improvement is due to the change in ratio of complex to simple carbohydrates that it brings about. I think it is the latter, and that these "fillers" reduce the intake of simple sugars and hence the call for insulin.

Where Do We Go from Here?

The saddest fact about diabetes is this: It cannot and will not be controlled until Western cultures such as ours first recognize the diabetes-causing patterns that we perpetuate from birth through the middle years—and then move to correct them.

The number of cases of diabetes can be drastically reduced. And we know how.

But the establishment simply refuses to buck the trend to technological food, to make a stand against the food industry and its lobbies. Sometime, somebody will have the courage to institute the type of public education that could save millions of Westerners from the scourge of diabetes.

The opportunity is yours, now. If you are diabetic, you can control your condition better than ever before because now you know what to do. And whether or not you are diabetic, you can keep your eye on those potential diabetics around you and spread the word to children, family, friends, and anyone else you can persuade to think nutritionally, *eat right*, and to consider a five- to six-hour glucose tolerance test.

A GTT will require your doctor's compliance. If your doctor objects, it may be because his office schedule is too crowded. Offer to have the test performed at a laboratory. I can think of no reason why a physician should object to a patient wanting to know about his potential for an illness *before* he becomes ill.

PART V
Reversing Vascular Disease

INTRODUCTION

I hope that by now you are aware that our ancestors didn't often die of coronary heart disease (CHD). In fact, the CHD and other cardiovascular disease that kills 50 percent of our population, often prematurely, is strictly a modern phenomenon. It is far and away the most serious epidemic of the twentieth century.[1]

Tension, anxiety, and inactivity have been held responsible for this scourge, and though I do concede that they are doubtless contributing factors, I am sure that tension, anxiety, and the sedentary life-style were prevalent in the 1800s too. We cannot blame all of our heart disease upon these factors.

Thus, if our forebears often led stress-ridden, anxious, or sedentary lives, we must look beyond these conditions for the roots of today's fantastic escalation in cardiovascular disease. In short, *we must identify those societal patterns that were not present in the past.*

It is obvious to me, and I assume to you, that the real culprit must be our diet.

I have already told you that many of my patients react to too much refined carbohydrate by producing too much insulin—a condition known as hyperinsulinism. There is more bad news about hyperinsulinism.

Recent studies evaluating risk factors in coronary heart disease show that high blood insulin levels have the greatest value in predicting who will, and who won't, get heart [2] and vascular disease.[3]

And just so you don't think I am going easy on smokers, "Smoking two packs of cigarettes per day results in a fourfold increase in the incidence of coronary artery disease." [4]

Cardiologists Are Not Trained in Nutrition

My initial training was in cardiology. I loved reading cardiograms and was absolutely sure I would specialize in treating heart disease. One of my responsibilities at St. Luke's Hospital in New York City was to set up the weekly conferences of the cardiology department. What strikes me now is that no cardiologist ever complained—or even noticed—that none of our meetings concerned nutrition.

Yet it is the cardiologist who dispenses most of the dietary advice that reaches patients. He may say, "No eggs and no animal fats." If you are taking a diuretic he may tell you to drink plenty of orange juice or eat bananas to replace potassium. He may tell you to use margarine and polyunsaturated oils.

Much of this advice has proved to be grossly erroneous.[5] And no wonder. Cardiologists were not, and still are not, trained in nutrition.

More than any other specialist, however, the cardiologist must perforce adopt the policy that prevention is the best medicine. After all, there is so little to offer a patient *after* the heart attack has occurred or the blood vessels are completely occluded.

The cardiologist knows that half the American population dies of cardiovascular disease and that he can do nothing whatsover about it except try to avoid complications after a coronary event. Though he talks about preventing problems, he tends in fact to wait until they occur. And when they do, out come the drugs.

Cardiologists have tinkered with such concepts as anticoagulation (that is, impairing the clotting mechanism to prevent vessel-obstructing clots, using vitamin K antagonists such as coumadin and its derivatives). This has met with unspectacular success.[6] They have toyed with cholesterol-lowering agents that have probably done more harm than good (especially since, as I will discuss later, cholesterol is not the issue in heart disease anyway). The current rage is drugs such as aspirin, sulfinpyrazone, and others which impair the function of blood platelets.

Platelets are involved in the process whereby blood vessel damage occurs, but nature has provided platelet control factors which make the use of drugs seem unnecessarily risky.

Aspirin, for example, is one drug that many authorities concede would not be approved for use today because of rather diverse side effects, such as gastrointestinal bleeding and ringing in the ears.

Much of our current "prevention" has involved cholesterol-lowering drugs. Playing with pharmaceutical fire has proven to be pathetically naïve and misguided—especially since cholesterol-lowering agents have *not* been shown to increase life-span. In fact, a recent study on the current anti-cholesterol best seller, clofibrate, showed that it produced a very significant increase in the death rate when its users were compared to the group that did not receive the drug's intervention.[7]

It seems obvious that the true preventive medicine should be based upon life-style change—with nutrition in the forefront.

I cannot understand how our scientists could have failed to realize that nature has provided prevention of heart disease throughout every culture man has ever developed, with only one exception: ours.

I Was Not Just a Cardiologist, but an Overweight Cardiologist

I am now thankful that at one point I had an appetite far too great for my bone structure. In other words, I was fat. I tried a balanced low-calorie diet and was so hungry that each day I completed the entire day's diet by 11:00 A.M. So when I tried a low-carbohydrate regimen, I not only lost weight but I learned much more than I had bargained for. It made me thankful that I was a cardiologist and could interpret the results.

After I had succeeded in losing weight, I began to recommend that my overweight patients try a low-carbohydrate regimen, too. Many of my overweight patients with angina—those oppressive, squeezing chest pains produced when narrowed blood vessels fail to deliver enough blood to the heart muscle—reported that they needed less nitroglycerin (a drug that reduces the symptoms of angina). And many patients' angina disappeared completely, eliminating the need for nitroglycerin.

Though it took me years to develop a theory about why this was happening, I became convinced that I had been using an effective new agent in treating angina.

I also noticed a remarkable improvement in my patients with congestive heart failure. And further, those patients who had heart rhythm disturbances (for example, paroxysmal tachycardia, or episodes of very fast, regular heartbeat) reported fewer attacks, if any, when they followed the diet. (Years later I discovered that Drs. D. Aldersberg and O. Porges described all of these beneficial effects of carbohydrate restriction in 1933.)[8]

Thus I saw for myself that a low carbohydrate diet was effective in many heart-related conditions. During the next decade I sought to find out why. Before I tell you what I learned, I would like to tell you what I had to unlearn, and what I fear too many in my profession will have to unlearn also.

Chapter 20

HEART RHYTHM

"Is my pulse faster than normal?" may be the first question you ask about your heart. The normal pulse rate tends to fall within a range of 50 to 90 beats per minute. In general, when the resting pulse rate exceeds 100 beats per minute, you may assume that something is amiss—but it is not necessary to assume that you have heart disease. There are many more common causes of rapid pulse. For example, you might have a food allergy (see Chapter 27), or if you are a smoker, you might be reacting to cigarette smoke. (Smokers tend to have higher pulse rates than nonsmokers.)

Dr. Arthur Coca, who first called attention to food allergy and its relationship to pulse rate, taught us that chronically elevated pulse rates may well indicate a food allergy or allergies.[1] The most common cause of an allergic tachycardia (racing heart) is cigarette smoking. In fact, Dr. Coca discovered that he couldn't do any kind of pulse testing in a patient who continued to smoke during his investigations.

There are other causes of rapid pulse, too; they include overactive thyroid, fever, chronic infection, anemia, and chronic anxiety. Rapid pulse may be a result of simply being out of shape and being unable to tolerate the mild exercise of getting around. Unfortunately, an abnormally rapid pulse may often go undetected.

I believe that most of the rapid pulse I see represents food and smoking allergies, "out-of-shapeness," and recurrent anxiety attacks secondary to low blood sugar. It is always worth considering all the possible causes of rapid pulse before jumping to the conclusion that heart disease is the problem. In general, I start out by treating rapid pulse as I do anxiety (see page 87). This approach starts with careful control of blood sugar, the "calming vitamins," and regular exercise.

The Slow Pulse

The slow pulse, on the other hand, may be a good sign or a bad one. It may be a sign of a sluggish thyroid or a heart block (also known as A-V block), where some beats are not being transmitted. It may also occur as a drug side effect.

Slow pulse also occurs among athletes and well-trained runners. If your pulse is slow, the first question you should ask yourself is, "Am I in good enough shape to have the pulse rate people in top condition have?" Unless you've been training actively, you can assume that this is not the case. (Many runners have resting pulse rates as low as 40 to 50 beats per minute.)

So if your pulse is slow and you are *not* a trained athlete, take stock. If you are taking any medications, then check with your doctor—that could be the answer. Perhaps your doctor will want to take an electrocardiogram and a thyroid function test and other studies to get to the bottom of why the EKG would show a slow rate or an A-V block.

Heart Rhythm Abnormalities

Rhythm disturbances (arrhythmias) are another of the prevalent heart conditions that today's doctors see all the time. The most common heart condition I see in patients under thirty-five is disturbance of the heart rhythm.

Traditional doctors seem to think that arrhythmias are caused by nerves and anxiety, so they often counsel their patients to relax. Usually, the doctor assumes that the patient cannot relax, so he prescribes a tranquilizer to treat the "underlying anxiety." The patient meanwhile may experience distressing palpitations—and he usually cannot be shaken from the belief that heart disease is the problem. It usually isn't.

Most rhythm disturbances are caused by an abnormality of the body chemistry, and not of the heart itself. This important distinction explains why nutrition measures can so often correct the problem.

Nevertheless, most physicians feel that it is more appropriate to prescribe propanolol (Inderal) or digitalis to slow the patient's racing heart, or drugs like quinidine or procainamide to reduce the irritability of the heart muscle. But don't forget that drugs work by poisoning or blocking one or more of the body's natural responses. The doctor reasons that this is preferable to allowing the heart to remain "unstable." I'd be surprised to hear of an orthodox cardiologist's entertaining the notion that the problem could be due to faulty diet. And I'd be even more surprised if that doctor would modify his patient's diet—even if only to see whether the patient's condition would improve.

Some drugs (such as many tricyclic antidepressants) may bring on arrhythmias. If you are on one of these drugs and experience a change in heart rhythm, report it to your doctor at once.

Some Arrhythmias Are More Common Than Others

Of the many types of heart rhythm disturbances a cardiologist may note, several types are more common than others.

Paroxysmal tachycardia is characterized by sudden onset of racing heartbeat—it may be double or triple the usual rate. Some patients describe this sudden racing of the heart, and sudden letup of the racing, as making them feel as though their heart had an on-off switch that was being flicked back and forth.

Atrial fibrillation is also quite prevalent, and it, too, may be of sudden onset. In this case, though, the heart beats with a grossly irregular rhythm. This problem carries with it some risk—namely that of insufficient heart muscle contraction because the ventricle of the heart doesn't fill completely between beats. There is also the possibility that some clots (thromboemboli) might be thrown off. These could lodge in a vital organ (lungs, kidney, brain) and cause severe damage. This condition is one which I still treat with medication (usually digitalis). If you have atrial fibrillation, your doctor's judgment has to be your guide to appropriate treatment.

Premature Ventricular Contractions (PVCs) and Premature Atrial Contractions (PACs): These arrhythmias are also referred to as "skipped beats." Often a patient may be unaware of them until an electrocardiogram or pulse check points them up. However, the PVCs can be experienced as a "skip" because they block the next scheduled beat.

These conditions are rarely serious. In point of fact, they are so benign that U.S. Air Force doctors don't hesitate to allow pilots with these rhythm abnormalities to fly.

Unfortunately, these episodes are sometimes quite frightening, and I feel that many doctors prescribe drugs simply to eliminate the frightening symptom and to allay the patient's apprehension. I wish they would just take the time to reassure their patients and let them know that there is really no need to worry.

Most patients with these conditions have normal hearts—*but they do not necessarily have a normal metabolism.*

I say this because these conditions so often clear up when my patients make the proper changes in their diets and start to take vitamin and mineral supplements—which leads me to believe that dysnutrition is behind many arrhythmias.

Paroxysmal Arrhythmias

When I talk about paroxysmal arrhythmias, I mean those heartbeat irregularities that come on suddenly rather than those that are always present. The clearing of these paroxysmal (sudden onset) conditions on a low-carbohydrate diet is so very predictable, that I can even speculate about their cause.

My hypothesis is as follows:

If diet can cause blood sugar level instability, then it may be the primary cause of these arrhythmias. The sequence may begin like this: A patient eats something imprudent, like a candy bar or coffee loaded with sugar, which immediately sends the blood sugar up and stimulates the release of insulin. If the patient has become susceptible because of a lifetime of junk food and coffee, he will release too much insulin which in turn causes the blood sugar to drop rapidly. This rapid fall in blood sugar provides the signal for adrenaline release. Adrenaline combats the falling blood sugar, and it stimulates the heart to beat more rapidly. Thus, tachycardia may follow sugar ingestion in susceptible individuals. When the heart cannot beat as fast as the adrenaline directs, the atria may fibrillate and a more irregular heartbeat will be the result.

What I Recommend for My Patients

Although there are mechanical techniques such as pressing on the carotid sinus in the neck or using the Valsalva maneuver (forcibly exhaling against a closed glottis), I will limit my discussion to those techniques which can help prevent further attacks. If you are subject to recurrent fast heartbeat, you should learn about the Valsalva maneuver and carotid sinus pressure techniques from your doctor.

Arrhythmias and Blood Sugar Control

In glucose tolerance tests of patients who get arrhythmias, I find that the majority of them show rapid drops in blood sugar. Sometimes the rhythm symptoms are repeated during the GTT, but more often they are not. In either case I start by stabilizing the blood sugar.

Most of my patients with arrhythmias tell me that their attacks become less frequent and less severe very soon after they begin their blood sugar control diet. And in many patients, the arrhythmic problem disappears completely.

Susan Black was a typical patient. She came to me after suffering with a racing heartbeat for eight years. The first thing I recommended was the lowest carbohydrate level of the Atkins Diet (in other words, virtually no carbohydrates) and the basic vitamin formula outlined on page 319.

Three days after starting her diet Susan no longer had her frightening arrhythmic episodes. The rare episode she now undergoes can usually be traced to some dietary indiscretion. Susan's heart has become the monitor of how well she sticks to her diet. If she tells me her heart's been acting up, then we both know she has cheated a little.

Of course, anyone with an irregular heartbeat should certainly consult a physician.

Mitral Valve Prolapse—A New Epidemic

When he consults a doctor nowadays, the person with palpitations may find a little more than he bargained for. The doctor, after careful listening to the chest (auscultation), may announce that he suspects a prolapse of the mitral valve and he may order a special test, the echocardiogram, to verify. Although the "echo" requires special equipment, the test is no harder on the patient than is the electrocardiogram, which in the case of mitral valve prolapse (MVP) is usually quite normal.

In this condition the leaflets of the mitral valve (the valve situated between the left ventricle, the largest of the heart's four chambers, and the left atrium), billow out or balloon into the left atrium. The net result is often an increased frequency of premature contractions, both PACs and PVCs. The key to understanding this condition may well be that the rhythm disorder is not constant, as one might expect, but intermittent. Obviously some other factor must also be present.

Although MVP had not even been described when I was arranging cardiology conferences in 1960, it is anything but a rare condition. It has been estimated to affect 10 percent of the population (it is more prevalent in women than in men), and one study found twenty-one cases out of a group of one hundred "normal" college women.[2] When MVP produces symptoms, the most frequently seen is palpitations, but light-headedness and fainting spells are also common. Chest pain, fatigue, shortness of breath, and anxiety have all been described, and most striking is the number of MVP sufferers who are thought to have psychoneurotic or hypochondriacal personalities.

To me, all this sounded very much like low blood sugar. When I studied the glucose tolerance test results of my patients with MVP, I was a little startled to find that the overwhelming majority of them did have hypoglycemia or a blood sugar irregularity. So even this seemingly "anatomical" heart valve condition may prove to be another one of the conditions of the modern epidemic caused by dysnutrition.

And There is More Proof

Recently, Dr. Harisios Boudoulas and the cardiology team at Ohio State University studied twenty patients with *symptomatic* MVP (most MVP subjects have no symptoms) and demonstrated what I had long suspected.[3] A three-hour GTT showed that the MVP patients ran blood sugar levels after glucose some 23 points higher than the controls. I am convinced that six-hour GTTs, which were not done, would show the usual hypoglycemic dip. One reason for my belief is that the adrenaline by-products (catecholamine) level, which is usually high in hypoglycemia, was significantly elevated among these patients.

Patients with MVP are often asked to go on drug therapy, usually propanolol (see page 232), and this could be for life. Or they may be asked to go on antibiotic prophylaxis (to take antibiotics whenever exposed to a dental extraction or the like). But for many there may be an alternative: Stay on one of the blood-sugar controlling diets (see page 270) and avoid the adrenaline reaction that seems to change this usually benign condition into a provoker of some rather frightening symptoms. Of course you should discuss these possibilities with your physician.

The Nutrients

Nutritional treatment of arrhythmias is not complete if it consists of diet only, and management is helped by appropriate supplements.

Although magnesium has long been known to be useful in treating heart rhythm disturbances,[4] magnesium orotate—the magnesium salt of orotic acid—has not received nearly the attention it deserves. Although magnesium is in my basic formula, I recommend an additional supplement in the form of 500 mg magnesium orotate, three times a day.

Inositol, the most reliable of nature's tranquilizers, is also useful in treating arrhythmias. I have been tempted to speculate that inositol may have other properties that make it clinically useful in heart rhythm disturbances, but I have not as yet found scientific data to corroborate this. Pantothenic acid and niacinamide, which have calmative actions, too, may be used as alternatives.

While most physicians may consider it counter to accepted medical dogma to suggest that diet might have something to do with arrhythmias, an eminent orthodox internist did, in fact, link arrhythmias to low blood sugar. Tinsley Harrison, the great internist and father of *the* textbook *Internal Medicine* (he compiled and edited it), related unstable blood sugar levels to cardiac arrhythmias in a paper published in 1943.[5] So even though cardiologists are reluctant to accept the thesis that heart rhythm problems relate to dietary factors, this idea may be more Harrison's heresy than mine.

Chapter 21

CHOLESTEROL–THE
PAPER TIGER

In dozens of interviews in the media, sooner or later I am always asked the same question: "Why do you allow eggs and saturated fats? Aren't you worried about raising your patients' cholesterol and creating heart disease?" My answer: "I've observed thousands of patients on all sorts of diets, and those who ate eggs and meat and cheese did very well *in all respects*. If anything, their heart disease improved."

The disturbing fact is that so many supposedly well-informed people ask the same question.

Cholesterol—the Buzzword

High cholesterol has been the great medical bugbear for the last generation. Intensive propaganda campaigns assert that high cholesterol levels are associated with greater risk of clogged blood vessels and all other forms of cardiovascular disease. This propaganda blitz was launched by the American Heart Association, the American Medical Association, and other medical groups. It is now the official line.*

* I think that my interest in the cholesterol controversy is partially due to what I see as the industry's organized, deliberate attempt to mislead the public. I have seen my own work repudiated by people from so-called authoritative sources (e.g., the American Medical Association) who nevertheless struck me as less than intellectually honest. Therefore, I dealt at great length with the cholesterol question in *Dr. Atkins' Superenergy Diet*.[1] Since that book was pub-

212

Thus, our well-intentioned allopathic physicians (with the full approval of the vegetable oil industry, of course) advocate limiting consumption of animal fats, including butter and other dairy products, forsaking the protein-rich, nutrient-packed egg and switching to margarine and unsaturated vegetable oils as sources of dietary fat.

How wrong they are.

It is, of course, true that in a large population sample, those groups with high cholesterol readings do have a greater likelihood of developing coronary heart disease. *What has not been proven, though, is that lowering individual lipid levels in any way prevents heart disease in that individual.*[3]

In fact, the whole cholesterol story boils down to one simple fact: *High cholesterol levels are statistically associated with heart attacks.*

The problem is that many authorities have given the wrong explanation. The common rationale is that a diet high in cholesterol *causes* heart disease. I don't believe this. I do, however, think that a high cholesterol level is an important finding, which should lead to a diagnosis of dysnutrition. And I also believe that this state of less-than-optimum nutrition—not a diet laden with cholesterol-rich foods or high blood cholesterol levels—is responsible for our rampant heart disease. In fact, Dr. Ian Macdonald of Guy's Hospital in London has demonstrated that serum lipids can be influenced by the amount and type of dietary carbohydrate you eat.[4]

Unfortunately, common thinking is simplistic. It holds that a diet high in cholesterol will raise the cholesterol level. And this, it is claimed, will cause greater deposition of cholesterol in the arteries and lead to heart disease. Ross Hume Hall, in his marvelous book *Food for Nought*, points out that the official dogma is itself the cause of the error, because all research out of line with the dogma is thrown away or discredited.[5]

The Role of HDLs

More significantly, recent studies have demonstrated that the high-density lipoproteins, which allow fats to be transported in the

---

lished, however, there have been many other scientific findings which strengthen my argument. Studies that show that eating eggs does not raise cholesterol levels are now commonplace, yet the media have yet to acknowledge this fact.[2] Further, it is particularly painful to note the frequency with which the Atkins Diet is repudiated in the media because of statements from our misguided establishment authorities—statements that run counter to all available scientific data.

bloodstream, are a key to cholesterol transport. High-density lipo-proteins (HDLs) even appear to be potentially protective against heart disease. So it is now recognized that a patient with a high blood cholesterol level is not necessarily at risk if he or she has an adequate supply of HDLs.

Stephen B. Hulley, M.D., MPH, associate professor of medicine at the Stanford University School of Medicine, asserts that "prelimi-nary evidence suggests that decreasing intake of simple (refined) carbohydrates increases the level of HDL." [6] In other words, carbo-hydrate control could, according to some researchers, have a bene-ficial effect on the blood lipid profile.

Cholesterol Is Necessary

It is really a shame that cholesterol is now such a dirty word, for it is absolutely essential to our bodies. Production of adrenal and sex hormones, of bile and of vitamin D, all depend upon it. Cholesterol makes up a large part of the brain and of the cell membranes. Bear in mind, too, that most of the cholesterol in your bloodstream, and most of the cholesterol your body in fact uses, is manufactured by the body as needed. Even if you were to avoid eating cholesterol, your body would still make as much as you need. And believe it or not, *any food in all major food categories can lead to production of cholesterol.*

The body has mechanisms for limiting the absorption of choles-terol and for restricting its manufacture. Further, a group of studies has demonstrated that if you take in more cholesterol than you need, your body will excrete it through the bile rather than deposit it throughout your blood vessels. [7]

The net result is that cholesterol levels tend to remain surprisingly constant, despite ordinary variations in the diet.

So lower is not necessarily better when it comes to cholesterol. In fact, according to the National Cooperative Pooling Project to study heart disease and death statistics, among those American white males ages thirty-six to fifty-nine who were studied, the death rate from all causes was lowest in the group whose serum cholesterols fell in the range of 225–249. Even those whose levels were below 175 had a higher death rate. [8]

---

* The immediate biochemical precursor of our cholesterol is the compound Acetyl Coenzyme A, which is a common point in the metabolism of proteins, fats, and carbohydrates. Thus, *any* food can lead to cholesterol manufacture.

Everybody Still Has Cholesterol on the Brain

You will probably not be surprised to learn that many patients who come to me are more concerned about their cholesterol levels than with their level of sugar intake or their blood sugar levels. Yet most studies confirm that high cholesterol is of less clinical significance than blood sugar disorders.

My particular rule of thumb is this: If one has to use drugs or other unnatural means to lower cholesterol and triglycerides (another very important blood lipid), I don't think the potential benefit justifies the risk, especially as *it has never been shown that cholesterol-lowering drugs prolong life-span*. In fact, several important studies (in particular the Coronary Drug Project, which was a multimillion-dollar, nationwide study) have shown just the opposite.[9]

I do believe, however, that when cholesterol and triglycerides are lowered through better nutrition and exercise, the improvement *is* significant. And I have yet to hear a formerly cholesterol-obsessed patient declare, after his options have been explained, that he would prefer the potential side effects of a cholesterol-lowering drug to a healthy diet that controls blood lipids and makes him feel better all over. (See page 23, on cholesterol-lowering drugs.)

Triglycerides

Blood triglyceride levels vary with carbohydrate and alcohol intake. Diets low in total carbohydrates and alcohol usually lower triglycerides dramatically. Simple sugars and refined carbohydrates seem to cause greater triglyceride elevation than do complex and unrefined carbohydrates.

Statisticians have struggled to determine whether triglycerides are more important than cholesterol or vice versa. I have seen good medical studies that support both views. I think it is fair to conclude that both contribute equally to heart disease potential.[10]

However, for those of you with extremely high triglyceride levels, there is one consolation: Extremely elevated levels may drop dramatically—and they usually do so promptly—when appropriate dietary changes, such as those I recommend, are made. Cholesterol levels are much more stubborn. They frequently remain very close to where they began, no matter how the diet is varied. The traditional low-fat, cholesterol-lowering diet recommended by the American Heart Association fails to lower cholesterol readings in one third of all patients who try it.[11] Fruthermore, the famed Framingham and Tecumseh studies show that there is no statistically valid relationship between dietary habits and high blood cholesterol and other lipid levels.[12]

I could recite case histories of individual patients whose cholesterol levels were extremely high—in the 300s (most doctors like to see cholesterol levels below 250)—and whose levels dropped to half of that. But then, all doctors have such patients. Instead, following is the actual data I have tabulated on one hundred consecutive patients, which graphically illustrates the difference a low-carbohydrate diet and improved nutrition make.

The irony of all this is that the medical profession in general sincerely believes that the results of eating a low-carbohydrate diet are precisely opposite to these, and to other reports that appear throughout the medical literature. (See page 315.)

ATKINS REDUCING DIET

100 Subjects	Mean Initial Reading	Mean Follow-up Reading
Cholesterol	227.4	212.7
Triglycerides	133.6	84.9

This can be subdivided into 3 groups.

GROUP A: Subjects whose cholesterol *dropped* more than 10 percent (38 subjects)

38 Subjects	Initial	Follow-up
Cholesterol	228.2	185.3
Triglycerides	176.0	83.8

GROUP B: Subjects whose cholesterol *remained* within 10 percent of starting level (53 subjects)

53 Subjects	Initial	Follow-up
Cholesterol	226.0	223.9
Triglycerides	119.7	88.7

GROUP C: Subjects whose cholesterol *increased* more than 10 percent (9 subjects)

9 Subjects	Initial	Follow-up
Cholesterol	218.9	263.2
Triglycerides	57.3	67.7

Notice that in only 9 percent of subjects did the cholesterol increase more than 10 percent. These subjects were all patients who began with *low* levels of triglycerides. If a dieter has a high triglyceride to begin with, the chance of a cholesterol level going up on a low carbohydrate diet is practically nil.

An additional 16 patients were studied who were not overweight, and were given the Meat and Millet Diet. Their findings were as follows:

16 Subjects	*Initial*	*Follow-up*
Cholesterol	224.8	217.8
Triglycerides	78.6	69.9

And don't think that the so-called prudent diet recommended by doctors is quite so innocuous as its proponents and the TV ads for margarine would lead you to believe. Some patients who follow it may experience a *rise* in their cholesterol levels; others may develop certain types of gallstones (cholelithiasis). (See page 222.) Further, a recent British study showed that the cholesterol-lowering drug clofibrate seemed to increase a patient's tendency to develop gallstones.[13] Worse yet, a Veterans Administration study demonstrates more cancer deaths in a group of patients who went on a diet high in polyunsaturated fats.[14] *

Nutrition Has the Most to Offer

If you are still worried about your blood cholesterol levels, there is good news for you. Since elevated cholesterol levels are a symptom of dysnutrition, if you correct the dysnutrition you will control your blood cholesterol.

The list of nutrients with a favorable effect on blood cholesterol is long. Keep in mind that cholesterol levels do not necessarily reflect the amounts or types of fat consumed.[15] They can be regulated by meganutrition.

For example, niacin is the nutrient best known for reducing blood cholesterol levels. In fact, it is the first one recognized by orthodox physicians as having a potentially beneficial effect upon blood lipids.[16] Although niacin, as well as the pharmaceuticals tested, was shown in the Coronary Drug Project to be ineffective in prolonging life, the study was another exercise in how *not* to use nutritional

* A further bibliography is included in *Dr. Atkins' Superenergy Diet*.

techniques.[17] One can hardly hope to succeed when using isolated nutritional agents. They were meant to act in concert with all other nutrients.

How I Use Niacin

In general, when niacin (B₃) therapy is indicated, I recommend niacinamide, because niacin (nicotinic acid) per se causes a flush that may be distressing and uncomfortable.

Some patients who fail to build up dosage slowly may also begin to itch, get a headache or tingling or stomach upset and even skin rash or allergies. Doctors using niacin as a drug (that is, individually, without regard to other vitamin therapy) found that niacin increased the possibility of developing diabetes, ulcers, liver problems, and glaucoma. But when niacin is used as part of a total vitamin plan and a good nutritional program, these complications seem not to occur.

Niacin itself seems to be a better cholesterol-lowering agent than niacinamide. Therefore I use both niacinamide and niacin in a ratio of 2:1.

Thus, when cholesterol levels are elevated, I might start with 50 mg of niacin three times a day and gradually build up to 300–500 mg, divided among three doses.

Lecithin and Cholesterol

Another nutrient that deserves early mention is lecithin. It has long been the center of a controversy over its effectiveness in controlling blood cholesterol levels.

I have very little doubt. I have given many of my patients lecithin —originally to see whether their elevated cholesterol levels would respond. Over the years I have seen such favorable responses in so many cases that I now consider it the most effective nutritional agent of all for cholesterol control.

Some patients' blood cholesterol levels have dropped as much as one hundred points. More proof comes from a frequently seen phenomenon: a subgroup of patients who for one reason or another have discontinued their lecithin, only to see their blood cholesterol rise. When they resume the lecithin, their cholesterol levels plummet again.

Scientific reports that detail the favorable effects of lecithin notwithstanding, some patients' blood cholesterol levels simply do not respond. These patients' results provide the basis for the erroneous conclusion that lecithin is "proven" not to work. Rather, it just won't work for everybody.*

Whether or not lecithin lowers cholesterol, nobody disputes that it is an emulsifying agent (that is, capable of "holding" globules of fatty material and making them unavailable for use in biochemical reactions). In fact, the food processing industry uses it to improve the "dispersion" of fats. Many have theorized that if lecithin does help ameliorate the possible effects of a high cholesterol level, it may offer some protection from coronary artery disease. But note that Dr. Edward H. Ahrens has said, "There is no evidence that lowering blood lipid levels reduces the danger of a myocardial infarction [see p. 225], although there is an association between certain high lipid levels and increased risk." [20]

This assessment of risk is based on the assumption that an individual's blood cholesterol levels relate to his likelihood of developing heart disease—a point that has not been fully demonstrated. I do not believe that excess blood cholesterol, by its mere presence, increases the likelihood that it will be deposited in the blood vessels.

PABA

Sometimes my patients respond so well that even I (who naturally expect a good response) am surprised. I have long speculated as to why my heart protection regimen is so successful. Perhaps Dr. B. Vessby at the University of Uppsala in Sweden provided the answer; he administered PABA (para-aminobenzoic acid) along with ascorbic acid (vitamin C) and ran a double blind crossover study on thirty patients. (Since he followed the most widely accepted scientific protocol, not even the establishment can fault his findings.)

Vessby divided the test group in two and gave one half the PABA preparation and the other a placebo for four weeks. Then he switched things around and gave the first group the placebo and the second the PABA. At no time did the experimenter handing out the capsules or the patients receiving them know what was being given.

---

* A recent report by Dr. A. K. Horsch at the International Symposium on Drugs Affecting Lipid Metabolism indicates that "long-term treatment of patients with type II and type IV hyperlipoprotenemia with polyunsaturated lecithin results in lower serum lipids, lower cholesterol." [18] (Other studies have also confirmed lecithin's cholesterol-lowering effects.)[19]

The results were quite favorable. Dr. Vessby and his associates showed the PABA compound reduced cholesterol and triglyceride levels while not affecting the levels of protective HDLs.[21]

Since I have found PABA extremely useful as a fatigue fighter and in a variety of other clinical problems, I had been using it in significant doses without being aware that it could be a factor that might lower my patients' cholesterol levels. After reading Dr. Vessby's results, I have made it a point to include even more PABA in any cholesterol-lowering regimen.

Vitamin C

The theory that vitamin C helps lower cholesterol probably got its start with Dr. Emil Ginter. He indicated that vitamin C reduces blood cholesterol in men and women whose diet is "seasonally deficient" in ascorbic acid. Dr. Ginter found that 300 mg of vitamin C a day substantially reduced serum cholesterol levels in individuals with high initial readings but had no effect on those with normal readings.[22]

Dr. Ginter's view is corroborated by Dr. Constance Leslie, a hematologist at Pinderfields General Hospital in Wakefield, England. She reports that vitamin C "has a controlling influence on all the factors that become abnormal in atherosclerosis." She believes that vitamin C is not only responsible for transport of cholesterol to the liver (so that it may be eliminated) but that it further acts to lower triglyceride levels.[23]

I have no doubt that adequate amounts of vitamin C are helpful in any cholesterol control program. Of course, vitamin C has so many benefits that I recommend it for a wide variety of conditions anyway—and my "everybody needs it" attitude about vitamin C may be yet another reason my patients' blood cholesterol levels tend to drop.

Vitamin B15 (Pangamic Acid)

Although there have not yet been many studies on B15 and blood lipids, there is preliminary evidence that it may be of some help in patients who are treated for a minimum of ten to thirty days with 120 to 300 mg of pangamic acid. Several researchers have concluded that the higher the initial serum cholesterol value, the greater the reduction of blood cholesterol after B15 therapy.[24] The problem here is that the studies were all done by Russian scientists and have not, to my knowledge, been corroborated in the West. American medicine is reluctant to accept otherwise unsubstantiated work done in other countries.

Other Nutrients

Guar gum, pectin, and bran (all good fiber sources) have also been advocated for lowering blood cholesterol. There are studies showing that garlic—which is available in tablets from which the odoriferous portion, allicin, has been removed—lowers cholesterol too.[25]

The Oily Situation: Polyunsaturates

Of all the food factors purported to have a cholesterol-lowering effect, the most widely publicized are the polyunsaturated oils. Numerous studies done in the 1950s indicated that they exert a cholesterol-lowering effect when used in place of the more saturated dietary fats.

At present, this view is coming under considerable scrutiny, and some researchers are testing polyunsaturates oil by oil to see if this is really so.[26] I see the polyunsaturates as a two-edged sword—and the bad edge is much sharper.

The unsaturated fats increase vitamin E requirements, so I insist that those of my patients who eat a lot of them supplement their diet with extra vitamin E. (Keep in mind, too, that lecithin granules are a very rich source of natural unsaturated fats.) Further, I insist that those vegetable oils that they do consume be cold-pressed (i.e., mechanically extracted), rather than chemically extracted.

In mechanical extraction, the seed is crushed, water added, and the "mash" then heated for half an hour at 230°F. In chemical extraction, the oil is treated with such substances as gasoline, benzene, carbon disulfide, and/or lye; it is boiled and subsequently deodorized by twelve hours at temperatures of 330–380°F, and an antioxidant such as BHA is added.

Ross Hume Hall, in his book *Food for Nought, the Decline in Nutrition,* sums up my reservations quite admirably. He notes that polyunsaturated oils and margarines present many more extraneous chemicals and modified molecular configurations than we bargain for.[27]

The oils sold in supermarkets meet the objectives of the refiner and marketer: light, clear, and bland, with good shelf stability.

But what about nutritional values? I'm sure you have a good notion that the vegetable oil refining process wreaks a nutritional havoc similar to that of the wheat refining process. The oil comes out of the grain, and probably not much else.

Margarine Versus Animal Fats

Without going into all the details, I would like to point out that margarines are made from vegetable oils. In order to get a butter-like consistency, the vegetable oils must be hardened, or hydrogenated. This involves tinkering with the fatty acids' molecular structure. The conversion of the naturally occurring *cis* isomer of fatty acids to the unnatural *trans* isomer, which occurs in the hardening of margarine, is a process requiring an understanding of physical chemistry, and is beyond the scope of this book. The major pitfall to be aware of is that these *trans* fatty acids get incorporated into the body's fat stores, where they are theoretically capable of inducing cellular damage. In fact, Dr. David Horrobin points out that the *trans* fatty acids will block the utilizaton of the *cis* fatty acids and thus must be considered an anti-nutrient.[28]

Since 1914, when margarine and hydrogenated cooking fat were first sold commercially, the American public has been subjected to a broad-reaching experiment. We don't know for sure what long-term effects these fats have, but some researchers wonder if they may be in some way related to today's health problems.[29]

In its enthusiasm to switch from animal fats to vegetable oils, the orthodoxy has failed to note that polyunsaturates are chock-full of free radicals which may hasten the aging and degeneration processes and increase our requirements for vitamin E.

Cholesterol and Thyroid

Last but not least, elevated cholesterol levels may be symptomatic of a sluggish thyroid. In my own evaluation of thyroid function, I think the basal body temperature correlates better with my clinical impression than do laboratory results. Perhaps this is partially because of the wide range of normal values for the blood tests and partially because we want to measure actual thyroid function rather than how much thyroid hormone is circulating.

When the thyroid is underactive for nutritional reasons, supplements of kelp may be useful, because kelp contains iodine, the element upon which thyroid activity depends.

Most cases of thyroid deficiency, however, are probably not due to iodine deficiency and are best treated by supplementation with natural or synthetic thyroid hormone. Nonetheless, I believe your doctor would agree that a trial of kelp is a relatively safe nutritional technique for cholesterol lowering when one suspects that a sluggish thyroid may be part or all of the problem. (In my practice, when an overweight patient shows a metabolic resistance to losing weight, my suspicion of thyroid deficiency is extremely high.)

How I Approach High Cholesterol

Often a patient comes to me taking such cholesterol-lowering medications as clofibrate (Atromid S) or probucol (Lorelco). However, experience with the low-carbohydrate diet in the overweight and with the low–refined-carbohydrate diet in the normal-weight person—and with the multitude of cholesterol-lowering nutrients—has given me great confidence in their effects upon blood lipid levels, and so I much prefer to treat my patients whose cholesterol levels are very high with dietary methods rather than medication.

As you saw on page 216, the Atkins Diet has a profoundly beneficial effect on triglycerides. The effect on cholesterol levels can best be described as "favorable but variable." I feel optimistic when I take my patients off cholesterol-lowering drugs and observe the effects of a low-carbohydrate diet for a month. It is inappropriate to check cholesterol levels during the first week, since they go up during fasting or on a low-calorie/low-fat diet or on a low-carbohydrate diet, because the body mobilizes its cholesterol stores. Certain authorities failed to appreciate this when they evaluated patients on the Doctor's Quick Weight Loss (Stillman) Diet for a week and found that cholesterol levels went up despite the fact that the diet is extremely low in fat.[30] Had they carried out the study longer, I am sure they would have seen an overall reduction in cholesterol, as did every other published study on a low-carbohydrate diet.

If the cholesterol level does not respond well to diet alone, I then recommend 1 to 2 ounces of lecithin granules per day as a supplement. The lecithin may be taken all in one dose or divided into several. Capsules are available but I find them less effective, because such a large number of them must be consumed. They seem to contain phosphatidyl choline as a separate chemical, rather than the "whole" lecithin. I much prefer and recommend lecithin granules or liquid. (Lecithin should be kept in the refrigerator after the container is opened—and you will probably enjoy the light, nutty taste.) Lecithin causes very few side effects, but some patients may experience bloating and other digestive difficulties—particularly with capsules.

After a month or two I repeat blood lipid studies to check my patient's profile. If it is still not where it should be, I might reevaluate thyroid function or institute a trial of kelp. Alternatively, I might step up dosage of vitamin C, niacin, PABA, or B15 and test the effect of each by doing more blood work a month after each addition, before going on to the next.

With this protocol, and *without* avoiding eggs and saturated fats, my patients have improved their blood fat profile, as the table on page 216 indicates. Rather than a high-fat "heart attack diet," as some of my more irrational critics have suggested, the Atkins Diet is really a regimen for treating patients with stubborn cholesterol elevations. The catch is that we are not sure if this achievement has any real meaning.

Occasionally, a major elevation in blood cholesterol *does* occur in patients on a low-carbohydrate diet. It seems entirely irrational for critics to suggest that the other 98 percent be denied the benefit of this remarkable diet in order to avoid a potential (and hypothetical) adverse effect in a small subgroup. In fact, in those subjects whose cholesterol levels go up, the nutritional supplements I have been discussing have, in most cases, brought the levels down without our having to resort to abandoning the diet.

Chapter 22

ATHEROSCLEROSIS

The cholesterol legend, like so many other forms of mythology, was advanced to provide a plausible answer to a riddle that cried out for solution. The riddle in this case: Why are so many people having heart attacks?

Most heart attacks come from a disease process called atherosclerosis—a buildup of plaque on the walls of our blood vessels that becomes deadly when it involves the coronary vessels—the ones that supply the heart muscle itself.

The major symptom of this condition is a chest pain called angina pectoris (Latin for "pain in the chest"), which is a symptom but is not a disease. Angina (also known as coronary insufficiency) arises when one or more of the coronary arteries is narrowed or in spasm, so that the heart muscle fibers supplied by that vessel don't receive enough oxygen-rich blood. Sometimes, the immediate cause is the heart's increased demand for blood above ordinary levels, as during exercise. Even though the impairment of blood flow may be only temporary, the angina of coronary insufficiency must be considered a warning sign that a coronary event (heart attack) could occur. *This pain cannot simply be ignored.*

In an actual coronary event (such as a myocardial infarction—also called a coronary occlusion) the blood supply is completely cut off from a part of the heart muscle for a period of time. This lack of blood supply (ischemia) may be caused by a blood vessel's being completely occluded by a clot or by plaque. It could also be caused by a partial occlusion complicated by a prolonged spasm. Whatever the cause, necrosis (cell death) of some heart muscle fibers occurs, and can be diagnosed by electrocardiogram or by laboratory tests. After a coronary event the heart must recover by replacing dead muscle fibers with scar tissue, or lose its ability to function efficiently. If there has been sufficient necrosis, recovery may not be possible. When this happens, a "pain signal" goes off as a warning.

How Can Coronaries Be Prevented?

Doctors bemoan the fact that there is so little they can do for a patient in the throes of a coronary occlusion—and precious little they can do for coronary insufficiency either. So they reason, and quite correctly, that the best treatment must be prevention. (Here is an instance where modern medicine has recognized the preventive instead of invasive treatment. But, as I will explain, the "experts" are barking up the wrong tree.)

For years, the cholesterol hypothesis provided a framework for preventive efforts. But the cholesterol story is only a small part of the whole truth—the part that doesn't work.

Yet I do believe that we are at the threshold of a new era in understanding coronary disease, with breakthrough after breakthrough in the offing, all because we have begun to look beyond the very limiting cholesterol theory to find things that *do* work. I now believe that we can not only prevent heart disease, we can also reverse it.

Let us start out by trying to understand the most up-to-date theories on the causes of atherosclerosis. At the risk of sounding like a textbook, I would like to give you some basis for understanding what is happening in the scientific world. (For those who like textbooks, I recommend the chapter by Dr. Jean Davignon in Genest's *Hypertension,* published by McGraw Hill, New York, in 1977.)

The Anatomy of a Plaque

One of the first and most significant discoveries was that the walls of our arteries are more than mere conduits for blood. They are biochemically quite active, and we are just beginning to understand some of this biochemistry and to learn the many ways nutrition can affect it.

Current theory about how atherosclerosis develops provides a pathologic description of several stages.

The first part is the penetration of toxic substances through the inner lining of cells of the arterial wall (the endothelium) into the next layer (the intima). The intimal cells are the ones that accumulate fatty substances (lipids such as cholesterol and triglycerides), fibrin (the clotting substance of our serum), and other substances.

Next, these intimal cells also grow in number and proliferate, thus beginning a buildup on the inner wall of the artery involved.* A very important step takes place when the blood's platelets (the circulating cell fragments that cause the blood to clot) are attracted to this area of injured intimal cells and debris, and in an effort to repair the wound they release some of the chemicals they contain. As the platelets stick like a bandage to the wounded area, the plaque grows, further nourished by the contents of the platelets themselves. Finally, all the constituents in the arterial wall react with the calcium circulating in the blood, to form insoluble calcium complexes. The plaque becomes solid and permanent.

When this calcification occurs there is no longer a chance for these substances to be reabsorbed by the blood, and atherosclerosis is said to be irreversible.

Now that you have heard the pathologist's description of atherosclerosis, most of which was learned from studying the cells of blood vessel walls under an electron microscope, you can see that it has very little to do with eating too much cholesterol or with cholesterol forcing its way into the arterial wall.

The Biochemist's Version

When you study the many chemical reactions involved, you will see why I think a breakthrough in preventing, halting, and even reversing heart disease is just around the corner.

The nutritional treatments available today are, in fact, so effective in reducing the *symptoms* of heart disease—especially those of angina pectoris—that I am able almost to assure my patients that they will see some noticeable improvement.

The Injury Factor

If an atherosclerotic plaque begins with a chemical break in the lining of the arterial wall, the first question is: What chemicals cause

---

* These cells may migrate to the intima from the next layer outward, the smooth muscle cells of the media. The media's muscle cells may be the same "monoclonal" cells discovered by Dr. Earl Benditt [1] and reported upon by Dr. Richard Passwater.[2]

the break? Researchers have discovered many substances that can cause injury, but there remains the question of which are the most important.

My candidate for enemy number one is a group of very active molecules called free radicals. These molecules are so unstable that, in seeking stability, they have to react with something—and it is often with the cells on the arterial wall. (Sometimes it is the lining of the joints, which helps to explain why so many treatments useful in cardiac disease are also effective in arthritis.) The free-oxygen–containing peroxides (superoxide, hydroxyl) and the lipid peroxides (which derive from our unsaturated fats) are among these natural "agents of chemical warfare," the free radicals. The peroxides are inhibited by the enzyme superoxide dismutase, and lipid peroxidation is prevented by vitamin E and the mineral selenium. Other chemicals which cause tissue injury are homocystine [3] (which can be countered by vitamin B_6), histamine (which is opposed by vitamin C), serotonin, adrenaline, and the products of an immune reaction.[4]

Thus we can view cholesterol in its true perspective: It is simply one of several chemicals that can produce injury to the arterial wall whenever too much of it is present (in association with too much of its carrier molecule, low-density lipoprotein—LDL). It may be that pure cholesterol is *not* atherogenic. Only when spontaneously oxidized, as in the case of dried egg yolk powder, is it angiotoxic, according to C. Bruce Taylor of Albany Medical College.[5]

The most important point of all, however, is that nature has provided many ways to protect us against the initial lesion of injury to the arterial wall. It is up to us to learn how to work with nature.

The Smooth Muscle Cell Proliferation

The smooth muscle cells that take up space on the arterial wall when they incorporate cholesterol, fibrin, and other complexes seem to have a nutritional mediator, too. It is insulin, which has been shown to accelerate their growth. Thus a diet high in refined carbohydrates, which promotes insulin overproduction, may well speed up damage to the arterial walls.[6] Conversely, the anti-insulin diets I recommend are ideal for controlling some of the factors underlying this phase of atherosclerosis.

Further, the fibrin that contributes to arterial thickening can be inhibited by vitamin C, which has been shown to have specific activity in breaking down the fibrin itself.

Those All-Important Platelets

Most of the prevention undertaken both by up-to-date ortho-doxists (who use aspirin and sulfinpyrazone) and nutritionists involves keeping the platelets from aggregating, or "clumping." This is considered important because platelets release several of the chemicals that break down the inner lining of the blood vessel wall and because they also stimulate the growth of smooth muscle cells. So, as the platelets heap up, a vicious cycle begins.

Platelets figure in most heart disease theories, because most substances implicated in causing heart disease seem to increase the "clumpability" of the platelets and/or shorten their life-span.

Smoking, for example, seems to have this effect,[7] and so does any dietary change that raises the triglyceride levels. Another factor would be sugar in the diet of the sugar-susceptible person. On the other hand, vitamin E,[8] garlic,[9] and bromelain[10] preserve the platelets, keep them circulating, and prevent them from piling on.

Prostaglandins Are the Key to It All

Prostaglandins are hormonelike messenger substances which seem to regulate vital metabolic processes throughout our bodies. They are a recent discovery, and there is a lot more still to be learned. But even the puzzle pieces we now understand would take volumes to explain and describe, so I will oversimplify and tell you as briefly as I can what these chemicals are and how they work.

Although there are more than thirty known prostaglandins, they occur in nature mainly in three major series (named series one, two, and three, according to the number of chemical double bonds). I would like to concentrate on two members of the "two" series, because they are fundamental to understanding how prostaglandins work, and because they are in greatest concentration in our bodies.

One is a very powerful "bad guy" called thromboxane (TXA_2) which circulates with the platelets and which can constrict your blood vessels or bronchial passages in an instant. Thromboxane is also the most powerful platelet aggregator the body has to deal with.

The other, the "good guy," is called prostacyclin (PGI_2) and is without question the most potent protector against platelet clumping and blood vessel and bronchial constriction. Prostacyclin stays in the blood vessel walls and the lungs and is the reason our platelets keep circulating as they should rather than breaking down all the time.

So you see that we are discussing two biochemical substances with opposing action. It is rather like the devil on one shoulder and an angel on the other.

If there were a way to increase our consumption of prostacyclin without increasing thromboxane, perhaps we could live longer. Unfortunately, like Cain and Abel, both of these substances have the same father. Both prostacyclin and thromboxane derive from the same fatty acid, arachidonic acid.

However, there are two parallel systems of prostaglandins, both slightly different in structure. One, the "three" series, is usually very sparsely present in our bodies, since it is derived from a fatty acid sparsely present in our diet—eicosapentaenoic acid, which we have all learned to know and love by the initials EPA. Its good guy prostacyclin (PGI_3) is active, but its bad guy thromboxane (TXA_3) is not.

So if you follow a diet with a high EPA content, you swing the balance of beneficial prostaglandins in your favor—or so claims Dr. Salvador Moncada, who is one of the experts in this field.[11] A high EPA diet means eating lots of fish (you can get 20 percent EPA in scallops, oysters, and red caviar) or taking cod-liver oil. In fact, doctors at London's famed Queen Elizabeth College were able to change the lipid content of the platelets in twelve young men enough to prolong their bleeding time 40 percent simply by giving them four teaspoons of cod-liver oil daily for six weeks.[12]

But from the standpoint of potential breakthroughs nutritionally, the most promising prostaglandins research, in my view, is now taking place under the worldwide influence of Dr. David Horrobin.[13] Dr. Horrobin explains that the "one" series prostaglandins, which derive from digammahomolinolenic acid (DGLA), are the most important ones for us to create through our nutritional building blocks because a) there are no "bad actors" in the "one" series and b) its most effective prostaglandin, PGE_1, produces an extremely varied list of beneficial effects. It dilates blood vessels, lowers blood pressure, prevents platelet clumping, inhibits cholesterol formation, stimulates immunity through the T-lymphocytes (see page 140), and can even relieve clinical depression.

What Does This Mean Nutritionally?

To create the optimal amount of PGE_1, we first need a liberal amount of *cis*-linoleic acid (not *trans*-linoleic, which occurs in margarine or hydrogenated oils). *Cis*-linoleic acid occurs in cold-pressed vegetable oils. Dr. Horrobin recommends that 3 percent of our total calories be in that form. Since we convert linoleic acid to DGLA quite slowly, we would be better off taking in gamma linoleic acid directly in our diet. The acid occurs in nature in only one substance known to date—the oil of the seed of the evening primrose.

Further, to create PGE₁ from linoleic acid or DGLA, the following nutrients have been proven necessary: vitamins C, B₆, and possibly niacin, plus the key trace mineral zinc. Dr. Horrobin is currently coordinating some sixty studies worldwide, evaluating this regimen in clinical problems ranging from psychiatric disorders through multiple sclerosis and heart disease to arthritis.

When I give evening primrose oil to my patients, I generally give three to four grams.

Calcification

The calcifying of the arterial wall is what makes the condition "irreversible," but it may not be irreversible after all. And when I tell you about chelation, you'll begin to see why.

These many biochemical/nutritional leads provide the basis for a genuine breakthrough in preventing or reversing heart disease. But does this mean you can now visit your cardiologist and expect to be placed on a program to achieve this? Not unless you are very lucky.

How Is Angina Treated?

A patient with angina who visits a cardiologist or other doctor is likely to receive a prescription for one of many medications—accompanied by not much nutritional advice other than that he should restrict his cholesterol and fat intake.

One drug very likely to be prescribed for relief of symptoms may be nitroglycerin or some other form of nitrite. Nitrites include amyl nitrite, pentaerythritol tetranitrate (PETN, Peritrate), erythrityl tetranitrate (Cardilate), and isosorbide dinitrite (Isordil), among others. Some are short-acting and are taken under the tongue when an attack of angina comes on; others are long-acting and are taken several times a day. Nitrites provide relief of chest pain because they dilate the coronary blood vessels. One of their better features is that the few side effects associated with their use rarely pose serious problems.

But nitrites also dilate blood vessels *all over the body*. Thus, when the drug dilates the vessels in the brain, a headache may result. And elsewhere they cause the blood returning to the heart to pool in the veins, thus causing the heart's output and the blood pressure to drop. This effect causes fainting in some patients.

Other nitrite side effects include a rash (which requires that the drug be discontinued), gastrointestinal distress, and other very rare, but more serious, side effects.

If there is a bad aspect to the nitrites, it's that they do not correct the fundamental problem—the thickening of the walls of the coronary blood vessels. And this means that the angina may continue even though the drugs are used conscientiously.

Propanolol to the Rescue

A new class of drug has recently hit the cardiology market with a bang. These are the beta blockers, of which propanolol (Inderal) is both the first to be widely marketed and the prototype for the class. The beta blockers are typical pharmaceutical blocking agents in that they inhibit certain metabolic functions in order to achieve the desired therapeutic effect.

These, too, do absolutely nothing to alleviate the underlying cause of angina, the clogged arteries.

I have watched another scene in the continuing drama of drugs versus nutrients, observing my patients go on and off beta blockers. The drugs do indeed relieve angina pains, lower the blood pressure, slow the pulse, and regulate the heart rhythm. They even occasionally improve migraines. But at what cost?

Fatigue occurs in many patients, and mental depression is often seen as well. Many of my patients report a decrease in their sex drive.[14] Propanolol patients may not complain of fatigue or depression when I first see them, but when, with the help of nutritional therapy, they agree to reduce their dosage step by step, they almost invariably report an upsurge in energy and a lifting of mood with each dosage reduction. Other side effects of beta blockers include diarrhea, weakness, asthma, poor concentration, even hallucinations and amnesia.[15]

Heart patients also have to be concerned not to aggravate congestive heart failure. And perhaps the most difficult problem of all is the fact that it is very difficult to get off beta blockers once you are on them. The very condition being treated—angina pectoris—often worsens if the drug is stopped abruptly, or even gradually. (This worsening on the rebound is one of the hallmarks of drug therapy in general—it applies to diuretics, diet pills, hypnotics, the newer ulcer drugs, and tranquilizers, to mention a few. It can be so easy to go on a drug and so hard to go off it.)

Add Tranquilizers for Good Measure

The hard-driving type-A personality has been recognized as being coronary prone. Unfortunately some doctors may approach this problem in their usual logical way and prescribe tranquilizers or sedatives to slow down the type-A drive. Hardly a technique that will accomplish much clearing out of the clogged coronary blood vessels. The net result of this therapy is often a sleepy patient with clogged coronary arteries!

And Another Nostrum—Why Not?

Cholesterol-lowering drugs have also received a fair share of play in patients with angina. It seems so logical. If the blood vessels are cholesterol-choked, why not lower the serum cholesterol and help alleviate the problem. In fact, drug-induced cholesterol-lowering rarely relieves angina, and the drugs that reduce serum cholesterol are the closest thing to what Dr. Carlton Fredericks bitingly calls the "perfect drug"—one that has nothing but side effects.

New, Possibly Better, Approaches Are on the Horizon

The most promising new drug approach to angina involves a group of calcium antagonists.[16] At present, these drugs (nifedipine, verapamil, perhexilene) are still experimental. The side effects reported thus far include dizziness, flushing, swelling of the legs, and reduced blood pressure when experimental subjects stood up. The good side, however, is that patients who tried the drugs reported a reduction in the amount of nitroglycerin they needed to control angina symptoms.

I wonder if the drugs' mode of action is similar to that of chelation (about which I'll have more to say later on), which also acts by decreasing the calcium concentration.

And Surgery, of Course

The most significant change in the treatment in coronary heart disease management involves surgery. Cardiac surgical techniques have improved to the point where most patients are being asked to consider a heart operation. In an open-heart procedure, the narrowed, clogged blood vessels are replaced by grafts of healthy vessels taken from other parts of the body. Even though surgical statisticians can present data to show that coronary bypass surgery can somewhat extend life expectancy, it is hard to consider as anything other than a last resort any surgery as risky and drastic as this technique. The more so, since the surgery does not correct the *propensity* toward clogged vessels. The same atherosclerotic process that led to the occlusions in the first place still continues. Given enough time, atherosclerosis develops in the other vessels—even in the newly grafted ones.[17]

So What's the Answer?

Nutritional changes seem to be the most logical answer. But more pertinently, what nutritional changes? Should we take as gospel the recommendations of the American Heart Association and limit our intake of dietary cholesterol and saturated fat? I don't think so, and my opinion is backed by a plethora of recent scientific studies that demonstrate that cholesterol restriction does not lower the blood cholesterol, prevent heart attack, or increase life expectancy.[18] In light of that sort of data, can such advice be recommended? And though proponents of the AHA diet claim it is prudent, I would have a tough time justifying that claim.

Apparently, at long last, so would a fifteen-man blue-ribbon panel of the Food and Nutrition Board of the National Research Council who announced in May 1980 that it found no evidence that reduction of cholesterol in diets will help prevent heart disease.[19]

Or should we do as Nathan Pritikin suggests?[20] The highly visible spokesman for the Longevity Institute recommends a diet of 80 percent carbohydrate, low in all fats (and marginal in the essential fatty acids our hearts so badly need), low in protein (marginal in essential amino acids, the building blocks of tissue), and certainly marginal in all vitamins, most notably the fat soluble vitamins A and E. Although Mr. Pritikin's devotees experience some rather striking short-term benefits, most nutritionists attribute these improvements to low intake of sugar and simple carbohydrates, high fiber intake, and Mr. Pritikin's enforced exercise program.

Further, I feel quite strongly that Pritikin is misleading when he asserts that low-carbohydrate (or high-fat) diets worsen diabetes. There are a world of scientific studies, and two centuries of experience, indicating that they have always been shown to improve it.[21] Or that dietary fats decrease oxygen in our tissues, a claim based upon a study done under extreme conditions—drinking a cup of heavy cream after fasting.

I simply cannot recommend the Pritikin type of "nutrition," because it subjects too many individuals to minimal intakes of protein, fats, vitamins, and trace minerals. My rationale is based on the major point made by Dr. Roger Williams, who proposes a "biochemical individuality" of nutritional needs.[22] Any diet that contains quantities of nutrients that are marginal for the average member of a group may in fact be deficient in those nutrients for many other members.

The Nutrition Breakthrough cardiovascular regimen does not depend on any principle so simplistic (and so inaccurate) as the restriction of fats or eggs. Rather it takes into account all the recent advances in understanding the biochemistry of our hearts and blood vessels. It is based on the well-known beneficial effects of the ketogenic diet, the harm of refined carbohydrates, the stresses initiated by excessive insulin response, the role of prostaglandins, of platelets, of free radicals, of peroxides, of calcium and calcium antagonists, of magnesium, of selenium, of nucleic acids—not to mention exercise and reduction of stress.

Before I propose some answers, let me first expand the arena to be discussed, since the entire vascular system can benefit from the nutritional approaches I use to treat my heart patients.

Chapter 23

PERIPHERAL VASCULAR DISEASE

Does anyone you know complain that walking just a few blocks produces severe leg pain? If so, then you have doubtless heard that the pain goes away after a few minutes' rest and may well come back again after walking is resumed. This is the main symptom of peripheral vascular disease (PVD) and is called "intermittent claudication." Its hallmark is that the pain occurs during exercise, but not during rest.[1]

Intermittent claudication could be described as angina of the legs, and its pain, too, results from narrowed blood vessels. The muscles send out a pain signal to protest receiving too little oxygen-rich blood. It is really another facet of the very disease process that occludes the coronary arteries.

Peripheral vascular disease is not confined only to the lower extremities. Similar vessel narrowing occurs in an even more serious condition, cerebrovascular disease (CVD), which compromises blood flow to the brain. When these arteries become clogged and blood is cut off from the brain, transient ischemic attacks (TIAs) occur. These "small strokes" are a sign that a cerebrovascular accident (CVA), or major stroke, could occur and cause permanent debilitation.

Other organs may also be at risk. For example, when the blood supply to the kidney is compromised, kidney failure and a severe but surgically correctible type of hypertension may arise.

Doctors diagnose peripheral vascular disease by first feeling for pulses in the knee, ankle, and groin areas. When the pulses are absent, then the physician may suspect that the vessels are occluded and order further laboratory testing to confirm or rule out his suspicions. He may test with equipment that measures the sound vibrations over the blood vessels (noninvasive testing) or with angiograms (invasive testing). (Angiograms are X rays of blood vessels injected with radiopaque dyes.)

Although many medical treatments for PVD have been offered, most experts agree that they are generally unsatisfactory. Drugs which dilate the blood vessels work only upon the smaller ones and are pretty useless in major vessel disease.

Surgery, which yields good results in the short term, may be disappointing over the long term. If most people with PVD had only one clogged blood vessel, then surgery might well do the trick. But unfortunately, a great percentage of patients with PVD have multiple clog-ups. Thus, in many patients, for surgery to be really successful would require multiple vessel grafts. Obviously this is not a practical approach to treatment.

A Pound of Prevention

Naturally I believe that a proper diet from the very beginning could well keep many from developing PVD. And I think that in early cases of PVD, proper nutrition might well, over a period of time, help undo the vascular havoc.

If you were my patient and came to me with PVD, the first thing I would ask is, "Do you smoke?"

If you said yes, I would tell you how dangerous it is to continue, for smoking constricts the blood vessels.

Diabetes and PVD

If your glucose tolerance test showed that you were in the diabetic ranges, I would concentrate my efforts on helping you reverse the diabetic state with appropriate diet and nutrients (see Chapter 18). Diabetics are especially likely to develop PVD. The poor healing and ankle swelling characteristic of the disease put the diabetic patient especially at risk for multiple-site vascular disease. Not only is this least amenable to surgical intervention, the diabetic per se is a patient surgeons tamper with as little as possible.

At the same time, I would tell my claudication patients to walk as much as possible to the point of tolerance, stopping when the pain comes and continuing as it goes away.

Vitamin E: Its Best Documented Use

Since I am a strong advocate of vitamin E for this condition, I often start patients with 600 units and gradually build up to 2400 units, all the while checking for improvement (or weight gain or a rise in blood pressure, which would be considered unwanted effects). Not everybody tolerates vitamin E in the same manner, so you will have to use vitamin E under your doctor's supervision.

Although some pooh-pooh the use of vitamins in intermittent claudication, Dr. Kurt Haeger of Malmö, Sweden, published a long-term study of forty-six male patients with total blockage of a major leg artery.[2] Those patients who received vitamin E in addition to following Haeger's other general recommendations improved markedly in the distance they could walk before pain stopped them.

Most patients with intermittent claudication should have some improvement with the following treatment plan: walking short distances, as tolerated, starting slowly and increasing distance as speed tolerance improves; along with the appropriate Nutrition Breakthrough diet, as well as the cardiovascular regimen (see next chapter) with an emphasis on vitamin E.

Recently Dr. Frank A. Oski of the State University of New York Upstate Medical Center demonstrated that vitamin E may have a beneficial effect on the "pollution of the vascular system" caused by certain metabolic wastes and might actually reduce the tendency of the platelets to clump, and help stem the buildup of plaque on the blood vessel walls.[3]

Chapter 24

THE NUTRITION BREAKTHROUGH
VASCULAR REGIMEN

From a nutritional standpoint, all vascular conditions can be approached in the same multiconceptual way. Whether the problem area is cardio-, cerebro-, or peripheral, the vascular system is responsive to many orthomolecular modalities.

Dr. Nieper's Approach

For example, one of the nutritional techniques I use was first proposed by Dr. Hans Nieper of Hannover, West Germany. He discovered the advantage of combining minerals with the metabolite orotic acid to form what are called orotates, which improve cell penetration.[1]

Orotic acid has been referred to as vitamin B_{13}. It normally occurs in the body as an intermediary metabolite, that is, one of the chemicals found in the chain of events as one biochemical substance progresses into another.* It is found in our diet in root vegetables and whey. When combined with a metal ion, orotic acid becomes a salt, called an orotate.

Dr. Nieper was able to transport the vital cardiac minerals magnesium and potassium directly to the heart muscle cells, providing maximum effectiveness.[2] The other element of Dr. Nieper's regimen is bromelain, the pineapple enzyme, which has been shown to have

* Specifically, orotate is a precursor of the pyrimidines in our nucleic acids.

239

anti-platelet-clumping effectiveness in its own right.* His reported results suggest that more than 90 percent of patients so treated can expect improvement in the course of their angina pectoris.

The Miracle of RNA

Another of my favorite nutritional aids for the vascular system is nucleic acids. The late Dr. Benjamin Frank devoted most of his career as a clinical research scientist to teaching us about these important constituents of the nucleus of every cell in our bodies.[3] RNA (ribonucleic acid) and DNA (desoxyribonucleic acid) are manufactured within the body, and orthodox nutritionists have long considered that we can manufacture all we need and therefore have no need to supplement them in our diets.

Dr. Frank proved (to my satisfaction, at least) that it simply isn't so. If we manufacture all we need, then why do so many people get such a dramatic response when RNA is given?

The Cold Hands Test

Whenever a patient of mine wants proof that RNA works, I say to him, "Start taking RNA, 400 milligrams three times daily, and see if you don't feel the warmth returning to your cold hands and feet."

In addition to being useful in heart and vascular diseases, nucleic acid therapy has been found to be useful in such diverse conditions as bronchitis and emphysema, osteroarthritis, aging skin, acne, cancer, and diabetes.[4]

I start with 1200 mg daily and build up to 4800 mg. (Caution— the uric acid level must be watched, as high doses can precipitate gout in the susceptible person.)

Allicin-Free Garlic

I have alluded to the value of garlic, and I will do so in greater detail when I discuss high blood pressure, for it has the greatest therapeutic (benefit/risk) ratio of any agent I have yet used to treat hypertension. In treating a vascular patient, it is one thing I almost always prescribe.

By now I think you see that there are many nontoxic natural

* Dr. Steven J. Taussig postulates that bromain inhibits the formation of thromboxane (see page 229).

agents to go along with the Nutrition Breakthrough diets I find so effective (presumably because of their anti-insulin effect) in the vascular patient.

There is no single protocol for the atherosclerosis patient. In the first place, there are more useful nutritional agents than most people need. Secondly, no two people respond alike. Remember biochemical individuality?

Let me give instead an example of how one patient was treated.

Meet Tony Castellani

As a cardiologist-turned-nutritionist, I get a great deal of satisfaction whenever my experience can prove helpful to a patient with a heart condition.

So when Tony Castellani, a fifty-seven-year-old diamond setter, came to me for the first time complaining of angina that overtook him on walking just two blocks, I readily agreed to take over his medical care.

Two years before, Tony had had to be hospitalized because of an erratic heartbeat; after that he was a virtual cardiac cripple, just barely able to make it to and from work because of chest pain, which would force him to stop and put a nitroglycerin tablet under his tongue.

Tony was a fighter, so he began to take, on his own, loads of vitamins and a breakfast drink containing lecithin and brewers' yeast. He followed the low-fat diet his doctor prescribed well enough to go down from 215 pounds to 190 (Tony is five feet eight) until he had to abandon it because it left him too weak.

Despite all his efforts his angina worsened, and his doctor kept adding medication. By the time he saw me first, Tony was taking a long-acting nitrate, a heart rhythm drug (disopyramide), and propanolol, each three times daily, plus requiring three or four nitroglycerin tablets every day. Tony could barely walk and sexual activity was hardly possible.

When I first examined him his electrocardiogram looked frightening, a pattern of severe ischemia (lack of oxygen) over the heart's left ventricle. His lab tests revealed that he was a diabetic, with blood sugars 160 fasting, and 295 two hours after glucose. His insulin levels were elevated and his cholesterol normal. Because his triglycerides were high (reaching 301), I was able to guarantee him that his lab tests would improve on the Atkins Diet.

On that diet, Tony lost ten pounds in the first seventeen days and over the next two months, he had shed eleven pounds more. More importantly, his angina got better week by week, until he could consistently walk a half mile to work without ever thinking about his nitroglycerin.

What treatment did Tony receive to accomplish this? Besides the Atkins Diet and the basic vitamin formula, Tony was given an extra gram of B$_6$, 6 mg of folic acid, 2 grams of inositol (at bedtime), 300 mg of B$_{15}$, 3 grams of magnesium orotate, 800 units of vitamin E (as D-alpha tocopherol), 150 mg of chelated zinc, 50 mg of chelated manganese, 600 mg of GTF chromium, 2 grams of allicin-free (deodorized) garlic, and 3 tablespoons of lecithin granules.

On successive visits, 1200 mg of RNA and 600 mg of bromelain were added. Later 8 tablets of superoxide dismutase were given. Meanwhile the drugs were gradually discontinued; first the disopyramide was cut to 2 a day, then 1 a day, then none. Next the propanolol, finally the nitrate. With each reduction of medication, Tony's vitality seemed to increase just a bit; certainly his sex drive and performance did.

Just three months later, when we reevaluated his progress, his lab values confirmed that we were on the right path. His blood pressure fell from 168/83 to 120/80, his sugar from 160 to 116, cholesterol from 211 to 185, triglycerides from 301 to 135, insulin from 46 to 11, uric acid from 7.1 to 5.4, and his electrocardiogram, although still showing an enlarged left ventricle, no longer showed the ischemic pattern.

Tony is not a special case; there are dozens like him. When I tabulated my results on angina pectoris, I confirmed that over 90 percent were clinically improved.

This comprehensive regimen that Tony received, element by element, is the real breakthrough—a way to treat heart disease aggressively and effectively—but without medicines.

If the Pains Remain

Suppose Tony's pain doesn't go away completely, or suppose the claudication patient's pain persists or his repeated noninvasive testing still indicates a block in the arterial blood supply? Must I tell the patient I've done all I can or that nutrition can only carry him so far?

Not yet, for I've yet to tell him about my most effective weapon—chelation therapy.

In fact, if my patient's problem was predominantly atherosclerotic in any of its manifestations (coronary, cerebral, renal, or peripheral), I would recommend chelation. In so doing, I would thrust my patient into the heart of the orthodox-versus-unorthodox, establishment-versus-antiestablishment, pharmaceutical-versus-nutritional struggle. The very struggle this book is about.

Perhaps you have never even heard of chelation. It is time we all learned a little more about this controversial technique, and the following pages will give you some understanding of chelation, what it can and cannot do, and why the heart specialists in your area may not *really* know about it.

Chapter 25

CHELATION THERAPY

The word *chelate* means to bind. Thus chelation is the administration of substances which bind certain of our body's minerals, allowing them to be excreted from the body. In a sense it represents the negative side of mineral administration.

Nutrition chelation is among the most underpublicized, least understood therapeutic measures in use today, perhaps because there is no single large industry or political group behind it. In fact, the establishment may even be threatened by chelation because it is a radical departure from currently accepted techniques.[1] (We must not lose sight of the fact that surgeons are taught to operate and allopathic doctors are trained to prescribe drugs. Since nutritional chelation therapy uses neither of these remedies, it comes as no surprise that the establishment doesn't accept the concept.)

A majority of the powers-that-be would have us believe the simplistic theory that atherosclerosis is the result of our dietary intake of cholesterol and fats. I hope I was able to make clear in the previous chapters that there is much more to the vascular disease problem than that. And there are many ways in which nutrition can enter into the biochemical picture to prevent, halt, or even reverse the atherosclerotic process.

The Role of Minerals

Perhaps the most direct way to intervene in the disease process is to restore the balance of minerals in our bodies to normal. The very functioning of the heart itself depends on a proper ratio between sodium and potassium and between calcium and magnesium. Most clinical problems arise when potassium and magnesium are too low. Metalloenzymes, those based on a trace mineral, are essential to many of the metabolic processes which take place in the arterial wall. On the other hand, toxic minerals can contribute to heart disease and hypertension.

Perhaps most important of all, the end stage of atherosclerosis involves calcification in the blood vessel wall (see p. 227).

Can Calcification Be Reversed?

The constituents of the blood vessel wall (mucopolysaccharides, lipoproteins, elastin, and collagen) are in a reversible chemical equilibrium *unless or until they calcify*. Before chelation therapy, once calcification occurred the plaques were there to stay, because calcium complexes are relatively insoluble. Ordinarily, therefore, you could not expect to reverse the atherosclerotic process. However, if calcium could be removed, then the dynamic biochemical processes taking place in the blood vessel wall could once again enter into a reversible state, and the atherosclerotic plaque might be resolved.

And that's where chelation comes in.

Disodium EDTA, which is administered by slow intravenous (IV) drip, is the chelating agent most commonly used. It binds heavy metals (such as lead) and removes abnormal calcium deposits from within the blood vessel, making it possible for the rest of the plaque then to disperse.[2]

What Chelation Actually Does

Chelation works by lowering blood calcium levels (by binding the calcium so it can be excreted through the kidneys) and forcing the body to release the calcium that is bound up in the blood vessel walls. As calcium is washed out of the blood vessels by repeated administration of a decalcifying agent, blood calcium levels are restored (under the influence of the parathyroid gland), and recalcification is more likely to take place in the bones, where it belongs.

(The bones are the residence of special bone-forming cells, osteoblasts, which direct exactly where calcium is to be deposited. Fortunately for us, these cells are not components of the blood vessel walls. If they were, our blood vessel walls would be more like lead pipe than flexible conduits for blood.)

Thus, the net effect of chelation is that calcium leaves those areas where it does *not* belong. This is the rationale for the claim that chelation provides an opportunity for a true reversal of the atherosclerotic process.

The main risk of chelation is that the "good" minerals are also chelated. Losses of chromium, zinc, manganese, and magnesium would be harmful to the body. So it is critical that the physician be sufficiently knowledgeable about trace mineral nutrition to replace those essential minerals lost in the chelation process.

Chelation Can Do More

One of the major breakthroughs in preventive cardiology involves the enzyme-activating function of magnesium which competes with the enzyme-inactivating function of calcium. Chelation therapy, by removing calcium and by replacing magnesium, can activate a lot of metabolic functions within the heart muscle. This may be extremely important in view of the fact that both magnesium-providing therapies (see page 239) and calcium-antagonist therapy (see page 233) have provided spectacular success in treating coronary conditions.

There Are Many Chelating Agents

Vitamin C, alfalfa, garlic, rutin, vitamin E, alginates, some legumes, and the sulfured amino acids (such as methionine, cystine, and lysine) have all been shown to act as chelating agents. Most chelation, however, is done by slow intravenous drip. In this procedure, disodium EDTA is administered in accordance with a protocol developed by the American Academy of Medical Preventics (AAMP). Chelation therapy cannot be accomplished all at one sitting (or dripping). Each session usually lasts about four hours; between twenty and fifty treatments may be necessary to complete the job.

Mineral Replacement

The critics of chelation therapy seem to have made the mistake of assuming that its scope was limited to the administering of

EDTA or some other similar compound. The term *chelation therapy* actually applies to the entire program of nutritional management based on such administrations. It demands regulating the mineral content of the body until an ideal balance is achieved. *Replacement* of minerals the body will need is just as much a part of chelation therapy as is the leaching out of calcium and toxic minerals with EDTA.

Do not be put off by reports that chelation may be toxic to the kidneys. EDTA compounds are extremely safe; only when EDTA combines with toxic minerals such as lead and mercury, and the therapy is administered too rapidly, is there any risk to the kidneys. Even that risk seems acceptable when reversing lead or mercury poisoning is at issue. AAMP's protocol calls for evaluation of lead and mercury levels (among others) before treatment. If they are elevated, treatment will proceed more slowly than usual. AAMP member physicians have administered more than two million treatments to over one hundred thousand patients with a remarkable record of safety and effectiveness.[3]

The Coronary Bypass

Heart surgery, with replacement of the blocked arteries, is today's popular treatment for coronary heart disease. However, Dr. Richard S. Ross, chief of surgery at Johns Hopkins, studied the long-term results and concluded that surgery is really of no benefit in lengthening the life-span.[4]

What Ross said rings true. The total cost of a triple coronary bypass ran about $37,000 in 1978, with much of the cost covered by insurance policies. Unfortunately, many of the grafted vessels themselves occlude, one study showing 80 percent doing so within two years.[5] You might think twice about having such major surgery if two years later you will be back almost where you started.

Chelation is not as risky as surgery, and it can easily be repeated —as it should be for proper maintenance of improvement. Furthermore, the cost is usually about one tenth that of a coronary bypass. The problem is that, since chelation is an unorthodox therapy, many insurance carriers have not been willing to pay for it. The total nutrition program that is part of a chelation procedure promises to do better than the bypass, simply because the emphasis is upon total and permanent life-style change.

Unless surgery is performed with this type of follow-up, how could it possibly bring about a lasting change?

Nutrition—the Coronary Bypass Bypass Bypass

Although I do advocate chelation, and though I am convinced it has much more to offer over the long term than surgery, my medical practice has taught me something. The Atkins Diet, supplemented with the right vitamins, minerals, and other nutrients, does what chelation can do in all but the most severe cases. My own office patients achieve such favorable long-term results that it seems they have been able to bypass not only the bypass, but the bypass bypass.

Chapter 26

HYPERTENSION

One cannot talk about heart disease without discussing hypertension, more popularly known as high blood pressure.

Hypertension is a scourge that strikes in epidemic proportions. Its later stages may include heart disease, loss of vision, and impaired kidney function, not to mention stroke. Worst of all, most people with high blood pressure don't feel it in the form of severe headaches until some damage has been done. The lucky ones find their hypertension before it's too late, as a result of routine screening.

The tragic cases are usually those patients who come in with symptoms, rather than those who have had their blood pressure checked regularly and have caught any untoward rise early. When hypertension is detected and treated early, there is far less risk of permanent damage to vital organs.

High blood pressure is the number one risk factor contributing to heart attacks and strokes. Thomas E. Ratts, M.D., summed up quite neatly the link between coronary heart disease and hypertension: "Next to age, blood pressure is the most potent factor known to contribute to the incidence of coronary artery disease." [1]

Smokers are more likely to have it than nonsmokers; so are one in four women who take The Pill. Obesity doesn't help either, because fat contains blood vessels and the heart has to work harder to pump blood through fatty tissue.

One of the major complications of hypertension is that the heart must pump against greater resistance to keep the blood flowing. This may cause the heart muscle to grow larger, to become inefficient and inelastic. On an electrocardiogram or a chest X ray, one may see "left ventricular hypertrophy" (LVH), in which the lower left chamber of the heart is markedly larger than normal. LVH in turn places a greater burden on the coronary circulation and increases the likelihood of heart attack.

In short, hypertension is bad news.

What Is Normal?

It is widely agreed that blood pressure readings of 120/80 (systolic/diastolic) are desirable. The New York Heart Association refers to a systolic of 140–160 over a diastolic of 90–95 as "borderline." They consider "moderate" hypertension to be in the 160–180/95–115 range, and "marked" hypertension as above 180/115. Whatever the case, most family physicians seem to feel that reducing the blood pressure to 140/90 is acceptable, and that an untreated patient with 140/90 to 150/100 should be carefully watched. Treatment is usually recommended for blood pressures that exceed these ranges.

Traditional Treatment of Hypertension

Most traditional physicians today prefer to treat hypertension in a stepwise fashion—adding medications as needed (usually a diuretic first, followed by other drugs which work differently) in an effort to keep the total number of drugs and the dosage as low as possible. When the orthodox physician states that hypertension is a disease amenable to dietary control, he invariably means a diet with a single feature. Salt restriction, for some reason, is the only dietary measure traditionalists think of when asked about diet in hypertension.[2]

A group of researchers from the University of Melbourne, Australia, cast serious doubt upon salt restriction, pointing out that most patients in their study did not achieve the desired amount of salt restriction, and that it is extremely difficult to eliminate salt completely anyway.[3] And Richard Gorlin, M.D., physician-in-chief of New York's Mount Sinai Hospital and editor-in-chief of *Primary Cardiology*, has asked, "Is there any real value in the utilization of such a strict low salt diet? I sincerely doubt it."[4]

I think that salt restriction is not of much use, because it doesn't always work[5] and because there are so many far more potent nutritional measures that really do the job.

After the traditional salt restriction, the physician usually prescribes a diuretic to reduce fluid volume by causing the kidneys to excrete the sodium that keeps fluid in the body. Potassium is of course lost along with sodium. Although doctors are usually aware of the risk of potassium depletion, very few have been taught to watch for loss of magnesium and other trace minerals.

Proof is not fully established, but the hair mineral analyses on diuretic users I have studied seem to indicate widespread deficiencies of many essential trace minerals. Apparently these minerals are washed out along with the sodium and potassium. Remember, there are specific biochemical reactions which are totally dependent on our having adequate amounts of *each* of these trace minerals.

I wonder how many doctors are aware that diuretics (as well as salt restriction) can actually raise the blood pressure. By lowering the blood volume and the sodium concentration, they stimulate the body to put out more renin and angiotensin, the very biological chemicals that *cause* hypertension.[6]

As I mentioned on pages 134–135, the diuretic is really a "poison" to the kidneys. Other undesirable side effects in some patients include high blood uric acid levels which could lead to gout or kidney stones. To me, the most undesirable side effect of all is that diuretics may aggravate diabetic and hypoglycemic hyperinsulinism.[7]

Then, if the diuretic doesn't bring the blood pressure near the goal of 140/90, most doctors progress to the next drug. Most also realize that overweight may increase blood pressure and usually recommend that their obese patients lose weight.[8] Unfortunately, they don't often give their patients much help in doing it.

The second step of drug therapy usually consists of propanolol (Inderal), methyldopa (Aldomet), or reserpine. And recently, newer agents such as clonidine (Catapres) and prazosin (Minipress) have been used too.

If the second step doesn't do the trick, there is still a third. The usual prescription at this point is for hydralazine.

All these highly potent drugs have heaven knows what metabolic interactions and side effects. The patient may be plagued with these drug-related problems and feel far worse than before. But if the blood pressure is still not down, there is one more, highly potent, line of defense: guanethidine, which itself may have the most frequent side effects of them all. Dizziness and fainting, dry mouth, stuffy nose, diarrhea, and inability to ejaculate are all quite common. This is why it is the drug to use last.

These taken-for-granted side effects are a major cause of lack of compliance with antihypertensive regimens. For when a patient reports back to his doctor that he feels terrible, the doctor often counters, "But you're better off now. Your blood pressure is under control."

I wonder if the patients who have to undergo the myriad side effects really believe their doctors' words.

Drugs Are Better Than Uncontrolled Hypertension

You might wonder why doctors so willingly prescribe drugs with such unpleasant side effects. The answer is really quite simple. *Untreated hypertension is far riskier than the side effects of the drugs.* The drugs are not ideal, but they may be lifesaving.

So don't be surprised if your doctor has told you that you will have to take your blood pressure medication for the rest of your life.

Even so, drugs may not be the best answer.

The Nutrition Alternative

Most doctors are unaware of an alternative that is effective in many cases.

It is time that situation changed.

A trial of nutrition looks truly worthwhile when you consider that antihypertensive drug side effects include impotence, depression, weakness, palpitations, menstrual irregularity, dry mouth, sweating, nausea, drowsiness, mental confusion, headache, insomnia, increased or decreased appetite, uncomfortable swelling of the breasts, nightmares, lethargy, twitching, and hyperexcitability.

The prescription-first practice can be a very dangerous one, as Dr. Harold W. Schnapper pointed out at a recent conference. He studied over a thousand mild hypertensive patients, using a perfectly designed double blind protocol in four medical schools, and found that "prompt pharmacologic treatment" may do more harm than good in younger patients with mild hypertension.[9]

And the young hypertensives are not the only ones who get into trouble. Graham Jackson and his colleagues described in *Lancet* a group of elderly patients on antihypertensive medication who had to be rushed to the hospital in various less than fully conscious states as the result of their drug intake.[10]

If a reasonable alternative to these drugs exists, then it would make sense to give it a fair try.

Nutrition Is a Powerful Weapon

Ellen Green came to me with a long history of high blood pressure.

Despite the fact that she was taking 40 mg of propanolol three times a day and hydralazine three times a day, her blood pressure was *still* 260/155. She also complained of severe headache, loss of memory, depression, and fatigue. At five feet three, she weighed 239 pounds, and she looked much older than her forty-three years.

An electrocardiogram showed left ventricular hypertrophy (one consequence of uncontrolled hypertension), and she had retinal changes consistent with severe hypertension. Her glucose tolerance test showed a minor diabetic-hyploglycemic curve and very high insulin levels—another risk factor in her already compromised condition.

Ellen had come to me because she had tried the Atkins Diet in 1972 after reading *Diet Revolution*.[11] At that time she had lost a lot of weight and felt great. But this time she felt she needed more help. Not being a paragon of self-discipline, she had gained all her weight back and more—and her hypertension was obviously completely out of control.

The first thing I did was to *add* methyldopa to Ellen's "pharmaceutical soup." Even though it's not my style, I did this because I was so concerned about her blood pressure that I felt it should be brought down to a manageable level before I tried to wean her from the medications.

Next I told her to discontinue the diethylstilbestrol she had been taking since her hysterectomy in 1971.

And then I put Ellen on the lowest carbohydrate regimen, both for blood sugar control and for its diuretic effect.* The other beneficial effect of the diet was that it would facilitate regular, lasting weight loss.

I also started Ellen on a vitamin regimen that included my basic formula (see page 319) plus 1 gram of vitamin B_6 with 2 grams of inositol each day.

By the end of the second week Ellen's blood pressure was down to a manageable 170/80, and I began to taper off the propanolol

---

* I am always baffled that the orthodox medical establishment regards the diuretic effects of a low-carbohydrate diet as "disastrous" when it has such obvious positive results—especially in the case of hypertension.

while adding a gram of calcium orotate and a gram of magnesium orotate to the daily regimen.

In the eighth week, her blood pressure pushed up again, but then it went down steadily as she dropped weight consistently. By the fifth month, we were able to cut out the hydralazine; by the seventh month, we eliminated the methyldopa. And by the ninth month, all the propanolol had been tapered out, and Ellen's blood pressure was 120/80. Her weight had come down to 164, and though she was by no means slim, she looked 100 percent better and years younger than she had nine months before.

Ellen showed other encouraging changes while she was on her diet. Her blood sugar returned to normal, her triglycerides went from 121 to 44, and her headaches (which were probably attributable to her high blood pressure) decreased in frequency and severity until they finally became very rare events.

Recently Ellen moved away, but I hear from her occasionally and am pleased that she has kept up her regimen and her newfound control of hypertension and weight.

As you can see from Ellen's case, my first line of defense is to control the blood sugar with an appropriate diet.

And then I add vitamins and minerals.

Nutritional Supplements Useful in Blood Pressure Control

Magnesium orotate is the nutrient I have found most effective. Magnesium (as in magnesium sulfate) has been a mainstay in treating hypertensive crises for nearly half a century. Dr. Hans Nieper, the prominent West German researcher, has shown that salts of orotic acid penetrate the cell membranes more effectively than other salts.[12] Calcium, potassium, and zinc orotates have all been used clinically with apparent success.

I mentioned earlier that orotic acid has been referred to as B_{13}. I doubt, however, that orotic acid will ever achieve true vitamin status, because it has no deficiency syndrome, and in addition, most of the research on it has been done in Russia and Germany rather than the United States.* But magnesium orotate has such obvious

* This strongly parallels the legal battles surrounding "vitamin" B_{15} (pangamic acid). Like B_{15}, orotic acid is a dietary constituent and a biologic substance normally found in the body. It even has its own enzyme—orotidylic pyrophosphorylase. The latter is an important point: The presence of an enzyme in the body indicates that the substance upon which the enzyme works is a normal and usual constituent of the body. Therefore, it is scientifically incorrect to classify the substance as a drug—i.e., a substance foreign to the body.

lowering effects on the blood pressure that I would anticipate that any controlled, double blind study (when and if performed) would corroborate this.[13]

The other agent that I gave Ellen—and which I give most of my hypertensive patients—is vitamin B6, the most effective nutritional diuretic of all the vitamins. The next most effective nutritional diuretic is vitamin C. I usually recommend 500 mg to 2 grams of B6 and 3 to 6 grams of vitamin C daily for this purpose.

The third line of defense is those nutrients that act as nature's tranquilizers. Clinical responses indicate that inositol (I usually give 1 to 3 grams) works best. Pantothenic acid (500–1500 mgs) also seems to have some effect. I reserve tryptophan and niacinamide for those cases where there is a specific indication.

Another nutritional agent is garlic, which can be taken either as a flavorable addition to foods or as deodorized tablets. The most plausible explanation for garlic's effectiveness is that it chelates toxic minerals and transports them out of the body. Dr. Henry Schroeder has shown that cadmium is one trace mineral that is toxic and seems to cause hypertension.[14]

Other nutritional measures include rutin (about 1500 mg per day) or alfalfa in tablet form. Although I sometimes prescribe them, their effect on the blood pressure is usually minor. These nutrients, too, seem to have a chelating effect.

My Results with Hypertensives

Hypertension is one condition I see quite often. Recently I tabulated thirty successive mild hypertensives who had been on no medications, and a much larger group who had already been on drug treatment.

Before their program was started, the average (mean) blood pressure for the group was 155/103. After a few months on the proper blood sugar control diet and nutritional supplements such as I have recommended, the mean blood pressure dropped to 135/85. Not a single patient failed to improve.

Among those on medication, almost all were able to decrease their dosage, and most could go off drugs entirely.

A Word about When to Use Drugs

After the nutritional techniques have all been instituted, and if the blood pressure is still not within the desired range, then the milder, nondiuretic antihypertensive drugs would be preferable to allowing blood pressure to remain elevated.

The list includes but isn't limited to reserpine, methyldopa, and propanolol.

Now the Proscriptions

In addition to nutrition, other life-style changes might help to control blood pressure. For example, I have already mentioned that many women on The Pill develop hypertension. If you take The Pill and tend to have high blood pressure, or if your blood pressure has gone up, then I strongly recommend that you find alternate contraception. And if you are on The Pill and your blood pressure is normal, I urge you to have your blood pressure checked at regular, frequent intervals.

This does not mean that I approve of The Pill for anyone. I believe that its metabolic effect is insidious. I further predict that we will one day realize that long-term use of The Pill has had an adverse effect on the life-span of those women who took it. I hope that by that time the Nutrition Breakthrough philosophy will have taken hold.

Alcohol, tobacco, and other unnecessary drugs—including the caffeine in coffee, tea, and cola beverages—are not much help either.

New Developments Implicating Sugar

Although many would not classify sugar as a drug, I cannot state strongly enough that it must be left out of your diet! It is no longer any secret that a high-sugar diet is a good way to increase risk of high blood pressure and atherosclerosis. Gerald S. Berenson, of the Louisiana State University School of Medicine in New Orleans, maintains that sugar is a factor in development and maintenance of hypertension. In an experiment with spider monkeys, the junk-food group averaged blood pressure readings about fifteen points higher than the monkeys fed ordinary animal-chow diets.[15] Dr. Richard Ahrens at the University of Maryland induced rises in blood pressure merely by feeding his patients sugar.[16] Dr. John Yudkin showed that sugar-susceptible people who regularly consumed sugar responded with high serum-cortisol levels (cortisol is an important adrenal hormone)—and one function of cortisol is to elevate blood pressure. The blood pressure elevations in Yudkin's sugar-consuming group dropped when the sugar was eliminated.[17]

In my own practice, blood pressures go up with such predictable regularity after sugar ingestion that whenever I see a patient whose formerly controlled pressure returns to a higher level, I can be almost certain that there has been some departure, however minor, from the no-sugar edict.

(One possible relationship between hypertension and blood sugar is that adrenaline release increases blood pressure, and when blood sugar levels drop abruptly, adrenaline and its by-products are released as compensatory mechanisms.)

There are several studies which indicate that 50 percent of diabetics also have hypertension[18]—so it would be prudent to control your blood sugar if you want to control your blood pressure.

My experience with hypertension makes it clear that the orthodox physicians' failure to consider the nutrition alternative constitutes medical mismanagement for millions of people. I firmly believe that their pharmaceutical reflex, which leads them to use drugs as the first rather than the last resort, has caused more than half of our hypertensives to take medications unnecessarily. The twenty-point decrease in blood pressure that the nutritional approach can achieve—and which my program did achieve—would save the majority of hypertensives from the necessity of taking these blocking agents and being debilitated by their side effects.

BOOK THREE

INTRODUCTION

If you have read this far, you know just how I feel about the way medicine is usually practiced. You are also aware that I do not believe in waiting for a diagnosable illness before starting to treat, especially since the diagnosable illness usually requires a pharmaceutical treatment that only substitutes one illness for another.

It is easy, of course, to criticize the way things are usually done, but I would not be so critical unless I had something better to offer.

Up to now, you have read about vitamins, minerals, and other nutrients that have helped my patients restore their health—without drugs. But you still have to learn to put it all together.

You need to be able to devise an eating pattern, with nutritional supplements, that gets your health back on the right track.

To do this, you must find a diet that balances your body chemistry (not necessarily a balanced diet, which of itself does not necessarily correct a system that is already out of balance), a mineral regimen that corrects your own pattern of deficiencies and overloads, and a program of vitamins and other nutrients that enables your body's various systems to achieve a new, more healthful equilibrium.

The chapters that follow will give you a step-by-step approach to setting up the nutritional regimen that is right for you.

Chapter 27

FOOD ALLERGY
OR HYPOGLYCEMIA?

Every week I see a number of new patients. They complain of depression, anxiety, fatigue, headaches, or even a prodigious appetite, among other things. And on each of them I perform a glucose tolerance test and order a complete battery of laboratory tests. Let us suppose that a typical patient's GTT comes back abnormal. (There is, of course, no "typical" patient, for all my patients are individuals —but it's a convenient term, because an abnormal GTT is a finding in so many of them.)

This patient's curve would show a steep rise in blood sugar after the glucose solution was drunk and then a precipitious drop into the obviously low blood sugar range.

Naturally I prescribe the appropriate blood sugar control diet. As often as not, the patient returns a week later reporting that all his symptoms have gone away, just as I had predicted.

So I would feel safe in assuming that I had just recognized, diagnosed, and treated a case of hypoglycemia.

But that is not always the case. Sometimes that conclusion would be wrong.

Food Allergy Often Mimics Hypoglycemia

Even the patient whose symptoms clear up in a week may have food allergies—also called "cerebral allergy" (brain sensitivity to food)—which produce many of the symptoms associated with hygo-glycemia.

Hypoglycemia and food allergy have a number of things in common:

1. Both are dietary. They are caused by an improper diet and corrected by an appropriate one.
2. Both may cause a broad spectrum of symptom-complaints, both psychiatric and physical.
3. Both food allergy and hypoglycemia symptoms may change by the minute or come and go on an hourly basis.
4. Food allergy symptoms and hypoglycemia symptoms are often time-locked and may bear a fixed relationship to mealtime.
5. Both conditions are seen more frequently in people with addictive food and drink patterns.
6. Both can present abnormal glucose insulin responses during the glucose tolerance test.
7. Both respond quite favorably to vitamin and mineral therapy—and most especially to the B complex vitamins.
8. Last, but most confusing of all, *both may clear up on a carbohydrate-restricted diet.*

It is on this last point that I feel I must expand.

What Is Food Allergy?

Food allergy is, as one might guess, a form of intolerance to specific foods. Not surprisingly, regular consumption of these specific foods may bring on symptoms. What *is* surprising, however, is that when these foods are not eaten, a set of worse symptoms—what might be called withdrawal symptoms—may develop, only to be relieved when the offending food is eaten again. And this sets the stage for the allergy-addiction pattern.[1]

Since the symptoms are worse when you don't eat the food, you never stay away from it long enough to get through the withdrawal and see how well you would feel without the stuff. Thus, food allergy could be said to be "masked," because people with the allergy-addiction pattern usually feel better immediately after eating the food that is not well tolerated.[2]

That is why I tell my patients to forget about eating those foods they are sure they couldn't live without. For it is just these foods that are the likely triggers of the allergy-addiction symptoms.

The Source of the Confusion

Why is food allergy confused with low blood sugar? It's simple, really. Most cases of masked food allergy are caused by such carbohydrate-rich foods as wheat, milk, corn (from which derives the very glucose solution used in a GTT), other grains, most sugars, chocolate, and several kinds of fruit.[3] And most alcoholic beverages come from grain or fruit, too. (Needless to say, alcohol is restricted on the carbohydrate-controlled diet, and this source of allergy is thus eliminated.) So even if the condition responds to the low-carbohydrate diet I recommend, it is hard to tell whether the problem was carbohydrate intolerance (a blood sugar disorder) or a food allergy.

Further, if I suspect that my patient is addicted to coffee or tea, I firmly suggest that these be given up, too, if only for the first few weeks of the new regimen.

Some patients, however, are allergic to some of the foods that *are* allowed on a carbohydrate-restricted diet. And most patients with allergies are allergic to more than one food, which complicates matters considerably. Common allergens among permitted foods include beef, eggs, chicken, lettuce, and artificial sweetener. A common offender is tobacco—and that may even include other people's smoke.

Most distressing, even the water we drink may be an offender. But spring waters, the bottled kind, are usually less allergenic than the water from municipal supplies which often contains chlorine and fluoride.

What About the Glucose Tolerance Test?

One would think that food allergy and carbohydrate intolerance (hypoglycemia) might be differentiated by a glucose tolerance test, because one would expect those with food allergies to have a normal GTT.

Unfortunately, it is not that simple. Dr. William Philpott, a pioneer clinical ecologist (the title adopted by doctors specializing in food allergy), painstakingly evaluates his patients by studying their blood glucose responses shortly after they consume a suspected food allergen. He has shown that some patients' glucose levels can go way up past the 200 mg percent range after an offending food is eaten—even if that food contains no carbohydrate whatsoever. Conversely, a corn-sensitive patient whose test results indicate diabetes after a glucose load may have perfectly normal results after an exposure to a differently derived sugar, such as maple syrup.[4]

Perhaps the assumption that a GTT delineates an individual's general response to *all* carbohydrates is not that valid after all.

How Do You Tell the Difference?

If the new diet makes you feel well, then the distinction between food allergy and hypoglycemia may seem academic. But is it really?

My practice has shown me that the blood sugar control diet helps nine out of ten patients who have hypoglycemia or food allergy.

For the 10 percent who don't improve, it is really essential to find out what food is causing the problem. And for the 90 percent who *do* improve, finding out exactly what foods cause the problem might mean a less restricted diet in the long run, because some of the eliminated foods could doubtless be eaten without risk.

There are many ways to test for food allergy. Some tests can be performed only in the medical offices of a trained food allergist, or clinical ecologist. Many types of testing can be performed by the clinical ecologist, and many by the orthodox allergist. Some allergy testing—if not most—can be very expensive and time-consuming. For a comprehensive discussion of the pros and cons of various allergy testing techniques, I suggest you refer to David Sheinkin and Michael Schachter's book, *The Food Connection.*[5]

Your Own Allergy Pattern

Because allergy testing in a physician's office can be so expensive and time-consuming, you may want to know what can be done to uncover hidden allergies. Dr. Richard Mackarness' book *Eating Dangerously* gives an easy-reading description of how you might go about the search.[6]

Keep in mind that food allergy is different from the usual wheezing, watery eyes, runny nose, and hives type of allergy in which you get a bad reaction whenever you come across the allergen. Classic allergy is mediated through antibodies, histamine, and the like. Food allergy, on the other hand, apparently depends upon the maladaption of some other system in the body—perhaps that involved with digestion. The underlying cause has not yet been fully explained, but clinical ecologists have observed that the maintenance of the allergic state requires repeated exposures—at least every four to seven days.[7] The good news, conversely, is that you can avoid the bad reaction and eat the food you like, by staying away from the offending item for four to seven days.

The Key to Allergy

The Four to Seven Day Rule is the key to coping with food allergy. It explains why a fast of ninety-six hours can wipe out all food allergy symptoms. And it explains why so many people feel so well when they fast. There are many, however—especially hypo-glycemics—who cannot tolerate fasting. Presumably, those who feel better when they fast are those with hidden food allergies, and the degree of improvement may be a clue to the extent of the allergies.

This determines how to proceed: Find the offending food or foods and eliminate them from the *daily* diet, relegating them to special treats to indulge in every four to seven days.

This procedure provided the basis for the first anti-food-allergy diet, proposed by the late Dr. Herbert Rinkel of Kansas City. Dr. Rinkel worked out a diet, the key feature of which was the rotation of foods so that none were repeated within any four days.[8] Contemporary versions of this diet appear in Dr. Marshall Mandell's book *5-Day Allergy Relief System*,[9] and in Sheinkin and Schachter's *The Food Connection*.[10]

These diets require tremendous discipline in preparation, and are far less desirable as a way of life than finding the foods to which you are allergic and simply avoiding them.

Rotational diets do, however, have a major positive feature: They enable you to prevent the emergence of new food allergies—a phenomenon that is all too common in the food-allergy susceptible patient.

How to Find Your Allergy Pattern

There are several techniques you and your doctor could use to discover your allergies.

Fasting is the first step. If you find that you feel better when you fast, then you may reintroduce specific foods, one at a time, so that you will know a reaction when you get one.

This technique heightens your sensitivity to offending foods, so when you return one to your diet the reaction might be dramatic. But at least you will find out which foods you should avoid.

I prefer what I call the "easy way." The first goal is to achieve the same well-being successful fasters experience—*without fasting*. (The reason you must feel well first is that you won't know when a food makes you feel rotten if you didn't feel well before you added it.)

Thus, your diet should exclude all those foods you crave, those you eat every day and rely upon, those you suspect you might be sensitive to, and those which are known to be the most common allergic triggers: wheat, corn, milk, and sugar.

I do not deny that this diet may be difficult for someone accustomed to eating as he pleases, but it has its rewards: It creates well-being in place of distressing allergic symptoms. And if you can manage to feel well for just a few days, you are then in a position to add all those foods you would like to reinstate (one at a time, of course) and see how you react to them. The technique for this reintroduction of foods is the same as the one I recommend after a fast.

Other Methods—the Pulse Test

There are other ways of determining what foods are your allergic triggers without resorting to expensive testing.

One is based upon the fact that after you consume a food you cannot handle, your pulse rate goes up for a short time. This phenomenon was first described by Dr. Arthur Coca a generation ago.[11]

Since tobacco increases the pulse rate and distorts the results of pulse testing, you must give up smoking before you begin.

The first step is to take your resting pulse rates (the resting pulse is taken after sitting calmly for a few minutes) before and after each meal, before you go to bed, and when you awaken in the morning. The first one in the morning, before you move a muscle, may be the slowest of all. Once you have this information, you are ready to see what effect individual foods have upon your pulse rate.

Before you eat the food in question, take your pulse, preferably when sitting. You need a resting pulse, because activity speeds the pulse rate enough to invalidate the test. Then eat the food you wonder about, and take your pulse—again when sitting—thirty to sixty minutes after eating.

Look for an increase of about six beats per minute or more. To be significant, the increased pulse rate should occur each time you repeat the test. But keep this in mind: If you have not been exposed to the food for four days or more, and your pulse rate does not rise, then the result isn't significant. You must repeat the test with that particular food the next day to see if a second exposure will trigger a reaction.

Keep a careful record of your testing.

Kinesiology Test

Another way to test for food sensitivity involves an obscure mechanism which underlies several systems of diagnosis.[12] It is called applied kinesiology.

To test kinesiologically, you will need a friend to test your muscle strength. One simple method is to have your friend apply steady pressure against your outstretched arm while you try to raise it.

First have your friend test your strength as it is under ordinary circumstances. Then put the suspect food under your tongue (if it's solid, chew it but don't swallow) and have your friend apply pressure again. If your arm seems significantly weakened after exposure to the food under your tongue, then you may well be sensitive to that food.

Once you have swallowed the food, don't test another one until your strength has returned to normal. If the test was negative, then you can try several foods in fairly rapid succession.

A Caution

Pulse testing and kinesiology testing can only provide guidelines to what foods you *might* be allergic to. The techniques are useful in confirming that possible triggers are indeed either highly suspect or probably innocent.

You can see how difficult nutritional detective work can be, and how confusing it becomes at times, especially in trying to differentiate between low blood sugar and food allergy.

In *Eating Dangerously* Dr. Richard Mackarness offers some pointers for recognizing food allergy.[13] Look for a set of symptoms that fluctuate. Look for evidence of food addiction and for other obvious local allergic reactions, such as hives, hay fever, morning headache, or asthma. And look for the following five symptoms that come and go: swelling, sweating, fatigue, fast pulse, and marked fluctuations in weight.

My own criterion, quite pragmatically, is whether or not a patient improves on the appropriate blood sugar control diet. If he does not, then he may well have food allergy.

It is still possible to devise diets that work for both low blood sugar and food allergy. I have done this for my patients. They are rotational versions of the Atkins Diet and the Meat and Millet Diet, and combine the principles of blood sugar control with the allergy-quieting advantages of rotational diets. Unfortunately, since the diets are so individualized, there would be little purpose in describing them here.

Chapter 28

HOW TO SELECT YOUR DIET

Those of you who read my first book, *Dr. Atkins' Diet Revolution*, knew what diet to follow—there was only one.[1] Millions of dieters simply called it the Atkins Diet. It was a very low carbohydrate reducing diet (not a high-fat diet, as many of my nonreading critics asserted). This is the diet I have used for virtually all of my overweight patients, and its safety and effectiveness records I can demonstrate most thoroughly. I still use it and I recommend it for the somewhat different clinical problems this book discusses.

For those who read my second book, *Dr. Atkins' Superenergy Diet*, there were two diets to choose from: the original Atkins Diet, for the overweight subjects, and a second diet, which allowed the protein foods *plus* the complex, unrefined carbohydrates, for subjects of normal or low weight.[2] That second diet is the one I have now labeled the Meat and Millet Diet. It provides blood sugar control without weight loss.

THE NUTRITION BREAKTHROUGH DIETS: THE ATKINS DIET

In the beginning of my nutrition practice most patients who sought my help were overweight, and so most of the sixteen thousand patients I have treated were given this diet. It is the same diet I wrote about in *Diet Revolution* and *Superenergy Diet*. And it is just as great today as it was then. Fads and trends in dieting may change, but human physiology does not. If a diet is the most efficient corrective for overweight patients in 1973, then you can bet it will be in 1983 as well.

I know what the Atkins Diet can and cannot do. In fact, I can generally predict quite accurately what its effect will be on a patient's weight, energy and mood levels, blood tests, sleep requirements, and the like.

I cannot help but conclude from all this experience that this diet is far and away the most appropriate cornerstone for nutrition therapy in the overweight patient. Don't think of it as primarily a reducing diet, but rather as the most nutritionally corrective diet for the individual whose basic metabolic tendency is to gain weight.

The objective of the Atkins Diet is to restrict total carbohydrate intake to the point where the body's stored fat serves as fuel. (This can be detected by testing the ketones in your urine with testing sticks called Ketostix, or in your breath with a ketone analyzer in some medical offices.) That achieved, the next step is the gradual restoration of some carbohydrates, primarily vegetables, to the point where the biochemical balance of the first dietary level is maintained.

How and Why It Works

1. The diet stabilizes the blood sugar, both by providing slow, steady fuel release through conversion of stored fat and by the directly protective effect of ketone bodies on the insulin-induced lowering of blood sugar levels.
2. It decreases insulin response, thereby bringing about a lowering of triglycerides, adrenaline (and adrenalinelike products), adrenal cortex hormones (cortisol and the glucocorticoids), glucagon, and gastric secretions.
3. The diet is the most direct technique for inducing stored fat to serve as fuel. This brings about weight loss, which continues as long as the diet is maintained.
4. It acts as a diuretic, inducing urinary excretion of fluid and minerals such as sodium and potassium.
5. It decreases motility of the stomach and the large intestine.
6. It decreases hunger dramatically.

The advantages of the Atkins Diet for overweight dieters are many:

1. It is the most luxurious and least restrictive of all reducing diets.
2. By abolishing hunger, it controls addictive eating behavior.

3. It provides a metabolic advantage; more fat is lost, calorie for calorie, than with any other diet plan.*

4. It has a favorable effect on blood fats (see page 216).

5. Its diuretic effect makes it effective treatment for edema and high blood pressure.

6. It can be useful in the management of stomach-esophagus-duodenal problems associated with excessive secretion or motility (ulcer, hiatus hernia, gastritis, dyspepsia, heartburn, flatulence, nervous stomach, and so on).

7. It can be useful for conditions associated with overactivity of the intestine (colitis, irritable bowel syndrome, diarrhea, and so on).

8. Most importantly, by decreasing the high insulin response and stabilizing the blood sugar, the diet can be useful for managing dozens of symptoms (such as those listed on pages 48–49), as well as such conditions as migraine, Ménière's syndrome, seizure disorders, schizophrenia, and other psychiatric disorders.

---

* This fact, which I reported in 1972 in *Diet Revolution*, was strongly denied by my critics. Since then, further proof of the metabolic advantage of very low carbohydrate diets has come from at least three different scientific studies.

Dr. U. Rabast of Wurzburg, West Germany, studied patients on 1000-calorie formula diets of two different compositions.[3] The following diets were used:
1. High carbohydrate (170 grams), low fat (11 grams).
2. Low carbohydrate (25 grams), higher fat (75 grams).
The study lasted over a month, and at the end, the low-carbohydrate group had lost an average of 30.8 pounds and the high-carbohydrate group, consuming the same number of calories, had lost only 21.6 pounds. The daily weight loss was 20 percent greater among those on the low-carbohydrate formula.

At Cornell University, Dr. Charlotte Young and her associates compared 30-gram, 60-gram, and 104-gram carbohydrate diets of 1800 calories.[4] Among their data are body composition studies demonstrating that whereas 25 percent of the weight lost on a 104-gram diet is nonfat tissue, only 5 percent is nonfat tissue on the 30-gram diet. In nine weeks, the 104-gram dieters lost 17.5 pounds of body fat whereas the 30-gram dieters lost 32.7 pounds.

And in another study, performed by Dr. Roger Unger and associates, they administered a 2870-calorie diet, similar in composition to the Atkins Diet (260 grams protein, 190 grams fat, 12 grams carbohydrate), and found that sixteen of the seventeen subjects lost between 0.66 and 6.4 pounds in a week.[5] The protocol of this study called for switching to a high-carbohydrate diet of the same number of calories, upon which there was, more often than not, a gain in weight.

The Rules of the Diet

The following food groups are unrestricted:

MEAT
FISH AND SHELLFISH
FOWL
EGGS

Watch out for carbohydrate fillers and additives, such as sugars in sweet pickling and curing, or cornstarch, corn syrup, bread crumbs, and the like. Other foods to avoid are bivalves (oysters, mussels, clams, and scallops) and organ meats (liver, sweetbreads, etc.), because they, too, contain some carbohydrates.

The following foods are allowed in controlled quantities:

CHEESE—Start with a 4-ounce limit on aged yellow cheeses. After the early stages of the diet, you may add up to 12 ounces of cottage cheese daily.

SALAD VEGETABLES AND OTHER VEGETABLES—These are the main regulators of the diet. When no vegetables are allowed, the diet usually contains less than 10 grams of carbohydrate. When 2 cups of lightly tossed salad are included (the usual starting level), the diet has 10 to 15 daily grams. If you want a 20-gram level, add ½ cup from the list of permitted vegetables below.

Asparagus	Spinach
Broccoli	Peppers
String or wax beans	Summer squash
Cabbage	Zucchini
Beet greens	Okra
Cauliflower	Pumpkin
Chard	Turnips
Eggplant	Avocado
Kale	Bamboo shoots
Kohlrabi	Bean sprouts
Mushrooms	Water chestnuts
Tomatoes	Snow pea pods
Onions	Sauerkraut

CREAM—usually limited to 4 teaspoons daily.

OLIVES—usually introduced in the second week; 6 to 12 daily, according to how much you enjoy them.

NUTS—usually added after the third week. Walnuts, pecans, Brazils, pignolia, butternuts, macadamias, are the best choices. No chestnuts or cashews. Nuts are usually restricted to 8 ounces per week. Peanuts, almonds, and pistachios, which contain somewhat more carbohydrate, may be eaten, but in smaller quantities.

Other permitted categories:

FATS AND OILS—These are permitted in moderate proportions. The best choices are cold-pressed—not chemically extracted—sesame, sunflower, and safflower oils. The worst choices are margarine, hydrogenated oil, shortening, coconut oil, and lard. Butter, olive oil, mayonnaise, and other oils are also permitted.

GELATIN AND DIET GELATIN—make sure the product you select contains no carbohydrate.

CONDIMENTS—You may use salt, pepper, paprika, onion salt, garlic salt, powdered or Chinese mustard, and any dried herb or spice except those containing sugar. Sugarless vanilla, chocolate, banana, or other extracts, horseradish, vinegar, and Maggi's seasoning are okay. Soy and Worcestershire sauces and regular mustard are allowed in quantities less than 1 ounce daily. No catsup or tomato products.

SWEETENERS—Saccharin and cyclamates are permitted. (Artificial sweeteners, despite recent controversy, are relatively safe, particularly when taken in moderation.) If the sweeteners are in packets containing 1 gram of carbohydrate, use them sparingly and remember to add the amount to your daily carbohydrate count. (And don't forget that diet chewing gum usually has 1 or 2 grams of carbohydrate per stick.)

LEMON OR LIME JUICE—The juice of half a lemon or lime is allowed daily.

BEVERAGES—Best choices are spring waters, bottled waters, club soda, and tap water. I find that the best hot drinks are noncaffeinated herbal teas. I also recommend clear broth, bouillon, and decaffeinated coffee. Regular coffee is an individual matter. If you are not addicted to caffeine, you may have up to 2 cups daily. In the same manner, I usually permit as many as 4 cups of weakly brewed tea.

No alcohol is permitted in the first stages of the diet.

Nothing else is permitted.

This diet *excludes* such favorites as fruit or juice, milk, yogurt, grains, and lentils. And it most emphatically excludes sweets and starches.

Further Levels

Beyond the 20-gram level, additions are made: usually vegetables and some fruits and grains to create the next level (25 grams of carbohydrate) and the following level (30 grams).

One can add carbohydrates gradually as long as the desired effect is achieved. (In the case of my overweight patients, the desired effects include a steady weight loss and usually some urinary ketone output, measured by Ketostix.) With gradual additions, the ideal level of carbohydrate intake is not likely to be missed. The other advantage of eating fewer grams of carbohydrate than necessary is that it rapidly induces mobilization of body fat. This shortens the sometimes difficult transition period when carbohydrate fuels (glycogen) are waning and fat fuels (ketones and fatty acids) have not yet reached peak levels. Further, it shortens the period of withdrawal symptoms for those who have carbohydrate addictions.

In case the sequence of diet levels gets interrupted, you should go back to the first level long enough to confirm that you are back in ketosis, and then shift directly to the last level you were following successfully.

THE MEAT AND MILLET DIET

This diet is the best blood-sugar-controlling diet I have been able to devise for the patient who cannot afford to be on a weight-losing regimen. It maintains most of the advantages of the Atkins Diet, except the advantages of being in ketosis. But it affords the many clinical advantages of a high ratio of complex (starch) to simple (sugar) carbohydrates, as well as a high ratio of unrefined carbohydrates. And it provides the added benefit of a high fiber intake.

Meat and millet are not the only components of the diet, but the term is used to remind you that although you are allowed to have carbohydrates, they must be complex and unrefined. (See chart on page 41). And the word *millet* might make you think to try complex carbohydrate sources you have neglected or left unexplored in the past.

The Meat and Millet Diet is not a ketogenic diet. You won't go into ketosis on it if you follow it properly, and you won't lose weight either. Rather, the Meat and Millet Diet will allow you to eat carbohydrates, but they will be starches instead of sugars, and they will be whole foods rather than partitioned ones. The no-sugars rule may mean that popular items such as milk and yogurt (lactose) and fruit and juice (glucose, fructose) will be curtailed, or even eliminated. But your insulin levels will be regulated; this is the cornerstone of an effective diet plan.

Principles: The main thrust is restriction of refined carbohydrates and simple sugars, replacing them with whole vegetables and grains. Further, it includes all the protein foods used in the reducing diet, as well as the essential fats our bodies need to be healthy and our foods need to be delicious.

Later, I allow many of my patients to restore gradually *some* of the sugar-type foods (fruit, milk, yogurt) and *some* refined starchy foods (bread and cereal) but only up to the point where the benefits of the strict diet are maintained.

How and Why It Works

1. It stabilizes the blood sugar. Enzymatic digestion of starches is a slow process, and the net effect is liberation of glucose (the ultimate fuel of starch) slowly and steadily. The natural fiber of unrefined carbohydrates has been shown to have a blood-sugar-stabilizing effect as well.
2. It decreases insulin response. It has been shown that the least—and thus most favorable—insulin response to a given amount of carbohydrate comes from complex carbohydrates, whereas the greatest—and thus least favorable—insulin levels come from glucose.
3. It provides the fiber, vitamins, and minerals inherent in whole carbohydrate sources.
4. It provides all the essential amino acids and essential fatty acids in the full spectrum of protein-containing foods.

The Rules of the Diet

The following foods are unrestricted:

MEAT

FISH AND SHELLFISH

FOWL

EGGS

CHEESES

The only exceptions are instances where sugar, corn syrup, or other natural sweeteners are added.

MILLET GROUP—This includes all whole vegetables and whole grains to provide adequate carbohydrate to prevent weight loss. Remember that many carbohydrate mainstays of most diets are suddenly removed in one abrupt change. Emphasis should be on the most starch-containing group of vegetables. Therefore, the best choices include millet, buckwheat, oats, groats, grits, bulgur, couscous, barley, brown rice, wheat, and rice bran, to mention a few. Potatoes, yams, and legumes (beans, peas, lentils) are acceptable. The less starchy vegetables like broccoli, Brussels sprouts, greens, onions, and carrots are also very much a part of this diet.

VEGETABLE PROTEIN SOURCES—Nuts, seeds, and soybeans (including tofu) are so perfect for this diet that they deserve a special mention, just for emphasis.

Foods Permited in Controlled Quantities

FRUITS—Perhaps half of the patients I place on this diet are allowed no fruits, except for avocado and olives. The other half may be permitted perhaps one whole fruit (such as an apple, orange, peach, or banana) per day, but no fruit juices. My decision is based on how severe I judge the blood sugar disturbance to be. If you have an abnormal glucose tolerance test or if your score on the Harper Index (see page 48) is 60 or more, then you should start without any fruit, except for avocado and olives.

MILK AND DAIRY PRODUCTS—Cheeses (but not cheese spreads or cheese foods) and cream (heavy, light, or sour) are allowed, but milk, yogurt, and buttermilk are usually limited to 4 to 8 ounces, so that foods and beverages which contain a small amount may still be allowed.

FATS AND OILS—These are permitted in moderate proportions. The best choices are cold-pressed—not chemically extracted—sesame, sunflower, and safflower oils. The worst choices are margarine, hydrogenated oils, coconut oil, shortening, and lard. Butter, olive oil, mayonnaise, and other oils are also permitted.

DESSERTS AND SWEETS—Since no simple sugars are allowed, you may have no sugar-containing item or dessert. You may, however, use artificially sweetened desserts, such as those made from recipes in the *Dr. Atkins Diet Cookbook* [6] or *Dr. Atkins Superenergy Cookbook.*[7] The most palatable sweeteners are a combination of saccharin (available in the United States) and cyclamate (available in Canada and Europe). Diet gelatin with less than 2 grams of carbohydrate per serving is available commercially.

CONDIMENTS—You may use salt, pepper, paprika, onion salt, garlic salt, powdered or Chinese mustard, and any dried herb or spice except those containing sugar. Sugarless vanilla, chocolate, banana, or other extract, horseradish, vinegar, and Maggi's seasoning are okay. Soy and Worcestershire sauces and regular mustard are allowed in quantities less than 1 ounce daily. No catsup or tomato products.

BEVERAGES—Consume liberally, but do not force fluids beyond your capacity. Spring water or mineral water is preferred. Club soda and tap water are allowed. Herbal teas (caffeine- and sugar-free) are the preferred flavored drinks. Caffeine is restricted. Therefore no coffee and no caffeinated sodas (colas, Dr. Pepper, coffee soda). Tea also containes caffeine; if it is allowed, it must be weakly brewed. Clear broth and dehydrated bouillons are generally allowed. Some contain up to 3 grams of refined starch or sugar, however, and would be limited to one serving per day. And diet soda can be used up to 3 glasses per day.

ALCOHOL—Not permitted.

BREADS AND CEREALS—Only certain stone-ground whole grain breads or cereals are permitted. Wheatless breads such as millet bread and oat bread are allowed, and when an allergy to wheat is suspected, they are the only types allowed.

Nothing else is permitted.

Note that although the total quantity of carbohydrate is unrestricted, those whose chief constituent is a simple sugar are sharply curtailed. Items which are refined from their natural state (flour, cornstarch, polished rice, potato starch, etc.) are not allowed either.

Quantities

Blood sugar is best regulated by frequent small feedings. Therefore, eat whenever you are hungry, or every four hours. If your symptoms disappear, then this interval may be stretched out.

Some people find that their symptoms are worsened by eating. This implies the presence of allergies to specific foods. To begin to track these down, keep a diary of everything you eat or drink and note *when* the symptoms occur.

Do not make the mistake of using so-called diet products, which may contain some form of sugar. Note that catsup, sweet relish, and many condiments and salad dressings contain sugar.

Liquid medications usually contain sugar, as do lozenges or cough drops, even though the label may not indicate any sugar content. However, an alternative can usually be found.

Further Levels

You will reintroduce the absent foods gradually. Start by adding small amounts of those starchy foods which contain *some* refined carbohydrate, such as ordinary bread, cereal, pasta, white rice, and so forth. Then try those foods with a sugar content: fruit and milk products. With each addition, evaluate how you feel. If you start to feel that you are losing ground or that the sequence of your diet has been interrupted, then it would be a good idea to go back to your starting point on the diet—the first level—long enough to confirm that you are back on the track. Then shift to the last level you were following successfully.

Selecting the Right Diet If You Are Overweight

The foregoing discussion should make your choice fairly obvious. If you are overweight, start with the Atkins Diet. If the results are as expected, and you feel considerably better, all you need do is follow the levels of the diet until one day you reach your ideal weight. By this time, the diet should have evolved gradually into a diet of somewhat higher carbohydrate intake, and it will be your maintenance diet.

If you cannot make the Atkins Diet work, due to persistent symptoms, then you will have to try a rotational version. Because a rotational diet depends on avoiding foods that you are allergic to, it is nearly impossible to give a rotational diet suitable for everyone. There are several books which describe a basic rotational diet as devised by Herbert Rinkel.[8] In these cases no provision is made to avoid the direct sugars found in fruits, milk, and the like, or to make the diet particularly low in carbohydrates. Therefore you must devise a diet that adds the principles of carbohydrate restriction to the principle of rotation (which avoids the repetition of the same food within a five-day span and the duplication of foods within a family).

The possibility that you will need a diet with a carbohydrate content is a remote one if you are truly overweight, but it should be mentioned. The Meat and Millet Diet with a ceiling on caloric quantities might be the best approach in that case.

If You Are Not Overweight

Those who are underweight or of normal weight should use the Meat and Millet Diet. This one can be suitable for a lifetime. When used in this way, there can be a possibility of occasional deviations, once the nutritional profile has been built up properly.

If the Meat and Millet Diet does not provide symptomatic relief, then try a rotational version (see above), combining the principles of a rotational diet with the principle of the restriction of simple and refined carbohydrates.

Some normal-weight people find that a ketogenic diet is the only answer to controlling their blood sugar symptoms. They may end up on a version of the ketogenic Atkins Diet, as long as they eat enough in all categories—protein, fat, and a little carbohydrate—to prevent unwanted weight loss.

You Must Make Your Own Decisions

I hope I have pointed the way to your initial dietary changes. If you follow these guidelines, your first diet decision should be the right one. If all does not go as hoped, you will have to work out a regimen based on your own personal observations. That is why it is a good idea to keep a notebook with a list of what you eat and drink matched alongside a column of how you feel. If symptoms persist or recur, you will then be able to study the food column to see if you can determine the reasons behind your setback. Did your symptoms come from not eating? From eating a simple sugar? From getting out of ketosis? Or from eating one of your favorite foods—to which you have become allergic?

This information will, step by step (and under medical supervision, if you have problems), lead you to the diet *you* should follow forever.

Chapter 29

HOW TO TAILOR-MAKE
YOUR OWN VITAMIN REGIMEN

Throughout this book I have stressed that although proper diet is fundamental to nutrition therapy or prevention, the right combination of vitamins and minerals is essential, too. Just which combination of vitamins and minerals a person needs is an individual matter, and it will take constant experimentation to arrive at a regimen that is just right for you. If you have problems or feel unsure, you should consult your doctor.

The First Step: Getting the Basic Vitamins You Need

Whenever possible, I recommend that my patients take the basic formula (see page 319) and then, building upon that base, supplement with vitamins and minerals geared for their specific needs.

There is a good reason for having a basic formula: I wanted all my patients to get a minimum dosage of all the vitamins and minerals they need, without overloading on any one or neglecting any other. I wanted my formula to be flexible enough to form the basis of a vitamin-and-mineral regimen for a complete spectrum of people with indivdual differences. And further, I wanted the formula to have enough of those vitamins that seem to be of most help to my patients—a feature that would make it superior to other formulas currently available. After much trial and error I devised my basic formula, and I have used it in my practice for the past four years.

Since it exists in pill form and has been used by over four thousand patients, I present it here as an example of a formulation which has been extensively tested clinically. The Atkins formula, as it now stands, differs from other good formulations in several ways—and these differences reflect my own clinical findings and experience. It is not necessarily the perfect formula, not even necessarily the best, since some patients cannot take it at all. But for the most part, my patients report to me that they can feel the difference when they switch to it or run out.

What's Different About It?

My formula, of course, places great emphasis on the water-soluble vitamins B and C, which happily are the two groups least likely to be overdosed. (The body, in its infinite wisdom, easily excretes via the kidneys whatever portions of these vitamins it doesn't need at the time.) The B complex vitamins are the nutrients most important in extracting the energy from proteins, fats, and carbohydrates.

My formula contains significantly higher amounts of all B complex constituents than those listed in the U.S. Recommended Daily Allowances (RDA). Any vitamin formula, like a chain, is only as good as its weakest link—and I wanted to be sure that there were no weak links in my patients' nutritional regimens.

The FDA's Folic Acid Problem

Despite my concern, there is a weak link nonetheless. All vitamin manufacturers in the United States (but not in Canada) have been limited in how much folic acid can be put in any formulation—and the amounts the FDA allows are disproportionately small—and quite foolishly so compared to the amounts of other vitamins permissible.

The limit now allows four tenths of one milligram (.4 mg) of folic acid in any vitamin formula, and that's nowhere near enough to supply the needs of most of us—particularly when the rest of the B complex is given generously. In *Dr. Atkins' Superenergy Diet*, I tried to overcome this obstacle by providing .4 mg (400 micrograms, the Recommended Daily Allowance) in each pill, which, if taken at the rate of nine per day (three pills, three times a day) *per doctor's instructions*, would at least provide you 3.6 mg of this remarkable vitamin.

In my own private practice, I usually added 3 mg or more of folate beyond that, so that most of my patients received between 6 and 10

mg of folic acid, *without a single instance of significant side effects.*
Yet if you see a product on your drugstore or health-food store shelf
labeled "Atkins formula," you will probably note that it contains
only 100 micrograms of folic acid per tablet. This is simply because
a company marketing to the public must obey FDA regulations,
while a practicing doctor is allowed somewhat greater latitude. The
manufacturers must conform to the limitations or risk product
seizure. Nonetheless, let me make it clear that the true Atkins formula should contain a minimum of 3600 micrograms (3.6 milligrams). *To duplicate it, you must add folic acid separately.*

To date, folate has been found to be essential to at least fourteen
different enzyme systems. Dr. Carlos L. Krumdieck calls it "the
most common hypovitaminosis of man." [1] I have been unable to
test this hypothesis, but I suspect that the optimal dose of folic
acid is greater than 15 mg daily.

The Other Bs

Specifically, I have emphasized the quantities of vitamin B_6, B_3
(niacin), and pantothenic acid. The basic formula provides 200 mg
of B_6, which is of critical importance because it acts as a cofactor
for an exceptionally large number of different types of enzymes
involved in various aspects of amino acid metabolism.[2] B_6, therefore, is especially important to people on high-protein diets. More
than any other single vitamin, it seems to correct the excesses and
deficiencies of a typical Western diet.

Similarly, vitamin B_3 (which I give as one-third niacin and two-
thirds niacinamide to prevent the flush that accompanies a stiff
dose of niacin) and pantothenic acid are emphasized beyond the
RDA. The formula provides a total 150 mg of the B_3 vitamins.

Just compare this dosage range both with the U.S. Recommended
Daily Allowance (15 mg) and with the dosages of niacin/niacin-
amide used by orthomolecular psychiatrists in treating schizophrenia
(often 10,000 mg) and you can see that the dosage range I employ
is neither standard nor megavitamin.

What About Metavitamins?

One of the most fruitful areas in contemporary nutrition involves a group of unnumbered B complex constituents which the
FDA and the food industry shrug off with the almost derisive phrase
". . . for which no recommended daily allowance has been estab-

lished." The fact that there is no "recommended" daily dosage doesn't diminish the *need* for these nutrients. They are known as metavitamins, a term given to a group of substances which have obvious nutritional qualities but which do not produce a deficiency state when they are absent.

Because the nutritional minimalists advising the food industry take the absence of an RDA as license to cut costs by not supplementing metavitamins—or by supplementing them only at a minimal level—they take on increasing importance in maintaining our health.

Despite the fact that deficiencies of these nutrients have not been shown to produce diseases in humans, these substances are nonetheless essential for good health. In fact, in most cases they are required in far greater doses than are the numbered B vitamins, especially since they have usually been refined out of our processed-foods diet. My experience tells me that if these metavitamins are to be useful, we must think of them in dosages of a gram or more rather than in milligrams.

The basic formula emphasizes three of these metavitamins: PABA, choline, and inositol. I have found PABA to be so useful to my patients that I have included 1200 mg of PABA per day, thus making it the second highest-quantity constituent of the formula, and perhaps the major reason why so many of my patients feel an obvious energy boost when the vitamins are taken.

The all-important "vitamin"—but the FDA says we cannot call it that—B_{15} (dimethylglycine) is a methyl donor [*] and should probably be classified as a metavitamin too. Legal restrictions prevent my incorporating it into the formula, but if they didn't, I would definitely add it. The metavitamin B_T, or carnitine, is one that I am currently investigating. Its metabolic action seems to be favorable to inducing ketosis; its deficiency slows down our ability to metabolize our fatty acids. It has been shown to be useful in angina [3] and in lowering the serum triglyceride levels in those patients whose levels were quite high.[4] (Those of you who want to learn more about this line of research will probably find news of it, as it comes out, in my newsletter.)

The basic formula also contains a healthy slug of vitamin C and the bioflavonoids. I consider vitamin C and the bioflavonoids a vitamin complex like the Bs, in that the various constituents com-

[*] See glossary.

plement each other's functions. Vitamin C (ascorbic acid) acts together with rutin and the other bioflavonoids to protect the capillary (small blood vessel) membranes and help prevent easy bruising, bleeding gums, and sometimes excessive menstrual bleeding. At 1500 mg it is the formula's single largest constituent.

In addition to the Bs, Cs, and minerals (which I will discuss in greater length in the next chapter), the basic formula also contains vitamins A, D, and E. I have kept the dosages of these fat-soluble vitamins especially low because, since they are stored in the body, there is a remote possibility of overdosage and resultant toxicity, particularly if one were to gobble down a large handful of vitamin pills.

Toxicity is quite rare at the dosage I recommend, but the formula is geared down to allow for flexibility in individual dosage, particularly as some people need far more of vitamins A and E than others.

Even the Basic Formula Must Have Some Disadvantages

Unfortunately, there are some individuals who have learned through their experience that they cannot take vitamins. These people usually do not do well with a comprehensive formula. But since their previous bad reaction may be to the source material (for instance, brewers' yeast, rice, bran, or wheat germ), it would be worthwhile to try the new formula, perhaps taking just one tablet. If they cannot tolerate this, I am forced to prescribe vitamins individually, one at a time, until I find out which ones are the offenders.

Not to belabor the synthetic-versus-natural vitamin controversy, one advantage of synthetics is the elimination of possible allergy sources. Another advantage is the ease of providing very large dosages when orthomolecular therapy is prescribed.

On the other hand, I have found many people who can take a natural vitamin but not the synthetic variant. Then, too, a natural-source vitamin is more likely to contain the companion nutrients that nature designed to be present along with the major vitamin. Some of these may be as yet undiscovered. Individuals do differ, however, and you should consult with the physician who knows your medical history.

I am convinced that virtually all of us could tolerate each vitamin if it were presented to us in the absolutely pure state. I find it hard to imagine that, unless we have an inborn error of metabolism, our bodies would reject a molecule that belongs in the body and is essential to our functioning, as are vitamins.

Of course, you don't have to use the Atkins basic formula, for you can piece it together, more or less, with a variety of other combinations. One such combination is a VM-75 type of formula plus extra folic acid, PABA, vitamin C, lecithin, and bioflavonoids. Ask your health-food store manager to show you the ingredients on the label of such a product.

Keep in mind that once a total daily dose has been estimated, it is far better to take this in divided doses rather than in one large dose. The main reason for this is that blood levels of some of the water-soluble B and C vitamins begin to drop within five to six hours. For example, half of the thiamine you take will be used up by your body within twenty minutes.

How to Supplement the Basic Formula

Time and again I have stressed that after my patients start on the basic formula, further supplementation is likely to be necessary.

When you are ready to put together your own vitamin supplement regimen, fill out the questionnaire at the end of this book. This will help you identify your main problem. And logically enough, your main problem is the one you tackle first. If your condition is serious enough to require medical help, then I am certain this will be the first question your doctor will ask you.

Once you have put your finger on your major complaint, turn to the chapter in which I discuss what I recommend for my patients with similar conditions. You will note that I start with a single nutrient or group of nutrients, like choline with inositol, for the first week. Add that and only that supplement in approximately the dosage I have recommended. (You can do this relatively safely only if you are taking an adequate basic formula. Otherwise you risk creating a vitamin imbalance by giving a single vitamin unmatched by those other vitamins that balance it out.) Wait for a week. If you feel better, you will know you're doing something right; if you don't, add the next step in the general regimen I have outlined.

Just be sure that you add no more than one variable at a time so you can tell which changes made a difference and which did not. Needless to say, I don't recommend making any major changes in your diet the same week you add or subtract a major nutrient in your regimen.

Once your primary problem seems to be clearing up, you can then start to tackle some of the others. It's a rare patient of mine who has only one complaint, and I'm sure that you, too, have a number of areas in which you would like to see some improvement.

There is a particularly interesting phenomenon among my office patients: Once a patient's blood sugar is stabilized and the basic vitamin formula has been started, there is usually a change for the better. And if a patient follows a regimen aimed at treating a major complaint, sometimes the minor ones simply evaporate without any further changes in the regimen.

The lesson is a simple one. Start with the diet and basic formula, add supplements gradually, evaluating carefully what effect you are getting—and don't be surprised if you feel far better than you ever dreamed you could.

Pitfalls

This book is not intended to be a substitute for sound medical advice. However, since it outlines some of the treatment regimens I recommend for my office patients, I think you should also be aware of some of the cautions I include in the advice I give my patients.

Pitfall 1: too little folic acid. This is a possibility if you rely upon a standard multivitamin without adding folic acid. If, for example, you supplement folic acid at the 400 mcg level (.4 mg) and take massive doses of vitamin B_1 (thiamine), B_3 (niacin), or B_6, you then risk a relative deficiency in folic acid.

Pitfall 2: too much folic acid. The lame pretext under which the FDA restricts folic acid goes something like this: Folic acid shares with B_{12} the ability to correct pernicious anemia, but unlike vitamin B_{12}, it cannot halt the neurological condition that occasionally accompanies it. Thus, the doctor who follows a patient's progress only by blood count could miss the neurological deficit in a patient liberally supplied with folic acid. To avoid this almost unheard-of sequence of events (since folic acid is almost always given with B_{12}) an entire populace is hard put to correct its number one vitamin deficiency. If you wonder why I feel the FDA does not play fair with us in our nutritional needs, I cite this example as exhibit A.

There is an explanation for why some people feel worse when they take folic acid. Folate raises the histamine levels. And there is a certain biochemical type, referred to by Dr. Carl Pfeiffer as the histadelic—high histamine—group, who tends to be ruminative, depressed, or subject to frequent headaches.[5] These patients do indeed often feel worse when they take the dosages of folic acid I recommend.

Another type of patient depends upon the drug diphenylhydantoin (DPH, dilantin), with which folic acid has a mutual antagonism. These patients' seizures could be made worse by folic acid—or, conversely, their DPH-induced symptoms could be made better.

So you see that folic acid dosage must be regulated individually. *Pitfall 3:* Vitamin B$_6$ dosage also must be regulated individually. A dose of 200 mg is exceptionally high for any standard multiple vitamin. Some natural vitamin formulations provide only microgram levels of B$_6$, and others provide less than the rather low RDA of 2 mg. For some individuals, 200 mg of B$_6$ may be excessive and lead to restlessness, nervousness, or other symptoms.

But for most of my patients, 200 mg seems to be not quite enough for optimal effect. Remember, we are always looking for the *optimal* dosage, not the minimal—and dosages of 2000 mg and more are often used by orthomolecular physicians.

The simplest way to find the ideal B$_6$ dosage is to note how often you are able to recall your dreams. B$_6$ intake may be considered optimal if you can remember in the morning something about your previous night's dreams at least half the time. (Dream recall also seems to relate to the minerals zinc and manganese and to the amino acid tryptophan.) It is fascinating to question those of my patients who report to me that they never, or hardly ever, dream before taking B$_6$, to see how many of them will not only have dreams but remember them after their B$_6$ dose is regulated. When this happens, B$_6$ works like a miracle drug for them, especially in the areas of mood, energy level, alertness, and memory.

Pitfall 4: too much or too little niacin and niacinamide. Both are forms of vitamin B$_3$. Both have the same important nutritional functions, though one may work better than the other in some conditions. But you have to watch out for niacin—also known as nicotinic acid—for it can cause an uncomfortable flush after you take as few as 25 mg.

Niacinamide, too, has been reported to cause several problems, including depression. I have not seen this in my clinical practice, however—in fact, my depressed patients seem to find niacinamide helpful. This may be due to the fact that the regimen I recommend is balanced and the niacinamide is given in conjunction with sufficient amounts of the other B vitamins.

Pitfall 5: allergy to brewers' yeast, wheat germ, rice, bran, and other natural substances in which B vitamins are found.

A patient who is allergic to natural-source vitamins may feel not quite right within an hour of taking them. Therefore, if a patient's response is not all it should be, I sometimes suggest he or she switch to the synthetic form of the vitamins I recommend, just to see if that will make a difference—and it often does.

Sometimes the techniques of muscle-weakness testing referred to as applied kinesiology (see page 268) can be used to determine which vitamins will cause unfavorable reactions. You may even be able to test for particularly helpful vitamins by using the same technique to find out which ones will *improve* your muscle strength.

Pitfall 6: allergy to a synthetic vitamin tablet. This allergy is usually not to the vitamin itself, for I believe that few of us are allergic to the pure vitamins, but rather to the filler (excipients) used to prepare the vitamin in tablet form. If you react badly to a synthetic vitamin tablet, then changing brands may solve the problem, because different manufacturers use different excipients and binders. Just changing brands cannot substitute for your physician's advice if you are having problems.

If you have arthritis, a heart condition, insomnia, fatigue, decreased sexual interest, depression, or an acute infection, then you might well benefit from taking a look at the Vitamins at a Glance section in the back of this book as well as checking with your own physician. There I outline suggested supplements to the basic regimens I recommend in those conditions. However, you must not make the mistake of assuming that this combination is perfect or that the proportions are fixed. You may require fewer or additional nutrients, and the proportions you need may differ greatly from the general recommendations. But they are a useful starting point, and I am planning to make these formulations available to my office patients so that they can get away with fewer tablets in these chronic conditions.

Now That I'm Perfect, What Do I Do?

Once you have reached a point where you're feeling better than ever, exercising like an Olympic contender, yet calm and peaceful, sleeping soundly, yet needing very little sleep, you will probably find you are taking dozens of vitamin pills every day. Your chief complaint may well be "all those vitamins I have to take."

Well, cheer up. You should be able, at that point, to cut down your vitamin intake. It's tapering-down time. Start by selecting those supplemental vitamins that seemed to make very little impact when you began them, or those which seem to be in disproportionately high dosages, and cut their dosage by one third to one half. As you stay on the reduced levels for about a week, ask yourself: "Do I feel just as well as I did before the cutback?" If the answer is yes, proceed to a similar reduction on the vitamins you take in the next highest dosage. If the answer is no, reinstate your old level; you probably need it.

Eventually you should be able to taper down to the basic formula, plus folic acid and some others that may be life-preserving, like vitamins E, C, brewers' yeast, garlic, etc.—pretty much the way I take my own vitamins.

What Do You Take, Dr. Atkins?

Often my patients will ask me what vitamins I take. I have reservations about telling any patient of mine—or anyone to whom I give nutritional advice—about the regimen I have devised for myself, just because the whole matter is so individual that what's good for me may not help anyone else. Over the years I have tinkered and experimented to arrive at a regimen that's just right for me.

But in case you are one of those who would ask the question if you bumped into me at a cocktail party, I'll tell you what I do in 1981. By 1982 it may be quite different, because I modify a little bit all the time, as needed.

I take six to nine tablets of my basic formula daily, and more still if I'm under stress. I also take an extra 20,000 units of Vitamin A, 400 units of vitamin E, 15 mg of folic acid, and extra C (with bioflavonoids) in variable amounts. I have found that three to six tablets of American ginseng seems to do something for me, along with three to six allicin-free garlic tablets, 1200 mg RNA and four tablets of superoxide dismutase. I supplement minerals based upon the results of my own hair analysis (three 50-mg tablets of magnesium orotate per day, chelated zinc, chelated manganese, and GTF chromium). If I feel tired, I'll take extra PABA, B_6 or thiamine, or some B_{15}, and if I feel too keyed up to sleep, I'll take extra inositol, pantothenic acid, and niacinamide. And when a cold threatens, I take 120,000 units of vitamin A plus extra pantothenic acid, zinc, and 1 or 2 grams of vitamin C every two hours.

Just remember that this is what I do today, as I write, and that tomorrow my regimen may change a little according to tomorrow's needs. Also, your needs may differ from mine. As my patients impress me with their successes, I often gain a greater appreciation of the potential value of various nutrients. And with tomorrow upon tomorrow, you can see that my regimen six months from now might be very different indeed.

Vitamins Are Not the Whole Answer to Supplementation

Vitamins do not always act alone. Sometimes they interact with minerals, or they may cause a mineral to be retained in the body or excreted in greater proportion. For example, vitamin B_6 causes a disproportionately greater excretion of copper than of zinc. And if a patient seems to be too high in copper or too low in zinc, one way to make the zinc/copper ratio more favorable might be to add more B_6 to the regimen.

So let us turn to the minerals and take a look at how to find out what they do.

Chapter 30

HOW TO DEVELOP
YOUR OWN MINERAL REGIMEN

If the clinical application of vitamins has been growing steadily of late, the clinical application of minerals has been undergoing a virtual explosion. Just visit your local health-food store, listen to any of the talk-show nutritionists, or attend a lecture or seminar; you will find that the conversation, which used to center around various vitamins, now involves the importance of zinc, chromium, manganese, magnesium, and other trace minerals.

Orthodox nutritionists had not, until recently, paid much attention to trace minerals other than to stress calcium and iron, because they assumed that our diets supplied sufficient quantities of most and because they didn't know much about mineral balance. As recently as 1974, Dr. Lawrence Lamb and other establishment voices were uttering such inaccuracies as "There doesn't seem to be any advantage in taking more magnesium to supplement your normal diet."[1] Zinc and chromium merited no mention whatever. The nutrition medicine community, on the other hand, always suspected that trace minerals were more important than anyone seemed to think, but only in the past few years has this suspicion been backed up by firm scientific evidence.

Mineral Deficiencies Are for Real

Dr. Henry Schroeder zeroed in on the problem when he pointed out that 85 percent of the magnesium, 86 percent of the manganese, and 78 percent of the zinc are lost when wheat, our major dietary staple, is milled.[2] And when you add to this the fact that virtually *all* nutritional factors are removed from sugar when it's refined, you can see how our modern, refined-carbohydrate diet routinely produces deficiencies of some very important minerals. And the more junk food in the diet, the greater the deficiency. For example, zinc levels of patients on high-sugar diets are often found to be low, whereas patients on high-protein diets, given identical amounts of zinc, have much higher levels. So it looks as though a mineral deficiency is related not only to intake but to composition of the diet as a whole.[3]

During the last decade, hundreds of scientific studies have demonstrated the importance of trace minerals in a wide variety of clinical problems. Much of the work centers around the essential minerals zinc, magnesium, chromium, manganese, and selenium as well as the toxic ones: lead, cadmium, and mercury.

But unlike vitamin therapy, for which the lab studies that establish blood levels or proper dosage are expensive, incomplete, and often misleading, proper mineral dosages can best be regulated with the help of a simple lab test—the hair analysis for minerals.

There are several reasons for choosing hair as a test tissue. To simplify, one could say that hair tends to represent the intracellular tissue levels of trace elements in the body, while blood tests reflect the extracellular levels, and that hair is a good measure of body stores. And if the hair sample is collected from a spot close to the scalp, there is every indication that the sample represents the recent status of the mineral balance in your body.

Best of all, hair analysis is a simple, painless procedure. All you need is a lock of hair. (Two tablespoons of hair is usually enough, and it's taken from the nape of the neck where the minimal loss will never show.) Depending upon the lab doing the studies, about twenty trace minerals can be quantified for a price that is relatively low (about $30–$40) considering how much information the money buys you.

You may wonder why your physician hasn't run a hair analysis on you, and the answer is simple. The interpretation of the results requires too much understanding of nutrition to fall within the province of the average non-nutritionally trained physician. But the test has achieved almost routine acceptance by the nutrition-oriented medical community, and for good reason too.

A Hair Mineral Profile Says a Lot About Your Body Balance

It is becoming increasingly clear that certain conditions are likely to be indicated by specific hair mineral patterns. Some may involve high copper and low zinc, others the reverse. Yet another may center on an imbalance between calcium and magnesium, and so forth. Many minerals compete with others of similar electronic charge, so that if you get too much of one mineral, it may completely counterbalance another which might be present in quantities adequate for ordinary needs. A hair analysis can point up this sort of problem quite effectively.

How Does This Benefit You?

Let us assume you have given your doctor a hair specimen for analysis. What kind of useful information will the results yield? Plenty, probably. The trouble is that even the experts have not yet discovered all of what this information means.

But going on what we *do* know, this is how I use hair mineral analysis in my day-to-day practice.

First, one of my nurses snips a hair sample and sends it off to the lab. A week or two later the results are back and I start my analysis:

Step 1: I look for toxic minerals. Are lead, mercury, cadmium, or copper levels too high? If so, I recommend further studies—usually blood, urine, and other tests to be absolutely sure. Lead poisoning is a real possibility, simply because our polluted environment contains a lot of it. For example, kids who live near major public highways have been shown to have higher blood lead levels than kids who live out in the country away from any great flow of traffic.[4] Hair studies may be more accurate than blood tests in ascertaining the presence of toxic minerals, but perhaps the most accurate test involves measuring the amount of lead excreted in the urine after a standard test dose of EDTA, the chemical known to chelate (bind) lead. If heavy metal toxicity is your problem, or a potential problem, you will certainly need your doctor's help to pin it down.

Calcium and Magnesium

Step 2: I study the calcium and magnesium levels—and this is where the confusion starts. Hair levels represent the mineral concentration *within* the cells, whereas the blood levels represent the concentrations *outside*, or between, the cells. When the blood calcium level is low, your parathyroid glands will be stimulated, and their effect is to drive calcium *into* the hair follicles. Thus, low hair calcium and magnesium usually represent low blood levels, as you might expect. But here's the trap: A high hair calcium level usually indicates an even *lower* blood level. By checking on the serum (blood) levels, the doctor can usually tell which is which. This is an example of how one can be misled by statistics on groups rather than individuals. Sometimes the findings are insignificant when a group's results are averaged. Yet the results may be quite meaningful when individuals at the high and low ends of the scale are studied.

Calcium and magnesium tend to maintain a relatively fixed ratio to one another—usually between 6:1 and 8:1. When they diverge, it can be significant. For instance, a high calcium/low magnesium ratio suggests a tendency toward atherosclerosis, kidney stones, or diabetes. When you see this, you may expect that magnesium supplementation can restore the ratio and bring about improvement in several types of conditions.

Zinc, Copper, and Manganese

Step 3: Next I take a look to see whether the levels of zinc, copper, and manganese are deficient. Most of the American population seems to be low in manganese, and a somewhat smaller percentage is low in zinc. But zinc has emerged as the number one trace mineral deficiency. (One sign of insufficient zinc is those white spots on your fingernails.) As in the case of calcium and magnesium, a high hair level of zinc can point to a low blood level. But any assessment of zinc status involves comparing the zinc level with that of copper, the mineral with which it competes.

Copper, unfortunately, is the most confusing mineral of all. It is involved in the metalloenzymes that are part of the processes necessary to form red blood cells, collagen, and RNA, as well as superoxide dismutase and some prostaglandins. Copper is therefore essential to many of our vital processes. But it can also be one of the toxic minerals, mainly when it interferes competitively with zinc and manganese. A high copper/zinc ratio is often seen in depression, schizophrenia, and learning disorders.

Zinc, on the other hand, is of extreme value and is often deficient. When its level is low, there may be a loss of sense of taste, poor wound healing, decreased sexual function, painful menstrual periods, decreased resistance to infection, psychiatric problems, and poor memory. It seems to be involved in most of the conditions this book discusses. But when the hair level is elevated it does not mean that we can feel secure that our zinc levels are adequate. Quite the opposite. High zinc usually means *deficiency*.

The Copper Problem

I repeat: Copper is confusing. A high copper level, especially when seen in arthritis, can also mean deficiency. But copper can be toxic and that high copper level may also mean *excess*. If the doctor decides to give copper to correct the deficiency, he is risking adding to the toxicity instead. For this reason, I personally tend to withhold copper in the presence of a high hair level.

Manganese is a companion to zinc in competing with copper, and its value parallels that of zinc. Next to chromium, it is the most common deficiency I see, at least in the eastern United States. Since it is among the least toxic of all the trace minerals, I frequently prescribe it when no hair analysis is available.

Another way to correct copper excess and zinc and/or manganese deficiency is to administer large doses of vitamin B_6. This is the basis of its use in orthomolecular psychiatry.

The Other Minerals

Step 4: Next, I study the levels of sodium and potassium. These major minerals are best studied by their serum levels, where they maintain a very narrow range of concentration. They are critical because they function as the major mineral interchange system through the membranes of all our body's cells. (The sodium is primarily outside the cells and the potassium mainly within them.)

The two minerals usually manage to maintain a fixed ratio to one another in the hair, frequently tending to run extremely high or extremely low. Both these variations imply that the subject is under a great deal of stress. After years of study, numerous diagnostic patterns have emerged, but most are beyond the scope of this book, and very few provide diagnosis with certainty.

Step 5: I take a look at chromium levels, because chromium is that element so closely tied to your glucose tolerance. It is now known to be the mineral part of a complex called the Glucose Tolerance Factor (GTF). I mentioned earlier that I believe GTF might well be a vitamin incorporating chromium, in the same way that vitamin B_{12} is built upon cobalt. The reason for attributing vitamin status to GTF is that it is effective in controlling high sugar levels, whereas the mineral chromium is relatively ineffective.

It is now known that GTF facilitates appropriate binding of insulin to the cells' membranes, thus regulating glucose transport. Low levels of GTF have been associated with impaired glucose tolerance and diabetes. Our diet is notoriously low in chromium, and our hair analyses almost invariably confirm that fact.

Step 6: Iron is often very low in hair specimens, but I don't feel comfortable in adding iron to a patient's regimen unless there is an actual iron deficiency anemia, or a low serum iron. Iron supplements can be harmful if too much is given, and some patients even find them constipating. Keep in mind that a diet high in meat and dark green vegetables provides more than enough iron to prevent iron deficiency.

Step 7: I look for patterns of disease. Enough work has been done computerizing hair analyses of patients with specific illnesses that certain mineral patterns can be distinguished in a variety of conditions.[5]

Although there are many more factors of hair analysis, most hair analyses come back with a computerized interpretation. So unless your doctor has definite expertise on this subject, order your analysis with the computer readout, which usually provides many suggestions for developing a mineral regimen in conjunction with your doctor.

One problem with hair analysis as it is practiced today is that its results may be altered by selenium-containing dandruff shampoos, by hair-coloring products, by recent washings, and other environmental factors, including swimming in chlorinated swimming pools. All may cause inaccurate results. These can generally be obviated by using an all-natural-ingredients shampoo.

Getting a Hair Analysis Done

If you cannot find a nutrition practitioner in your area, and if your doctor denies that he has access to the technique, then I may be able to help you. Please let me know if you would like to have the test done when you fill out the questionnaire at the end of the book. I can then help arrange for you to have it done.

How to Use Your Hair Analysis to Develop Your Mineral Program

Before you do anything, keep one fact in mind: Minerals are not vitamins. *Unlike vitamins, they may be toxic if taken in excess.* In most cases we don't have license to take them in massive doses. With each mineral, there is an ideal therapeutic range, so if you're taking mineral supplements, it is prudent to repeat the hair analysis every six months as a way of tracking your mineral status and as a guide to regulating dosages.

For example, if a patient whose zinc and chromium levels are low takes extra amounts of both minerals, another hair analysis must be made after a few months. Sometimes there is very little improvement in the levels of deficient minerals, and we may then presume that dosage should be increased. If, however, the level switches from too low to too high, this might provide a warning to stop the mineral in question. Unfortunately, we are not completely certain of this, because too high a hair level may well mean too low a blood level. So if your hair analysis indicates a mineral is too high, you might well get a blood test for a truer picture of which situation applies in your case.

There Are Universals in Each Culture

Every culture has different dietary patterns and, not surprisingly, every culture has different mineral patterns. Hair analyses can be used to evaluate the mineral pattern of a geographic region or a homogeneous group. The American diet produces a fairly characteristic pattern, so that there are mineral recommendations that might well apply to most Americans.

Since my patients (who seem to be typical of other Americans when I compare my office patients' hair-analysis results with those of other groups) are so often low in manganese, chromium, and zinc, I often supplement these minerals even before I get the hair analysis back. It is uncanny how often the results confirm that this is exactly what should be done. A detailed analysis of the typical American diet will show plainly why most of us are deficient in these three minerals.

Back to Basics

My basic formula contains minerals as well as vitamins. You will get some zinc (45 mg), magnesium, manganese, calcium, iron, and iodine, but no copper. The mineral dosages are too low to have much impact on most hair or blood levels, so you should not hesitate to supplement your mineral intake if your levels test out too low.

My basic technique for regulating minerals often goes something like this: Start with the basic formula and supplement chromium, the best sources of which are derived from brewers' yeast. At the same time, have a hair analysis (with computer printout) performed properly. With the help of the computerized analysis, I can then add the more important minerals that are the greatest proportion below standard.

For example, when manganese is low, I give 20–50 mg of chelated manganese, because absorption is better when the mineral is chelated, or bound, to an amino acid. When zinc is low, or if the zinc/copper ratio is lower than ideal, I will give 50–150 mg of zinc chelate. Zinc salts with orotate, aspartate, ascorbate, or even the more commonly available gluconate are all good sources of zinc. Make sure that the milligram amount in question refers to the *elemental* mineral and not the mineral salt. There is a big difference between 50 mg of elemental zinc from zinc gluconate and 50 mg of zinc gluconate, most of which is gluconate, not zinc.

Magnesium is an extremely important mineral. It activates over five thousand different enzymes in our bodies and can be used to raise serum calcium levels because calcium tries to stay in proportion to magnesium. It is particularly desirable to supplement magnesium when the calcium/magnesium ratio is too high. Further, magnesium is also very useful in preventing, or treating, atherosclerotic heart disease, and magnesium orotate is my nutrient of choice in treating high blood pressure.

Selenium, too, is becoming increasingly recognized as an extremely critical trace mineral. It potentiates vitamin E, acts as an antioxidant, and seems to play a favorable role in protection against heart disease and cancer. But it can also be toxic in high doses. I usually give between 50 and 200 mcg per day, depending on whether the hair levels are normal or low.

What If the Mineral Levels Stay Low?

Often six months or a year of taking the right minerals will show very little effect on the hair levels when the test is repeated, and the same low readings persist. This means that the minerals in question are not being sufficiently absorbed through the gastrointestinal tract. The fault may lie with the products themselves. Inorganic salts are not always absorbed, and the biologic availability of some amino-acid–mineral chelates is quite variable, depending on the manufacturing techniques used by each company. You cannot learn about this quality problem by reading labels; you will need to consult an expert.

The fault may also lie with your stomach. You may need to take digestive aids such as hydrochloric acid (usually given as betaine HCL) or the pancreatic enzymes in order to absorb your minerals.

What to Do If Your Minerals Are Too High

When lead, cadmium, or mercury levels are too high, the treatment is not so simple because it involves removing these minerals from the body.

The treatment of choice is chelation (EDTA therapy, see page 244) and is, quite obviously, a medical decision. (This technique for eliminating toxic minerals is also part of orthodox practice, for the orthodoxy is only too ready to acknowledge that the potential risk of toxicity from overloads of certain minerals far outweighs the risks involved in chelating them out of the system.) If the elevations are mild and not associated with high blood levels, and if you have no adverse symptoms, then EDTA is probably not indicated and nutritional chelating agents such as garlic, vitamin C, sulfur-containing amino acids (methionine, cysteine, lysine), alginates, pectin, alfalfa, rutin, and fiber may be used.

I wish I could be sure that this brief treatise on minerals would cover your specific mineral imbalances, but since no two of my patients are alike, I am certain no two readers are alike. I know you will have unanswered questions, but I hope I have at least showed you how complicated—and how effective—the procedure of mineral balancing can be. If you are patient, you can gradually work toward idealizing your individual mineral levels.

As the levels begin to improve, there is usually a distinct lessening of any symptoms you may have. The improvement is usually so gradual that you are really not sure what made the difference. But it points up the value of the hair analysis in providing a personal reading that will allow you to adapt the general advice that nutritionists dispense to those needs which are specifically yours.

Chapter 31

HOW TO GET WHAT YOU NEED

Any information about nutritional techniques and the virtues of orthomolecular therapies—those that change the concentrations of substances *natural* to the body—would be useless without corresponding information on how and where you can obtain many of the enablers I discuss.

They are not all available in the usual sources, and when they are, it is not always in the dosages and forms nutrition doctors like to prescribe. But the nutrition movement is steadily gaining ground, and health-food stores are popping up like mushrooms after a rain, many of them carrying just the substances I recommend. Further, the traditional drugstore nowadays carries a wider stock, and many of the more progressive ones carry some, if not all, of the supplements discussed in this book.

Since nutrition applied in this way can change our body chemistry, it is fair to call it "nutritional pharmacology." It is a rapidly developing frontier that promises to find natural cures to our society's unnatural illnesses.

The Obstacle of the FDA

One of the difficulties in obtaining the nutrients recommended by nutrition doctors and orthomolecular physicians is that some of these agents have not been approved for use by the government on the grounds that they are still experimental or that they are too new and there isn't enough data to ascertain their effectiveness. Yet they are being used by the nutrition people because they are substances natural to the body.

I predict that as the popularity of nutritional medicine increases, there will be a greater swing away from pharmaceuticals toward nontoxic therapies, and an increasing number of nutritional substances will become unavailable as the Food and Drug Administration seizes and embargoes vitamins, minerals, enzymes, and metabolites, substances which are normally found in our bodies. This "contraband," or class of illegal substances, will have in no way been found dangerous. It will be seized because of FDA policy on therapeutic claims.

Before I go on, there is a distinction to be made. The FDA is apparently trying to position itself to rule that *any* substance for which therapeutic claims are being made is a drug or a food additive and thus subject to the FDA's food or drug regulations and to every provision the goverment can invoke to control usage and distribution.

Only if no claim is made could the substance be considered other than a drug or an additive, and thus be distributed freely. This means that the seller can say very little about what the substance can do, for that would constitute a claim.

When Is a Vitamin Not a Vitamin?

According to the FDA position, if one were to make therapeutic claims for a vitamin or mineral, the government would consider it a drug. Just assume for a moment that a vitamin distributor labeled all his bottles of vitamin C with the line "Good for Colds." This would constitute a claim, and the government would be in a position to seize all the vitamin C so labeled. A possible exception is that substances which can be considered food might be excluded from this ruling, so that though the government might be able to ban over-the-counter sale of vitamin C, they would be less able to ban rose hips, a food source of vitamin C.

A good example of a nutritional compound under FDA seizure is pangamic acid (B_{15}), which many believe to be a vitamin but which the government refuses to allow distributors to label as such. B_{15} is certainly an intermediary metabolite and an important source of nutritionally essential methyl groups.* It was originally named *vitamin* B_{15} because it is a nutritional substance which is found in bran and the grits of several of the grains. Its synthetic variant, dimethylglycine, which has been shown to have many of the char-

* See glossary.

acteristics of a nutrient, has nonetheless been seized by the government and considered not fit for distribution.

The Jurisdiction of the FDA

The FDA is determined to gather popular support for this anti-nutrition stance with an ongoing propaganda campaign. The campaign currently involves their appointment of a blue-ribbon panel to issue opinions on the lack of efficacy of vitamins. Judging from the gross inaccuracies emanating from this handpicked group (i.e., "There is *no evidence* of vitamin C's effectiveness against the common cold. Vitamin E is ineffective."), this panel seems ready to do a thorough job.

Look at it this way: Government agencies are always attempting to expand their sphere of influence. That seems to be an inevitable feature of a bureaucracy. The FDA wants jurisdiction over any substance involved in treatment of disease. And they seem to have it. But since prevention is really a form of treatment of disease (their reasoning, not mine) the FDA would like to have jurisdiction over that, too.

It is through this "therapeutic benefit" approach that the FDA attempts to gain control over the entire field of nature's vitamins and minerals.

The FDA has been determined to limit available dosage forms to something only a bit beyond the recommended daily allowance—amounts sufficient to prevent the deficiency diseases, but far short of the quantities my colleagues and I have found desirable in using vitamin therapy clinically. Obviously it is not in the better interests of the American people to have vitamin dosages under FDA control. An overwhelming wave of letters to Congress led to the passage of the Proxmire Amendment, which in effect eliminates the restrictions on dosages of most vitamins.[1] I believe this was an important development and can teach us that if we are firm in our convictions and make our beliefs known, perhaps we can stem the ever-increasing tide of government intervention in our free choice of personal health care.

The FDA and the Public Interest

FDA-watching can be a fascinating pastime. Whenever a nutritional substance is found useful, the FDA seems to remove it from the market. It may sound as if the FDA is functioning *against* the public interest, but when you understand that the FDA considers the public interest best served by the maintenance of a healthy drug industry, you can see that useful vitamins would pose a severe threat to the present balance of economic power.

After all, what would happen to the tranquilizer business if everyone knew that such vitamins as inositol or such amino acids as tryptophan could do the same job, and with far fewer side effects?

When a research report indicates that a vitamin regimen is useful therapy, the FDA interprets this as a therapeutic claim. And, finally, it becomes the rationale for the FDA to regulate that substance. Neat, isn't it?

When the FDA takes over regulation of a previously unregulated substance, to all practical purposes it is removed from the marketplace. For to be brought back into commerce, it must be registered as an Investigational New Drug (IND) which then must go through expensive, time-consuming testing protocols to establish both safety and efficacy. The costs have escalated to the point where at least 20 million dollars may be required to obtain FDA-acceptable proof. And it's hard to find a manufacturer willing to invest that kind of money on a nonpatentable natural substance that is already in the public domain.

The net result is litigation between the vitamin manufacturers, who assert (rightly) that their products deserve vitamin or nutrient classification, and the government, which insists that the vitamin in question is just another illicit drug or food additive.

How does all this affect you? Directly, unfortunately. For while these court battles go on, the nutritional substance is usually unavailable.

The Demand for Proof Can Cost Your Life

The demand for "proof of efficacy" is a major deterrent to the use of nutrition medicine techniques. In America it is assumed that most medical research will be done by the private sector. This creates a bias in favor of the patentable, toxic drugs. Nutrition becomes the orphan that nobody wants. This is how it works: I think we all know that vitamin C is safe. And I think every one of us suspects that it can be effective in many instances. But who would pick up the tab to *prove* that it is safe and effective? Vitamin C is generic, widely distributed by vitamin companies, and inherently cheap; who could profit from proof of its efficacy?

Proof like this would have to come through government funding, but I doubt that our government is about to undertake such studies.

Of course, when we talk about serious illnesses such as cancer or heart disease, the problem is magnified greatly. Suppose that vitamins A, C, and B_{17} (laetrile), in combination with other nutrients, comprised a safe, effective treatment against cancer. Who would prove that in our free economy? There isn't a single manufacturer that could afford to do it. Does this mean that people will die of cancer and heart disease merely because a simple, inexpensive, readily available cure was a possibility but nobody would test it?

It seems to mean just that.

Beyond the Scope of This Book

Sometimes there are ways to get around all this. If you keep in touch with me (by filling out the questionnaire), I'll tell you how. I shall be putting out a newsletter that will keep you updated on the latest nutrient availabilities, in addition to detailing the latest advances in the rapidly booming field of nutrition medicine.

I believe that my responsibility to you doesn't end when you've read this book. Once I get you started on the path to the nutritional alternative, I want to guide you along by giving you the very latest news and helping you to improve your health. New research is pointing to new techniques for treating some of the so-called incurable diseases and finding ways to prevent others from developing. Nutrition is growing so fast that it is hard even for someone in the field to keep abreast of the newest developments. You should know the latest advances, just as I pass them on to my office patients.

Where to Buy Nutrients

There are actually four separate distribution systems for nutrients, although there is some overlap between them. The first supplies pharmacies, the second takes care of health-food stores, the third goes direct to the consumer via mail order, and the fourth is sold to and dispensed by nutrition doctors. Megadoses can usually be purchased through health-food stores, while most drugstores carry a less extensive line of vitamins and rarely offer the high dosages needed for megavitamin therapy. This is largely because the prescription-drug industry and its vitamin-marketing branches have yet to participate in the megavitamin movement. Which is not surprising if you think of megavitamin treatment as in competition with drugs.

Thus, if you are looking for vitamin B₆ in 500-mg tablets, you may not find any in stock in the drugstore, but you would locate several brands in a health-food store or mail-order vitamin catalogue. And don't be discouraged when you ask for a large-dose vitamin formulation if a druggist tells you "they don't make that." It just doesn't appear in the catalogues from which *he* orders, and because his wholesaler doesn't carry the items, the druggist may be unaware that these formulations exist.

You will probably save yourself a lot of time and annoyance if you look for your supplements in a health-food store first. Once you find a vitamin formulation you like, you might then, if you prefer, ask the pharmacist at your favorite drugstore if he can order the product for you.

Vitamins bought at drugstores and health-food stores are usually not quite as cheap as those obtained through mail-order sources. In some cases, the nutrition doctor may give you the best price. He certainly should know which products are of high quality.

Another way to save money is to find a comprehensive basic multivitamin and mineral formula that you tolerate well. It can reduce the number of pills you take while providing much of what you need (as does my basic formula, on page 319). You can then supplement from there if you need additional amounts of any single nutrient. There is no question that a good basic multivitamin-and-mineral formula can save you time and money, compared to taking each and every vitamin in individual tablets.

Labs and Doctors

The question of where you go for laboratory work is secondary, of course, to the question, "Where can I find the right doctor for me?" There are nutrition-oriented medical groups, of which I am a member, and at the end of this chapter you will find the addresses where you can obtain the rosters of the International Academy of Preventive Medicine, the Orthomolecular Medical Society, the American Academy of Medical Preventics, the International College of Applied Nutrition, and the International Academy of Metabology.

Any of these groups may be able to supply you the name and address of a nutrition-oriented doctor in your area who can perform, order, and interpret your laboratory work in addition to treating you as an individual patient.

This can in no way be construed as an endorsement of medical practices as performed by all members. Bear in mind that there are no real requirements for membership in these groups, with the exception of the American Academy of Medical Preventics, which requires that a doctor must pass a comprehensive exam on the use of chelation therapy before he or she may become a member. Nonetheless, mere presence on the roster of one of these societies indicates that the physician in question is open to learning more about nutrition medicine.

Drug-Oriented Philosophy Is Built into Our Health Insurance System

Perhaps the greatest single deterrent to nutrition medicine and the foremost supporter of drug- and surgery-oriented medical care is the third-party carrier—the insurance companies. They almost dictate that medicine be practiced along toximolecular (drug-usage), rather than orthomolecular (nutrient-usage) lines, by paying only for drug-oriented care.

Thus, insurance offers a bonus for dangerous drugs and a penalty for safe ones. It reimburses you for prescription-only items but not for over-the-counter ones. I do not mean to say that *all* patent medicines and nonprescription drugs are safe, but the implication is that they are safe enough to be taken without medical supervision—as are vitamins.

Look at the irony here. If you are willing to take something that is risky, your insurance carrier will probably pay for it, but if you take something quite safe, chances are it won't.

Often the doctor is forced to treat the "wrong" way if he wants to be paid. Let me present a letter from a major insurance carrier to one of its own paid-up policyholders, in this case a woman with hypertension, angina, and a blood sugar disorder:

> As you know, your contract covers the usual and customary treatment of a non-occupational illness or injury. It appears that Dr. Atkins' course of treatment is nutritional which is not considered a customary treatment within the limits of your policy. . . . Therefore, . . . we cannot cover the charges incurred in connection with the treatment by Dr. Atkins.

Personally, I do not believe that an insurance carrier has the legal right to pronounce that nutrition is not a "customary treatment." Therefore I suggested to my patient's husband that he sue the carrier, asking punitive damages. Instead, this indignant policyholder saw to it that all five hundred employees in his firm changed to another carrier.

The irony is that nutrition techniques are cheaper and, because they so often lead to the patient's getting well, actually can *save* the carrier a lot of medical payout over the years.

ORTHOMOLECULAR SOCIETIES IN THE UNITED STATES

These societies can provide you with the names and addresses of physicians in your state who are dedicated to using nutritional methods to maintain their patients' health.

International College of Applied Nutrition
Box 386
La Habra, California 90631

American Academy of Medical Preventics
2811 L Street, Suite 205
Sacramento, California 95816

International Academy of Metabology, Inc.
P.O. Box 15157
Las Cruces, New Mexico 88001

International Academy of Preventive Medicine
10409 Town and Country Way, Suite 200
Houston, Texas 77024

Orthomolecular Medical Society
2698 Pacific Avenue
San Francisco, California 94115

Chapter 32

GETTING A DOCTOR'S HELP

The implication of a self-help book is that you read the book and then you are ready to help yourself. Not so in this case. Many of the medical conditions I have discussed in this book *must* be overseen by a doctor. You should always be in touch with your own physician as you experiment with your body chemistry and make significant changes in your diet.

Your logical first choice is a doctor who practices nutrition medicine. But there are two kinds of nutrition doctors. The traditional, or orthodox, nutritionist is very different from the orthomolecular nutrition doctor (which is what I am). If you find yourself visiting a traditional nutritionist, you will soon learn that he or she is still wedded to the concept that adequate nutrition is achieved merely by choosing foods from the four basic food groups, and that if you don't have a deficiency you don't need vitamins. Although the traditionalist understands the biochemistry of nutrition very well, he is still not making the most of its practical applications. So he may not be up on the techniques for using nutrition as a treatment for your arthritis, your emotional ups and downs, your menopausal symptoms, or your insomnia.

The orthomolecular nutrition doctor thinks in terms of changing your diet and life-style, cutting out coffee, tea, alcohol, along with adding large doses of specific vitamins and minerals to treat illness. Although a rare and endangered species, his ranks seem to be growing nonetheless. The traditionalist is threatened by the new nutritionists, because they have a different treatment philosophy which seems to undermine the doctor-patient relationship that is based on the doctor as a dispenser of drugs. After all, in most states, doctors are the *only* ones who can prescribe—and many try to set themselves apart from other health professionals by emphasizing this special privilege.

Whose Patient Are You, Anyway?

If there are no suitable nutrition doctors within easy reach, you will have to rely upon the more orthodox ones instead. Traditional doctors tend to come in two varieties—one of which you may be able to deal with, the other of which you probably won't.

The doctor most likely to give you a rough time is the one we'll call the Rigid Antinutritionist. He or she really believes that nutrition is some sort of quackery and that vitamins and therapeutic diets which depart from tradition are undesirable. He may even think they are somehow harmful.

If you arrive in his office with vitamins in hand, he is likely to tell you to get off those dangerous vitamins and take your medications. And if you tell him you would rather try to do without your pills, he may insist that you take them anyway, reassuring you that *he* is the doctor, and that he, after all, knows best.

And please, please, do not tell him you want to try nutrition because you read a book aimed at the lay public, like this one. That is like waving a red flag, and it might jeopardize your relationship. After all, you may need him—especially if he is the only doctor in your community who makes house calls!

Let's call the other type of doctor the Flexible Clinician. He or she is more likely to work with you on a give-and-take basis. He will recognize your right to make choices, to eat what you think best, and to pursue an interest in physical fitness. He will also recognize your right to be well. In fact, he may even sincerely sympathize with your interest in nutritional techniques.

Thus, despite his own skepticism he just may humor your idiosyncrasies, your strange desire to improve your health by cooperating with nature.

Even if he is not an expert in nutrition, the Flexible Clinician will probably maintain an open mind and be willing to learn. He can be valuable, even essential, in your quest to improve your health. He can order appropriate laboratory tests to appraise your health and arrive at accurate diagnoses. He is also in an ideal position to evaluate your improvement or backsliding, and he may even save your life in insidious conditions such as diabetes and hypertension—

because you cannot always be aware of what's going on by the way you feel. He will be able to help you monitor your blood sugar, your blood pressure, your cholesterol, and a variety of clinical findings that are likely to change.

In case you are still not sure which category your doctor falls into, keep in mind that the Flexible Clinician, unlike the Rigid Antinutritionist, would probably be willing to explain *why* you should take your medications, rather than say, "Just take them. I know what's best for you."

If you continue to wonder about your doctor's orientation, ask him what medication he has prescribed for you and why he has ordered it. If his answer tells you nothing, you will have a good clue as to where he stands. The Flexible Clinician, of course, will tell you as much as he can. He respects your intelligence and your desire to participate actively in managing your case.

There is yet another way to assess what kind of doctor you have seen: At the end of the office visit, ask yourself whether what your doctor is treating is an underlying condition, or only a symptom, with little or no attention paid to the underlying cause.

How to Present Your Case to the Flexible Clinician

If your doctor seems to be a Flexible Clinician, you are still faced with getting his or her effective cooperation. Make sure you let him know that you want to improve your health by improving your lifestyle. Offer to cut out your junk food, your coffee, your booze, your smoking, and your late hours. Tell him you'll get more exercise.

Who could argue with this approach? Even the Rigid Antinutritionist would probably admit that this course of action could in no way *hurt* you, so long as he approved of the exercise you had in mind.

Your flexible doctor, of course, may be a little amused and perhaps a bit skeptical. But chances are he won't object to your giving it a try. He might even be willing to do a glucose tolerance test simply because he might learn something significant from it. If nothing else, it might pique his curiosity.

How to Get Permission to Embark upon a New Diet

By indicating his or her willingness to see you give up junk food, your doctor has, in effect, given you permission to find the diet in this book that is most appropriate to you, and then to follow it.

This is because each diet in this book is precisely based on the elimination of junk food.

If your doctor tries to help you by pulling out some diet sheet neatly prepared for him by some food or drug company, you would do well to point out that you have given the matter a great deal of careful thought and would really like to sink your teeth into a new diet that you feel is *nutritionally oriented*.

Assuming that your doctor has relatively few preconceptions about nutrition, he should be inclined to go along with your preferences.

An Ongoing Dialogue with Your Doctor

Once you and your doctor have agreed that you will change your diet, be sure to arrange for follow-up. Although most people are taught that nutrition takes months to exert its effect, the techniques I have used tend to work quite rapidly; you may not have long to wait for results. For instance, if you are trying to clear up dry skin, you might space your visits six weeks or more apart. But if you have hypertension, diabetes, an arthritic flare-up, or anything serious, potentially debilitating, or relatively acute, an appropriate interval between visits might be just a week or two. I have noticed that things my patients take for granted—moods, energy levels, and sleep patterns—often change within a week or two. Thus, if your symptoms are those which tend to change rapidly, by all means schedule your follow-up accordingly.

Although one purpose of a follow-up is to oversee your progress and to safeguard against any unforeseen problems, another equally valid purpose is to help you stay committed to your diet. After all, you will soon learn that you must give up something you previously relied upon—and that you must make up your mind to do without it permanently. With your doctor's help, you will know there is someone with an interest in holding you to a promise which I'll wager is almost as often broken as it is made.

Defending Your New Philosophy

Let's go back a step for a moment and assume that you can find neither the nutrition doctor nor the Flexible Clinician in your immediate area. This means that you might have to rely upon the orthodoxist.

It also means that you may have some differences of opinion. I feel bound to give you some of the arguments I use that may be of help to you in defending your right to try some of my recommendations.

How to Argue with an Orthodoxist

Suppose you were innocently to seek help from a dietician who belongs to the American Dietetic Association, or from an orthodox nutritionist or hard-line traditionalist physician. You would probably find that they totally reject just about every premise I have presented here, simply because these ideas are not what has traditionally been taught. Or if you are in a hospital and find yourself in the stronghold of nutrition's enemies—where they confiscate your vitamins and put you on a junk-food-filled diet—you may want to have a chat with the person in charge and try to get the diet you think is right for you. You would be likely to find that your pleas and protestations would get you nowhere. Nowhere at all.

I have tried to anticipate some of the orthodoxists' arguments so that you can be prepared when you find yourself on the firing line.

Suppose the person in authority takes away your vitamins or tells you not to take them—because "you don't have any deficiencies."

How to Counter the No-Deficiency Fallacy

You might answer this way: "Well, I probably don't. But I certainly *do* feel better when I take my vitamins, and if, as you claim, they're just a waste of money that can do me no harm anyway, why not humor me and let me have 'very expensive urine.'" You could add this: "I admit that you may not see any data that proves to *your* satisfaction that vitamins and minerals can make me feel better, but the fact that I feel better when I take them is proof enough for me."

Having thus set the stage for the upcoming battle, you might then get to the fundamental misconception: "And what makes you cling to the concept that all nutrients can do is correct deficiencies? Haven't you considered that nutrients can have regulatory or corrective functions and that they might even act as unusually safe pharmaceuticals?"

Be prepared to give examples to prove your point. You might point out that the concentration of the brain's major transmitters of nerve impulses is affected by nutrient intake; that a body chemical called acetylcholine can be built up by giving lecithin or choline, and that serotonin levels increase when tryptophan intake increases. *And this has nothing to do with deficiency.* Even a "normal" individual can increase his brain levels of these neurotransmitters by taking the appropriate nutrients.

And you might want to go on to point out that many harmful oxidation reactions in the body can be inhibited by vitamins C and E, or that the even more harmful peroxidation reactions can be countered by a newly discovered, naturally occurring substance, superoxide dismutase. No deficiencies involved here, either.

More Ammunition Against the No-Deficiency Mentality

If your physician shows signs of weakening (or even if he doesn't), ask him if he is aware that vitamin B_6 can improve the copper-to-zinc ratio and restore a high one to normal. You might add that when that happens, many psychiatric problems vanish. Or you might tell him that many schizophrenic patients must take in massive amounts of vitamin C before they spill any in their urine—and that once they are tissue-saturated (in other words, passing the excess in their urine), they often get better. And these patients are not ones you would call classically vitamin C deficient by any means.

If you need more ammunition, you could mop up with a few assorted facts such as, "Toxic heavy metals can be chelated out of the body with vitamin C, garlic, methionine, and other nutrients," or, "Cholesterol levels can be brought down with niacin, PABA, vitamin C, and lecithin, among others."

Or you might want to slip in the news that "the clumping of platelets can be inhibited by vitamin E; the pineapple enzyme, bromelain; or the papaya enzyme, papain." Or how about, "Vitamin C has been shown to have an antihistamine effect, and it enhances the body's production of substances vital to the immunity mechanisms (such as interferon) and has been shown to prolong the life of patients with metastatic cancer if the immune system hasn't been previously knocked out with chemotherapy?"

Another, if you want to be particularly erudite, runs, "Are you aware that cod-liver oil, because of its high eicosapentaenoic acid level, can favorably affect the type of prostaglandins in the body and improve the anti-clotting prostacyclin to pro-clotting thromboxane ratio?"

There's more, of course, and much of it is in this book.

But if you have used any of these arguments, your authority person should be more than just a little angry—and he may be confused and visibly shaken as well. So use your kindest manner to summarize:

"I hope by now you can see that it was this very concept—that vitamins are to prevent deficiencies—that has held back clinical nutrition for the first four fifths of the twentieth century."

The Anti-Low-Carbohydrate Argument

Just as often, the attack may be directed at your new or proposed diet. To some orthodoxists, the low-carbohydrate diet (or even the name Atkins) is a red flag. It invariably means high fat, which to them means high blood cholesterol readings, which in turn means heart attack.

You might answer this objection with, "That's strange. I seem to be eating even less fat than I used to because my appetite is so much better controlled. And I no longer eat ice cream, doughnuts [which are about 30 percent fat or vegetable oil of some sort], or french fries. I stopped raiding the refrigerator at night, and I now have genuine control over my eating. Based on Dr. Atkins' patients' results and on eight published studies in the medical literature, I fully expect my cholesterol level to go *down*." [1] If you are a betting person, you might even offer this sucker bet: "And I'll wager five to one that my triglycerides have gone down, too." You're pretty safe here, because the odds are more like twenty to one! [2]

Throughout this book you should find more arguments than these I have briefly given you. Use the Notes in the back of the book so that you can cite references; this is the most effective technique to counter the medical mentality.*

The Dangerous-Ketosis Fallacy

If your particular authority figure happens also to be disturbed by the supposedly harmful effects of ketosis, you may suspect that you are about to have a discussion with someone who is not well-informed. So respond by announcing: "Why, then, is it that whenever I'm strict on my diet and my Ketostix are purple, I feel better than ever, and when I cheat enough to go out of ketosis, I'm my old tired, cranky self again? Show me where in your medical training they teach you that when you feel great, you're really sick, and when you feel rotten, you're really well."

---

* I have recently found it necessary to counter some rather glaring inaccuracies concerning the Atkins Diet. My comments, and a 44-reference bibliography, appear in the December 1979 *Medical Times*. [3]

You might then add, "Why is it that all the experts in ketone body metabolism agree unanimously that ketones are simply a normal fuel of metabolism, the one the body entrusts with the responsibility of providing fuel to the brain cells whenever we have to rely upon our fat stores to supply our energy—the very reason we have a fat-storing mechanism in the first place?" [4]

The Doctor-Knows-Best Argument

Another argument you will have to deal with is based upon the high regard in which modern medicine holds itself. The argument goes something like this: "If all the greatest professors at Harvard or Hopkins or Mayo or Cornell have agreed that the treatment of choice in hypertension, or diabetes, or arthritis, or whatever, is drug therapy and I am prescribing it to you because all the authorities agree it is the proper approach, how can you listen to some crackpot author whom these very authorities have discredited?" And the companion argument is: "Remember that these unproven therapies keep you away from standard, proven-effective ones."

This last argument can end in nothing but a standoff, because it threatens the very basis of the orthodoxist's belief system. To convince the orthodoxist of your point, you would have to convince him that the orthodoxy itself is all wrong. And you know how unlikely that would be.

If you wanted to take on the argument, you would probably have to say something like this: "Couldn't it be that modern medicine has a failing? After all, the condition I have [or whatever condition you're discussing] still exists in me and in many others, and it's not cured by the drugs you prescribe. It's merely being controlled after a fashion. So all that medicine is doing is substituting a set of drugs for a set of symptoms and biochemical imbalances—and creating other biochemical imbalances. Remember, if modern medicine's on the wrong track, then its most eminent physicians must be on the wrong track, too. Therefore, we must dismiss our preconceived notions about whom we should listen to, and consider the basic logic. Aren't you taught to try the safest therapy first, and to rely upon the riskier ones only if the safer treatments fail? And since you must know something about the side effect and risk potential of the drugs [or surgery or radiation] you propose to me, wouldn't you agree that vitamins, minerals, and the elimination of bad dietary habits would be safer, and therefore the most logical first step?"

If he won't concede that point, you will have to conclude that you've really picked a lemon. A hopeless case.

The most likely answer from this orthodoxist, however, would probably run, "Safe, yes, but therapy, no. Otherwise the great medical minds would have made your vitamin therapy the treatment of choice. And they haven't, have they? And that must be because it doesn't work."

At this point, you can answer, "I rather think the real reason they ignore nutrition is because the antinutrition bias is the hand-me-down legacy of medical education, or because they, too, feel insecure enough over their position in the medical hierarchy to risk aligning themselves with a movement that's politically unpopular. At any rate, I prefer to stick to an approach where the safest therapy is tried first. I'll come back in a few weeks, and then you'll be able to see whether or not I've improved."

Orthodox Treatment Keeps the Patient Away from Treatment That Works

If you are feeling aggressive, you might also point out that *drug therapies act as a deterrent to nutritional therapies*. This is not a statement made merely for shock value. Rather, it represents the most salient problem most of my patients have had to face—the suffering and prolongation of illness simply because patients are given drug therapy first and have not been exposed to the *definitive* nutritional treatment—treatment which proved the drug therapy both unnecessary and fraught with risks that need not have been taken.

So when you argue with an orthodoxist, keep *his* perspective in mind. Be aware that he is bombarded by the medical media. That the information he gets is selectively filtered to tell him what the FDA and the pharmaceutical corporations want him to hear. Bear in mind that the news about vitamins and more natural therapies cannot seem to get through. Pity the poor guy; he doesn't know what he's missing. But my real sympathies go to those who trust in him, to those whose illnesses continue because they have faith in their doctor, even when he tells them, "There's nothing else that can be done."

If Your Doctor Is a Flexible Clinician

On the other hand, if you find an open-minded physician, try to get him to read this book. There are ample references in it to show him that I have derived much of what I say from within the professional literature. Perhaps he will go to the library and check out some of the references himself. Caution him, though, that because of the ideological embargo against nutrition imposed by most medical journals (especially those that carry pharmaceutical advertising), he may have to go to a pretty comprehensive library to dig out all my references.

If he tells you that he doesn't have time to look up all the references, assure him that the Notes are quite accurate and that when I refer to a text or article, the conclusion is not taken out of context. I have made every effort to report fairly. But if your doctor is willing to read this book, he may see its logic and try some of its suggestions on his problem patients. As he learns that nutrition can work he may begin to put his prescription pad aside and gradually adopt the nutrition alternative. And you might have contributed in no small way to his conversion.

How Flexible Are You?

Don't fall into the trap of assuming that your doctor is alone. I may have led you to believe that your ills are caused by our society, by agribusiness, by a conspiracy of the AMA, FDA, and the food and drug industries, or by previous doctors you have seen. But I must point out that you yourself may be the greatest obstacle of all. You may be one of those people who is able, but not willing, to make a major improvement in your health.

When a patient walks into my office, the problems of the past end and the real responsibilities and potentials begin. True success can only come to those whose value system allows for it. Health restoration cannot begin until you have placed a higher value upon your health than upon the immediate gratification you might get from food or your other pleasurable bad habits.

The greatest single determinant of your health is you. What *you* do to restore, preserve, and enhance your health will dictate the final outcome. Value your health and your behavior will reflect that value. And so will your health!

VITAMINS AT A GLANCE

Below is the basic vitamin-and-mineral formula I have been prescribing for most of my office patients. It is listed according to total
daily dose so that you may more easily devise your own formulations. The actual tablets are sugar- and starch-free, with no fillers or
chemical dyes. Each tablet contains one ninth (11.1 percent) of the
total daily dose; that way they can be taken three after each meal,
to make a total of nine daily.

BASIC FORMULA

Vitamin A	10,000 IU
Vitamin D	400 IU
Vitamin B_1 (Thiamine)	100 mg
Vitamin B_2 (Riboflavin)	75 mg
Vitamin C	1500 mg
Niacin	50 mg
Niacinamide	100 mg
Vitamin B_6 (Pyridoxine)	200 mg
Choline	750 mg
Inositol	450 mg
Biotin	300 mcg
PABA	1200 mg
Calcium pantothenate	150 mg
Folic acid	3.6 mg
Vitamin B_{12}	750 mcg
Vitamin E	200 IU
Calcium	600 mg
Magnesium	300 mg
Manganese	6 mg
Zinc	45 mg
Rutin	45 mg
Bioflavonoids	300 mg
Iron (as ferrous fumarate)	18 mg
Iodine (as kelp)	225 mcg

The following formulations are being used for specific purposes by some of my office patients. I designed them to meet the need for safe and effective drug-substitutes drawn from available nutritional supplements. They were meant to be used in addition to the basic multiple vitamin-and-mineral formula. These formulations work for many people, but, obviously, not for everyone. You should not simply start taking these vitamins if you have problems. Remember, these are part of a whole nutritional regimen. There are no magic solutions. *Be sure to check with your doctor first.*

SLEEP FORMULA

L-Tryptophan	200 mg
Inositol	300 mg
Pantothenic acid	200 mg
Niacinamide	100 mg
Calcium gluconate	200 mg
Magnesium gluconate	200 mg

Usual dose: 1 to 6 before bedtime

ANTI-FATIGUE FORMULA

Vitamin B_1	150 mg
Vitamin B_6	100 mg
Folic acid	400 mcg
Vitamin B_{12}	75 mcg
PABA	400 mg
Choline	250 mg
RNA	150 mg
B_{15} (Dimethylglycine)	50 mg
or L-Methionine *	200 mg

Usual dose: 1 or 2, three times daily

ANTI-HYPERTENSIVE FORMULA

Magnesium orotate	400 mg
Allicin-free garlic	250 mg
Inositol	300 mg
Vitamin B_6	200 mg
Pantothenic acid	150 mg

Usual dose: 4 to 8 daily, in divided doses

* The FDA attack on B_{15} may lead to its unavailability at some times. Therefore I suggest as an alternative the amino acid L-methionine, which shares with B_{15} the metabolic function of providing necessary methyl groups.

CARDIOVASCULAR FORMULA

Magnesium orotate	250 mg
Potassium orotate	100 mg
Allicin-free garlic	250 mg
RNA	100 mg
Choline	100 mg
Inositol	100 mg
Vitamin B_6	100 mg
Niacin	25 mg
Niacinamide	75 mg
Vitamin C	150 mg
Vitamin E	100 IU
Bromelain	75 mg
Selenium	15 mcg
Folic Acid	400 mcg
Vitamin B_{12}	75 mcg
GTF chromium	50 mcg

Usual dose: Start with 4 daily, in divided doses, and progress gradually to 8 to 10 daily

ANTI-ARTHRITIC FORMULA

Pantothenic acid	200 mg
Niacinamide	100 mg
Vitamin B_6	100 mg
PABA	200 mg
Vitamin C	200 mg
Bioflavonoids	75 mg
Vitamin E	50 IU
Chelated zinc	10 mg
Chelated manganese	5 mg
Chelated copper	5 mg
Superoxide dismutase	50 mg

Usual dose: 4 to 8 daily, in divided doses
Caution: Do not maintain this dosage beyond one month without checking copper levels.

Immune System (Anti-Viral) Formula

Vitamin A	12,500 IU
Vitamin C	750 mg
Bioflavonoids	150 mg
Vitamin B_6	75 mg
Pantothenic acid	150 mg
Chelated zinc	15 mg
Folic acid	400 mcg

Usual dose: 6 to 8 daily, in divided doses
Caution: Do not maintain that dose beyond a week without your doctor's permission.

Anti-Depressant Formula

Vitamin B_6	150 mg
Niacinamide	100 mg
Niacin	25 mg
Vitamin C	300 mg
Choline	100 mg
Chelated zinc	15 mg
Chelated manganese	5 mg
Folic acid	400 mcg
Vitamin B_{12}	100 mcg
L-Tryptophan	300 mg

Usual dose: 4 to 8 daily, in divided doses

Pre- and Post-Operative Formula

Vitamin C	600 mg
Bioflavonoids	250 mg
Rutin	300 mg
Vitamin A	15,000 IU
Chelated zinc	20 mg
Chelated manganese	5 mg
Pantothenic acid	200 mg

Usual dose: 3 to 6 daily
Post-operatively only—add 400 to 1000 units of Vitamin E per day

GLOSSARY

Adrenal cortex: The outer part of the adrenal gland which elaborates cortisonelike hormones.

Adrenaline: A neurotransmitter from the adrenal glands which is released in response to fear, heightened emotion, or physiologic stress.

Alginate: A salt extracted from marine kelp.

Allicin: The sulfur-containing principle obtained from garlic; the chemical that gives garlic its odor.

Allopathic medicine: A system of medicine that utilizes drugs to combat disease; i.e., traditional medicine.

Amino acid: An organic acid containing a nitrogen group. Amino acids are the chief components of proteins.

Analgesic: A drug that relieves pain without loss of consciousness.

Anemia: A condition resulting from an abnormally low number of red blood cells; symptoms include pallor, weakness, fatigue.

Angiogram: A diagnostic tool for examining the blood and lymph vessels by means of X ray after injection of a radiopaque dye.

Angiotensin: A hormone that plays an important role in the reabsorption of salt by the kidney. It also acts as a vasoconstrictor and increases the heart rate and blood pressure.

Anhedonia: A condition of chronic lack of pleasure in acts that normally give pleasure.

Antibodies: Any of various proteins in the body that are generated in reaction to foreign bodies and which neutralize them, with specificity by producing immunity against certain microorganisms or their toxins.

323

Anticoagulant: A substance that retards or prevents blood clots or coagulation.

Anticonvulsant: An agent that suppresses convulsions.

Antidepressant: An agent that prevents or relieves depression.

Antihistamine: An agent used for treating allergic reactions by blocking or opposing the action of histamine.

Antihypertensive: An agent that reduces high blood pressure.

Anti-inflammatory: An agent that counteracts or suppresses the body's usual response to noxious stimulus.

Antioxidant: A substance that prevents oxidation or inhibits reactions promoted by oxygen.

Aorta: The largest artery in the body, through which the blood leaves the heart.

Arachidonic acid: A fatty acid, precursor of the "two" series of prostaglandins.

Arrhythmia: Abnormal heartbeat rhythm.

Arthritis: Inflammation of the joints due to infectious, metabolic, or constitutional causes.

Ascorbate: The ion of vitamin C which can be combined with calcium, sodium, or other minerals.

Atherosclerosis: A disease characterized by waxy buildups within the arterial walls; the single most prevalent cause of death in Western cultures.

Atherosclerotic plaques: Hardened deposits in the walls of the arteries which narrow the artery opening.

Atrial fibrillation: A heartbeat that is irregular in both rate and rhythm.

Basal temperature: The temperature of a healthy body after at least eight hours of sleep.

Beta blockers: A class of drugs that block one aspect of the sympathetic nervous system, used in the treatment of heart disease, migraine, and so forth.

Biochemical individuality: The concept developed by Dr. Roger Williams which states that the biochemical needs of individuals vary greatly and that general guidelines cannot be strictly adhered to for individual treatment.

Bioflavonoid: A constituent of the vitamin C complex.

Blood sugar control mechanism: The mechanism that regulates the amount of sugar in the bloodstream. It includes the pancreas, insulin, glucagon, and adrenaline.

Bromelain: An enzyme found in pineapple.

Calcification: Inflexibility caused by the formation of calcium salts.

Carotid sinus: The slight enlargement of the large artery on each side of the neck which contains nerve bundles that can slow the heart or regulate the blood pressure.

Catecholamines: Breakdown products of adrenaline.

Cerebrovascular accident: A brain hemorrhage or blood clot of the cerebral vessels which can cause alterations in consciousness, seizures, and neuromuscular incapacity; also known as "stroke."

Chelate: A mineral bound to a protein for better absorption by the body.

Chelation: The bonding of a mineral or metal with two positive charges to an organic compound that holds the mineral in its structural "claws." Chelation therapy is used to remove toxic metals from the body.

Chemotherapy: The use of toxic chemical agents in an attempt to halt the growth of cancerous tissue. The term may be applied to any form of drug therapy.

Cholesterol: A solid atomic alcohol, a precursor of a form of vitamin D and a universal tissue constituent found in oil, brain tissue, blood cells, plasma, liver, kidney, adrenal glands, milk, egg yolks, and seeds.

Clinical ecologist: The title adopted by physicians who specialize in allergy from chemical and environmental causes.

Congestive heart failure: The relative inability of the heart to pump blood that has been returned to it.

Coronary heart disease: Diseases pertaining to the blood vessels supplying the heart itself; also known as ischemic heart disease.

Coronary occlusion: A blockage or clot in a coronary artery that prevents the blood from reaching the heart for its own use.

Cross-addiction: The body's tendency to switch from one addiction to another.

Cysteine: A sulfur-containing amino acid.

Cystic breasts: A condition affecting women characterized by large, generally benign, cysts in the breasts.

Cystitis: An inflammation of the urinary bladder.

Degenerative disease: A disease which causes permanent deterioration of the tissues such as atherosclerosis, cancer, arthritis, diabetes.

Diethylstilbestrol: A drug possessing estrogenic activity, prescribed for pregnant women.

Digammahomolinolenic acid: The fatty acid which is the biochemical precursor of the "one" series prostaglandins, the precursor of PGE$_1$.

Digitalis: A drug employed in heart disease to increase the heart's ability to contract.

Disodium EDTA: The chelating agent used to remove toxic minerals from the body.

Diuretic: An agent that promotes the excretion of urine.

Dysinsulinism: A malfunctioning of the insulin response in the body, with the result that blood sugar levels vary between too high and too low.

Dysnutrition: A condition in which specific nutritional requirements are undersupplied by a diet that is otherwise plentiful and in some ways oversupplied. Dysnutrition implies specific nutritional imbalances which can be corrected only with specific nutrients.

Electrocardiogram: The recording of changes in electrical potential occurring during heartbeat; used in diagnosing abnormal heart action.

Electrolyte: A mineral ion which, when dissolved in a suitable liquid, becomes a molecular fragment with either a positive or negative charge.

Enteric: Relating to the intestine. An enteric-coated medicine is treated so that it can pass through the stomach unchanged and disintegrate in the intestine.

Enzymatic reactions: Biochemical reactions that take place in the cells due to the presence of particular enzymes.

Enzyme: A protein capable of producing or accelerating a specific biochemical reaction at body temperature.

Ergotamine: A blood vessel-constricting drug used in the treatment of migraine headaches.

Estrogen: Any of the several female steroid hormones produced chiefly by the ovaries and responsible for female secondary sex characteristic development.

Fibrin: A fibrous protein that helps to tangle blood cells and form a blood clot.

Free radicals: Highly reactive molecular fragments generally harmful to the body.

Gallstone: A hard inorganic mass formed in the gallbladder or bile ducts.

Gastritis: Inflammation of the mucous membrane of the stomach.

Generic: Said of a group of drugs not protected by trademark registration and often sold at a lower price than the brand-name drug.

Gingiva: Medical term for the gum.

GI series: A series of X rays to determine any abnormal conditions occurring in the upper or lower intestinal system. The initials stand for *gastrointestinal.*

Glaucoma: A disease of the eye marked by increased pressure within the eyeball and gradual loss of vision.

Glucagon: A hormone of the pancreas which increases the sugar content in the blood. It is considered an antagonist to insulin, which lowers blood sugar. The relationship between glucagon and insulin helps to maintain a steady blood sugar level.

Gluconate: A salt of gluconic acid, most often used to facilitate the absorption of a mineral into the bloodstream.

Glucose: The simple sugar, half the molecule of sucrose, that is the usual form in which carbohydrate exists in the bloodstream.

Glutamine: An amino acid.

Glycine: An amino acid.

Glycogen: The principal form in which carbohydrate is stored in the body, for ready conversion into energy. It is found especially in the liver and muscle tissue.

Gout: A disease marked by an excessive amount of uric acid in the blood and painful inflammation of the joints.

Hair mineral analysis: A test to determine the extracellular minerals in the body by measuring the amounts of minerals present (or absent) in a lock of hair.

Hepatitis: An inflammatory disease of the liver.

Hesperidin: A constituent of the vitamin C complex that provides protection against fragility in the capillary blood vessels.

High-density lipoprotein (HDL): A protein combined with a fat (which enables fat compounds to be transported in the bloodstream) that carries cholesterol from tissues to the liver for eventual excretion. Studies now indicate that high-density lipoproteins protect against heart disease.

Histadelic: Referring to the biochemical state of excessive levels of histamine, said to produce suicidal depression, obsessive thinking, and loss of contact with reality.

Histamine: A compound, found in many tissues, that is responsible for the increased permeability of blood vessels and plays a major role in allergic reaction.

Homocystine: A compound capable of replacing methionine in the diet if choline is present.

Hyperinsulinism: An excessive secretion of insulin which can result from overconsumption of carbohydrates.

Hypertension: Persistently high blood pressure; the systemic condition accompanying high blood pressure.

Hyperventilation: Excessive rapid, deep breathing which leads to symptoms including dizziness.

Hypoglycemia: A low or falling concentration of glucose in the bloodstream (low blood sugar), often caused by an excessive intake of refined carbohydrates in the diet; symptoms include nervousness, anxiety, headache, dizziness, fatigue, and mental confusion.

Hypotension: Low blood pressure.

Idiopathic edema: Retention of water in the tissues, with the cause unknown.

Immunology: The science that deals with the phenomena and causes of immunity, i.e., resistance to disease.

Inositol: A member of the B complex found in fruits, nuts, whole grains, milk, meat, and yeast.

Insulin: A protein hormone secreted by the pancreas into the blood, where it regulates carbohydrate, lipid, and amino acid metabolism; a preparation of the active principle of the pancreas used in treating diabetes.

Interferon: A protein formed by the cells themselves in response to a virus or other foreign body; considered the latest breakthrough in cancer research, because of its potential value in treating the disease

Intermittent claudication: Cramplike pains in the legs on walking, caused by insufficient arterial blood supply to the legs.

Intima: The innermost coat of a blood vessel.

Ischemia: Reduced blood supply to some part of the body.

Isomer: A compound having the same constituents as another compound but a different structure or shape.

Kelp: Any of various large brown seaweeds; in condensed form, a dietary source of iodine.

Ketones: Two-carbon molecular fragments that derive from the breakdown of stored fat (triglyceride). Ketones comprise one of the primary normal fuels of the body, and one of the two fuels which can be utilized in brain metabolism.

Ketosis: Physiological condition in which ketones are present in the body, indicating that the body is burning its own fat supplies for energy.

Ketostix: Dipsticks used to measure the amount of ketones that are being passed in the urine.

Kinesiology: The study of the principles of mechanics and anatomy in relation to human movement.

Labile hypertension: High blood pressure that fluctuates.

Laetrile: Also known as vitamin B_{17}; found in the seeds of bitter almonds, apples, apricots. Some researchers have attested to its usefulness in treatment of cancer.

Lecithin: A waxlike substance, found distributed in animals and plants, that has emulsifying and antioxidant properties.

Lesion: A wound or injury, any morbid change in an injury to tissue; a patch of plaque in a blood vessel.

Lipid peroxidation: The combining of a fat with oxygen.

Low-density lipoprotein: A lipoprotein fraction that unloads cholesterol into the tissues. See also *High-density lipoprotein.*

Lymphocyte: A white blood cell, produced in the lymph tissue, that is a constituent of human blood.

Lysozyme: An enzyme present in saliva, tears, egg whites, and other animal fluids. It functions as an antibacterial agent.

Medulla: The central part of certain organs, as in the adrenal gland, where it is responsible for the secretion of adrenaline.

Megadose: A larger dose of vitamins and/or minerals than is needed to prevent deficiencies, used by orthomolecular physicians for the treatment of physical and mental diseases.

Metabolic pathways: The body's natural "routes" for the transformation of food into energy.

Metabolic physician: A physician who practices metabolic therapy.

Metabolic therapy: A term used to describe treatment of cancer and other patients with a combination of vitamins, minerals, and other nontoxic substances (laetrile, autogenous vaccines, and so on).

Metabolism: The sum of the processes in the building up and destruction of protoplasm; the chemical changes in living cells by which energy is provided for vital processes and activities and new material is assimilated to repair the waste; the sum of the processes by which a particular substance is handled in the living body.

Metabolite: Any chemical normally found in the body as a result of normal metabolic processes.

Metalloenzyme: An enzyme which has combined with a metal as part of its structure.

Metastasis: A transfer of a malignant tumor from the original site of the disease to another part of the body.

Metavitamins: A group of substances with obvious nutritional qualities which, however, do not produce a deficiency state when absent.

Methionine: A sulfur-containing amino acid that must be obtained in the human diet.

Methyl donor: A compound that, in living tissue, is capable of supplying methyl groups for transfer to other compounds.

Methyl groups: Groups of atoms that include a carbon atom with three hydrogen atoms and one empty atom for combining with other atoms.

Micronutrient: An organic compound, such as a vitamin or mineral, essential in minute amounts for growth and the maintenance of normal functioning.

Monilia: A type of fungus.

Myocardial infarction: Damage to the heart due to the loss of blood supply in a region of the heart muscle.

Narcolepsy: A disease characterized by a sudden uncontrollable desire to sleep which occurs at irregular intervals.

Necrosis: Death of a living tissue.

Neurologic: Having to do with the nervous system.

Neuropathy: An abnormal or degenerative state of the nervous system.

Neurotransmitter: A substance that transmits nerve impulses across a synapse; brain chemicals that are involved in carrying messages to and from the brain.

Nitroglycerin: A drug that acts quickly to expand the heart vessels so that blood flow is unimpaired; often used in the treatment of angina.

Noradrenaline: The precursor of adrenaline, a hormone given off by adrenal glands. A potent stimulator that increases heart rate and the force of contractions, and causes other physiological effects.

Oncology: The study of tumors.

Orotate: A salt of orotic acid; said to be a most effective molecule for transporting a mineral through a cellular membrane.

Orotic acid: Vitamin B_{13}; a metabolite in the pyrimidine series.

Orthomolecular medicine: The treatment of human illness by varying the concentration of substances normally present in the human body.

Osteoarthritis: A degenerative joint disease.

Pangamic acid: Vitamin B_{15}. Dimethylglycine bound to calcium.

Paroxysmal tachychardia: Periodic reappearance of an abnormally rapid heartbeat.

Pathogenesis: The causation of a disease.

Peripheral vascular disease (PVD): Disease characterized by a reduction in blood supply to the smaller blood vessels.

Peroxide: A compound containing a higher proportion of oxygen than the usual form of the compound.

Placebo: A pill having no medicinal value, often used to satisfy a patient's psychological need for medication or as a control in an experimental situation.

Platelets: The disc-shaped structures in the blood known chiefly for their role in blood clotting.

Prodrome: A warning symptom of a disease or abnormal condition.

Propanolol: One of the *Beta blockers.*

Prophylactic: Tending to prevent or ward off disease.

Prostacyclin: One of the prostaglandins which protects against platelet clumping and blood vessel and bronchial constriction.

Prostaglandin: One of several compounds formed from essential fatty acids and whose activities affect the nervous, circulatory, and reproductive systems and metabolism.

Psychoactive: Said of drugs which act on the individual's mental and emotional functioning.

Psychopharmacology: The study of the effects of drugs on the mind and behavior.

Reagins: Antibodies, found in the blood of individuals with some form of allergy (hay fever, asthma), which sensitize the skin.

Renin: An enzyme in the kidneys that plays a major role in the release of *angiotensin.*

Retinoids: Vitamin A and similar compounds.

Rheumatoid arthritis: A chronic systemic disease of unknown origin in which inflammatory connective tissue changes predominate. Pain, limitation of motion, and joint deformity are common.

Rheumatologist: A doctor who specializes in treating arthritic conditions and joint disorders.

RNA: Ribonucleic acid; a compound of nucleic acid.

Rutin: Part of the vitamin C complex which acts to decrease capillary fragility.

Serotonin: A substance present in many tissues, especially the blood and nerve tissue, which stimulates a variety of smooth muscles and nerves and is believed to function as a neurotransmitter.

Spilling sugar: Sugar is spilled in the urine when there is an excess in the bloodstream and the kidneys cannot reabsorb it. This is one of the first signs of diabetes.

Steroid: Any of numerous compounds and various hormones containing a carbon ring system of sterols. Included are the male, female, and adrenal cortex hormones.

Superoxide dismutase: A natural substance found in living cells (an intracellular enzyme) that inactivates the superoxide radical.

Superoxide radical: A harmful substance produced inside the cells by oxidation; suspected of initiating atherosclerosis and arthritis.

Tachycardia: Abnormally rapid heartbeat.

Teratogen: An agent that produces developmental deformities in fetuses.

Thromboembolism: The blocking of a blood vessel by a blood clot that has been transported in the bloodstream to a new location.

Thromboxane: One of the prostaglandins which circulates with the platelets and which can constrict blood vessels instantaneously; the most powerful platelet aggregator the body has to deal with.

Thyroid: An endocrine gland at the base of the neck responsible for regulating the rate of metabolism.

Tranquilizer: A drug used to reduce mental disturbance (such as anxiety and tension) in humans and animals.

Transient ischemic attacks: Spasmodically occurring attacks that reduce the blood supply of the heart because of atherosclerosis.

Tryptophan: An essential amino acid useful in treating sleep disorders and depression.

Tyramine: An amino acid formed from the breakdown of tyrosine, found in such foods as ripe cheese.

Uric acid: A product of protein metabolism present in the blood and urine.

Valsalva maneuver: Forced exhalation against the closed vocal folds to increase the pressure within the chest and to impede the release of blood to the heart.

Vascular disease: Referring to diseases of the blood vessels.

Vasoactive: Affecting the blood vessels with respect to their degree of relaxation or contraction.

Vitamin: Any of various organic substances that are essential for normal metabolic functioning of the body.

NOTES

BOOK ONE

Chapter 1

1. See: Hall, Ross Hume. *Food for Nought* (New York: Harper & Row, 1974).

Chapter 2

1. See: Helmholz, H. F. "Ten Years Experience in Treatment of Epilepsy with the Ketogenic Diet," *Archives of Neurology and Psychiatry*, vol. 29 (1933), p. 808.
2. See: "Anticholesterol Drug Withdrawn," *Journal of the American Medical Association*, vol. 80, no. 4 (1962), p. 25.
3. See: Fleischmajer, Raul. "Hypolipidemic Drugs," *American Family Physician*, vol. 17, no. 2 (February 1978), pp. 188–90. See also: "Clofibrate and Gallstones," *New England Journal of Medicine* (August 5, 1978), p. 8084.
4. See: "Clofibrate: A final verdict?" editorial, *Lancet*, vol. 2 (1978), pp. 1131–32. See also "Cooperative trial on primary prevention of ischemic heart disease using clofibrate to lower serum cholesterol: mortality follow-up," *Lancet*, vol. 2 (1980), pp. 379–85.
5. See: Beaver, William, and Thomas Kantor. "Putting aspirin to its many good uses," *Patient Care* (September 15, 1979), pp. 70–84.
6. See the Boston Collaborative Drug Surveillance Programme report, "Oral contraceptives and venous thromboembolic disease, surgically confirmed gall-bladder disease, and breast tumors," *Lancet* (June 23, 1973), pp. 1399–1408.
7. See: King, Janet, "Nutrition during oral contraceptive treatment," *New York State Journal of Medicine* (April 1978), pp. 840–41.
8. See: Wynn, Victor. "Vitamins and oral contraceptive use," *Lancet* (March 8, 1975), pp. 561–64.

Chapter 3

1. See: Williams, Roger. *Biochemical Individuality* (Austin: University of Texas Press, 1969).

Chapter 4

1. See: Burkitt, D. P., A. R. Walker, and N. S. Painter. "Dietary fiber and disease," *Journal of the American Medical Association*, vol. 229 (August 19, 1974), pp. 1068–74. See also: Trowell, H. "Ischemic heart disease and dietary fiber," *American Journal of Clinical Nutrition*, vol. 25 (1972) pp. 929–32.
2. See: Schroeder, Henry. *The Trace Elements and Man* (Old Greenwich, Ct.: Devin-Adair, 1973).
3. See: Minot, George R. "The role of a low-carbohydrate diet in the treatment of migraine and headache," *Medical Clinics of North America*, vol. 7 (1923), pp. 715–28.
4. See: Roberts, H. J. "Migraine and related vascular headaches due to diabetogenic hyperinsulinism. Observations on pathogenesis and rational treatment in 421 patients," *Headache*, vol. 7 (1967), pp. 41–62.
5. See: Abrahamson, E. M., and A. W. Pezet. *Body, Mind and Sugar* (New York: Holt, Rinehart & Winston, 1951).
6. See: Pfeiffer, Carl C. *Mental and Elemental Nutrients* (New Canaan, Ct.: Keats, 1975), p. 382.
7. See: Brennan, R. O. *Nutrigenics* (New York: New American Library, 1975), p. 42.
8. See: Yudkin, John. "Dietary factors in arteriosclerosis: sucrose," *Lipids*, vol. 13 (1978), pp. 370–72.
9. Ibid.
10. See: Antar, M. A., M. A. Ohlson, and R. E. Hodges. "Changes in Retail Market Food Supplies in the U.S. in the Last 70 Years," *American Journal of Clinical Nutrition*, vol. 14 (March 1964), pp. 169–78.
11. See: Cleave, T. L. *The Saccharine Disease* (New Canaan, Ct.: Keats, 1978), p. 8.
12. See: Sussman, Karl, et al. "Plasma insulin levels during reactive hypoglycemia," *Diabetes*, vol. 15, no. 1 (1966), pp. 1–4. See also: Hofeldt, Fred, and Edward Lufkin. "Are abnormalities in insulin secretion responsible for reactive hypoglycemia?" *Diabetes*, vol. 23, no. 7 (1974), pp. 589–95.
13. See: Roth, Jesse. "Insulin Receptors in Diabetes," *Hospital Practice* (May 1980), pp. 98–103.
14. See, for instance: Kunin, Richard. "Ketosis and the optimal carbohydrate diet: basic factor in orthomolecular psychiatry," *Orthomolecular Psychiatry*, vol. 5, pp. 3203–11.

Chapter 5

1. Atkins, Robert, and Shirley Linde. *Dr. Atkins' Superenergy Diet* (New York: Crown, 1977, hardback; New York: Bantam, 1978, paperback).
2. Harper, Harold. *How You Can Beat the Killer Diseases* (Westport, Ct.: Arlington House, 1977)

3. See: Harris, Seale. "Hyperinsulinism and Dysinsulinism," *Journal of the American Medical Association*, vol. 83 (1924), p. 729.
4. See: Kryston, L. J. "Diabetes and Reactive Hypoglycemia," in *Endocrinology and Diabetes*, Kryston and Shaw, eds. (New York: Grune & Stratton, 1975), p. 473.

Chapter 6

1. See: Burkhardt, Rainer, and Gerhard Kienle. "Controlled clinical trials and medical ethics," *Lancet* (December 23/30, 1978), pp. 1356–59.
2. See: Hoffer, Abram. "An examination of the double-blind as it has been applied to megavitamin therapy," *Journal of Orthomolecular Psychiatry*, The Double-Blind Studies Reprint, pp. 7–14.
3. See: Danilevicus, Zenonas. "The power of unbiased observation," *Journal of the American Medical Association*, vol. 231 (March 31, 1975), p. 966.
4. See: Williams, Roger. *Nutrition Against Disease* (New York: Bantam Books, 1971), p. 8.
5. Ibid.
6. See: Yudkin, John. "Low Carbohydrate Diet in Treatment of Obesity," *Postgraduate Medicine*, vol. 51, no. 5 (1972), pp. 151–59.
7. See: Stunkard, Albert. "Dieting and Depression Reexamined," *Annals of Internal Medicine*, vol. 81 (1974), pp. 526–33.
8. Dr. Herbert has stated: "There is some evidence that megadoses of vitamin C may have a mild antihistamine effect; however, taking a mild antihistamine for relief rather than megadoses of vitamin C would be preferable." From: Herbert, Victor. "Megavitamin Therapy," *New York State Journal of Medicine*, vol. 79 (February 1979), p. 278.
9. See: Cameron, Ewan, and Linus Pauling. *Cancer and Vitamin C* (Menlo Park, Cal.: Linus Pauling Institute of Science and Medicine, 1979).

BOOK TWO

PART I

Chapter 7

1. Pauling, Linus, and David Hawkins, eds. *Orthomolecular Psychiatry* (San Francisco: Freeman, 1973).
2. See: Osmond, Humphry. "The Background to the Niacin Treatment," in *Orthomolecular Psychiatry*, D. Hawkins and L. Pauling, eds. (San Francisco: Freeman, 1973), p. 194. See also: Hoffer, Abram. "Nicotinic acid an adjunct in the treatment of schizophrenia," *American Journal of Psychiatry*, vol. 120 (1963), p. 170.
3. See: Hansen, J. "Vitamin B_{12} deficiency in psychiatry," *Lancet* (October 29, 1966), p. 965.
4. See: Stein, S. I. "Some observations on pyrodoxine and L-tryptophan in a neuropsychiatric medical regimen," *Annals of the New York Academy of Sciences*, vol. 166 (1969), p. 210. See also: Binder, D. A.

"Tryptophan and serotonin in schizophrenia," *Lancet* (August 21, 1976), p. 427.

5. Ward, Jack. *Emotional Aspects of Hypoglycemia in Endocrinology and Diabetes* (New York: Grune & Stratton, 1975).
6. See: Salzer, H. M. "Relative hypoglycemia as a cause of neuropsychiatric illness," *Journal of the National Medical Association*, vol. 58, no. 1 (January 1966), pp. 12–17.
7. See: Smythies, J. R. "The biochemistry of psychosis," *Scottish Medical Journal*, vol. 15, no. 1 (1970), p. 34.
8. See: Hoffer, Abram. "Treatment of Schizophrenia," in *A Physician's Handbook of Orthomolecular Medicine*, Roger Williams and Dwight Kalita, eds. (Elmsford, N.Y.: Pergamon Press, 1977), p. 83.

Chapter 8

1. See: Kales, Anthony, et al. "Rebound insomnia—a potent hazard following withdrawal of certain benzodiazepines," *Journal of the American Medical Association*, vol. 241, no. 16 (April 20, 1979), pp. 1692–93.
2. See: "Insomnia confuses patients and physicians," Medical News, *Journal of the American Medical Association*, vol. 239, no. 25 (June 23, 1978), pp. 2637–46.
3. See: Kripke, D. R., et al. "Average Sleep, Insomnia and Sleeping Pill Use," *Sleep Research*, vol. 5 (1976), p. 110.
4. See: Pfeiffer, Carl. *Mental and Elemental Nutrients* (New Canaan, Ct.: Keats, 1976).
5. See: Cooper, Alan J. "Tryptophan: Antidepressant Physiological Sedative—Fact or Fancy?" *Psychopharmacology*, vol. 61 (1979), pp. 97–102.
6. Hartmann, Ernest. *The Sleeping Pill* (New Haven: Yale University Press, 1978).
7. See: Goldberg, Philip, and Daniel Kaufman. *Natural Sleep (How to Get Your Share)* (Emmaus, Pa.: Rodale Press, 1978), on magnesium, p. 249; on calcium, p. 111; on niacin, pp. 105–6.

Chapter 9

1. See: "1977 Top 200 Drugs, Total Number of Prescriptions Slumps Again for Fourth Year in a Row," Continuing Education, *Pharmacy Times* (April 1978), pp. 41–48.
2. See: Garber, A. J., et al. "The role of adrenergic mechanisms in the substrate and hormonal response to insulin-induced hypoglycemia in men," *Journal of Clinical Investigation*, vol. 58 (1976), pp. 7–15.
3. See: Philpott, William H., and D. K. Kalita. *Brain Allergies* (New Canaan, Ct.: Keats, 1980), pp. 115–25.
4. See: Perrick, Jeffrey, et al. "Abrupt withdrawal from therapeutically administered diazepam," *Archives of General Psychiatry*, vol. 35 (August 1979), pp. 995–98.
5. "Senate Unit Is Warned of Danger in Valium Abuse," *New York Times* (September 12, 1979), p. A21.
6. See: Salzer, H. R. "Relative hypoglycemia as a cause of neuropsy-

chiatric illness," *Journal of the National Medical Association*, vol. 58, no. 1 (January 1966), pp. 12–17. See also: Fredericks, Carlton. *Low Blood Sugar and You* (New York: Grosset & Dunlap, 1969). And: Abrahamson, E. *Body, Mind and Sugar* (New York: Holt, Rinehart & Winston, 1951).

Chapter 10

1. See: Ravoris, C. L., et al. "Use of MAOI antidepressants," *American Family Physician*, vol. 18, no. 1 (1978), p. 109.
2. See: Stewart, Richard. "Tricyclic antidepressant poisoning," *American Family Physician*, vol. 19, no. 5 (May 1979), pp. 136–44.
3. See: Bigger, Thomas J., Jr., et al. "Effects of tricyclic antidepressants on the heart and blood," *Practical Cardiology* (January 1978), pp. 64–75.
4. See: Adams, P. W., et al. "Effect of Pyridoxine Hydrochloride (Vitamin B_6) upon Depression Associated with Oral Contraception," *Lancet*, vol. 1 (April 28, 1973), p. 897.
5. See: Chouinard, G., et al. "Tryptophan-Nicotinamide Combination in Depression," *Lancet* (January 29, 1977) pp. 249–51.

Chapter 11

1. See: Jones, J. F. "Magnesium balance studies in chronic alcoholism," *Annals of the New York Academy of Sciences*, vol. 162 (1969), p. 934.
2. See: Shive, William. "Glutamine as a general metabolic agent protecting against alcoholic poisoning," in *Biochemical and Nutritional Aspects of Alcoholism*, symposium (Austin: University of Texas, 1965), pp. 17–25.
3. See: Smith, Russell. "A five-year field trial of massive nicotinic acid therapy of alcoholics in Michigan," *Orthomolecular Psychiatry*, vol. 3, no. 4 (1974), pp. 327–33.
4. See: Brody, Nathan. "Guidelines in Treating the Alcoholic Patient in the General Hospital—Orthomolecular Therapy," *Journal of Orthomolecular Psychiatry*, vol. 6, no. 4 (1977), pp. 339–412.
5. See: Pfeiffer, Carl. *Mental and Elemental Nutrients* (New Canaan, Ct.: Keats, 1976), pp. 377–78.

PART II

Chapter 12

1. See: Waters, W. E. "Prevalence of Migraine," *Journal of Neurosurgery and Psychiatry* (1975), pp. 613–16.
2. See: Kobayashi, R. M. "How to get to the root of your patient's headaches," *Modern Medicine*, vol. 46, no. 21 (1979), p. 12.
3. See: Friedman, A. P. "Headache," in *Clinical Neurology*, A. B. and L. H. Baker, eds. (New York: Harper & Row, 1976). See also: Graham, M. R. "Migraine: Clinical Aspects," in *Handbook of Clinical Neurology*, P. J. Vinken and G. W. Bruyn, eds. (Amsterdam: North-Holland Publishing, 1968), vol. 5, pp. 45–58.

4. See: Brown, K. "Migraine and Migraine Equivalents in Children," *Developmental Medicine and Child Neurology*, vol. 19, no. 5 (1977), pp. 683–92.
5. See: Grant, Ellen. "Oral contraceptives, smoking, migraine and food allergy," *Lancet* (September 9, 1978), p. 581.
6. See: Brainard, John B. *Control of Migraine* (New York: Norton, 1977).
7. See: Anthony, Michael. "Role of individual free fatty acids in migraine," *Research in Clinical Studies in Headache*, vol. 6 (1978), pp. 110–16.
8. See: Dalessio, Donald. "Classification and Mechanism of Migraine," *Headache*, vol. 19, no. 3 (1979), pp. 114–21.
9. Graham, John. "Migraine Headache—Diagnosis and Management," *Headache*, vol. 19, no. 3 (1979), pp. 133–41.
10. See: Diamond, Seymour, et al. "Cluster: the Headache that Attacks Men," *Current Prescribing* (April 1979), pp. 44–54.
11. Ibid.
12. See: Grant, Ellen. "Food Allergy and Migraine," *Lancet* (May 5, 1979), pp. 966–68. See also: Monro, J., et al. "Food Allergy in Migraine," *Lancet*, vol. 2 (1980), pp. 1–4.
13. See: Dexter, James, et al. "The Five Hour Glucose Tolerance Test and Effect of Low Sucrose Diet in Migraine," *Headache*, vol. 18, (May 1978), pp. 91–94. See also the article by H. J. Roberts in *Headache*, vol. 7 (1967), pp. 41–62, cited above in note 4, Chapter 4.
14. See: Sicuteri, Federigo. "The ingestion of serotonin precursors improves migraine headache," *Headache*, vol. 13 (April 1973), pp. 19–22.
15. See: Kangasniemi, P. "Levotryptophan in migraine," *Headache*, vol. 18 (July 1978), pp. 161–65.
16. See: Brainard, John B. *Control of Migraine* (New York: Norton, 1977).
17. See: Dalton, Katharina. "Food Intake Prior to Migraine Attacks—Study of 2,313 Spontaneous Attacks," *Headache*, vol. 15 (1975), pp. 188–93.

Chapter 13

1. See: Spellacy, W. N. "Glucose, insulin and growth hormone studies in long-term users of oral contraceptives," *American Journal of Obstetrics and Gynecology*, vol. 106 (1970), p. 170.
2. See: Behall, K. M., et al. "The Effect of Kind of Carbohydrate in the Diet and Use of Oral Contraceptives on Metabolism of Young Women, III, Serum Glucose, Insulin and Glucagon," *American Journal of Clinical Nutrition*, vol. 33, no. 5 (1980), pp. 1041–48.
3. See: Cooper, Alan J. "Tryptophan: Antidepressant Physiological Sedative—Fact or Fancy?" *Psychopharmacology*, vol. 61 (1979), pp. 97–102.
4. See: Fredericks, Carlton. *Breast Cancer: A Nutritional Approach* (New York: Grosset & Dunlap. 1979).

Chapter 14

1. For similar cases, see: Thorn, George. "Cyclical Edema," *American Journal of Medicine*, vol. 23, (1957) p. 507.
2. See: Mostow, J., et al. "Cyclic edema and reactive hypoglycemia," *Psychosomatics*, vol. 3 (1962), pp. 17–27. See also: Kryston, L. J. "Small-vessel disease and cyclical edema in diabetes mellitus," in *Endocrinology and Diabetes*, Kryston and Shaw, eds. (New York: Grune & Stratton, 1975), pp. 443–50.
3. MacGregor, G. A., et al. "Is idiopathic edema idiopathic?" *Lancet* (February 24, 1979), pp. 397–400.
4. Lewin, Sherry, "Evaluation of Potential Effects of High Intake of Ascorbic Acid," *Comparative Biochemistry and Physiology*, vol. 47-B (1973), pp. 681–95.

PART III

Chapter 15

1. See: Newberne, P. M. *Malnutrition and the Immune Response*, R. M. Suskind, ed. (New York: Raven Press, 1977), p. 375.
2. See: Leibovitz, Brian, and Benjamin Siegel. "Ascorbic acid, neutrophil function and the immune response," *International Journal of Vitamin and Nutrition Research*, vol. 48 (1978), p. 159.
3. See: Dreizen, S., in the *International Journal of Vitamin and Nutrition Research*, vol. 49 (1979), p. 220.
4. See: Tryfiates, G. P., ed. *Vitamin B-6, Metabolism and Role in Growth* (Westport, Ct.: Food & Nutrition Press, 1980), p. 205.
5. See: Chandra, R. K., and B. Au. "Single Nutrient Deficiency and Cell-Mediated Immune Responses. I, Zinc," *American Journal of Clinical Nutrition*, vol. 33, no. 4 (1980), pp. 736–38. See also: Golden, Michael H., et al. "Zinc and immunocompetence in protein energy malnutrition," *Lancet* (June 10, 1978), pp. 1226–27.
6. See: Horrobin, D. F., et al. "The Nutritional Regulation of T-Lymphocyte Function," *Medical Hypothesis*, vol. 5 (1979), pp. 969–85.
7. See: Dreizen, Samuel, "Nutrition and the Immune Response—a Review," *International Journal of Vitamin and Nutrition Research*, vol. 49 (1979), p. 220.
8. See: Leibovitz, Brian, and Benjamin Siegel. "Ascorbic acid, neutrophil function and the immune response," *International Journal of Vitamin and Nutrition Research*, vol. 48 (1978), p. 159.
9. See: Dreizen, Samuel, "Nutrition and the Immune Response—a Review," *International Journal of Vitamin and Nutrition Research*, vol. 49 (1979), p. 220.

Chapter 16

1. See the section What's New, "Are Patients on Aspirin More Vulnerable to Bacteria?" *Geriatrics* (June 1979), p. 14.

2. See: Hoelzel, F. "Diet and Resistance to Colds," *Science*, vol 86 (1937), p. 399.
3. See: Nesbit, R. M., and C. H. McDonnell. "Low-calory, low-fat ketogenic diet for treatment of infection of the urinary tract," *Journal of the American Medical Association*, vol. 105 (1935), p. 1183.
4. See articles about Linus Pauling in the *Medical Tribune* (March 24, 1976), pp. 18–19, and (April 7, 1978), pp. 37–38.
5. See: Dykes, Michael, and Paul Meier. "Ascorbic acid and the common cold—evaluation of its efficacy and toxicity," *Journal of the American Medical Association*, vol. 231, no. 10 (March 10, 1975), pp. 1073–78.
6. See: Morishige, F., and A. Murata. "Vitamin C for prevention and treatment of viral diseases," *Proceedings of the First International Congress of the Microbiological Society*, Japan, vol. 3 (1975), pp. 432–42.
7. See: Siegel, B. V., and J. I. Morton. "Vitamin C and the immune response," *Experientia*, vol. 33 (1977), pp. 393–95.
8. See: DeChatelet, L. R., et al. "Ascorbic Acid: Possible Role in Phagocytosis," paper read at 62nd Meeting, American Society of Biological Chemists, San Francisco, June 18, 1971.
9 See: Korant, Bruce, in *Medical World News* (June 7, 1974), p. 12.

Chapter 17

1. See: "A Survey of Unorthodox Cancer Treatments," in *The Encyclopedia of Common Diseases* (Emmaus, Pa.: Rodale Press, 1976), pp. 357–70.
2. See: Gerson, Max. *A Cancer Therapy: Results of Fifty Cases* (New York: Whittier Books, 1958).
3. See: Moss, Ralph. *The Cancer Syndrome* (New York: Grove Press, 1980), pp. 91–92.
4 Bailey, Herbert. *A Matter of Life or Death: The Incredible Story of Krebiozen* (New York: G. P. Putnam's Sons, 1958).
5. See: Moss, Ralph. *The Cancer Syndrome* (New York: Grove Press, 1980), pp. 155–71.
6. Ibid.
7. See: Null, G. "The suppression of cancer cures," *Penthouse* (October 1979), pp. 91–96.
8. See: Livingston, Virginia W. *Cancer: A New Breakthrough* (San Diego: Reward Books, 1979).
9. See: Manner, Harold. "Amygdalin, Vitamin A and Enzyme Induced Murine Mammary Adenocarcinomas," *Journal of Manipulation and Physiological Therapeutics*, Chicago (December 1978). See also: Nieper, Hans. "Problems of early cancer diagnosis and therapy, particularly amygdalin in cancer prophylaxis and therapy," *Agressologie*, Paris, vol. 11, no. 1 (1970).
10. See: Issels, Joseph. *Cancer: A Second Opinion* (London: Hodder & Stoughton, 1975).

11. See: Bradford, Robert, and Michael Culbert, eds. *The Metabolic Management of Cancer* (Los Altos, Cal.: Bradford Foundation, 1979).

12. Ibid., p. 129.

13. See: Cameron, E., and L. Pauling. "Supplemental ascorbate in the supportive treatment of cancer: Reevaluation of survival times in terminal human cancer," *Proceedings of the National Academy of Sciences*, vol. 75, no. 9 (1978), p. 4538.

14. See: Morishige, Fukumi, and Akira Murata. "Prolongation of Survival Times in Terminal Human Cancer by Administration of Supplemental Ascorbate," *Journal of the International Academy of Preventive Medicine*, vol. 5 (1978), p. 47.

15. See: Moss, Ralph. *The Cancer Syndrome* (New York: Grove Press, 1980). See also: Bradford, Robert, and Michael Culbert, eds. *The Metabolic Management of Cancer* (Los Altos, Cal.: The Bradford Foundation, 1979). And: Dilman, V. M. "Metabolic immunodepression which increases the risk of cancer," *Lancet*, vol. 2 (1977), pp. 1207–9.

16. See: Moss, Ralph. *The Cancer Syndrome* (New York: Grove Press, 1980).

17. See: Livingston, Virginia W. *Cancer: A New Breakthrough* (San Diego: Reward Books, 1979).

18. See: Gutterman, J. U., et al. "Active Immunotherapy with BCG for recurrent malignant melanoma," *Lancet* (June 2, 1973), p. 1208.

19. Passwater, Richard. *Cancer and Its Nutritional Therapies* (New Canaan, Ct.: Keats, 1973).

20. See: Cameron, E., L. Pauling, and B. Liebovitz. "Ascorbic Acid, Neutrophil Function and the Immune Response," *Cancer Research*, vol. 39 (1979), p. 633.

21. See: Sporn, Michael B. "Vitamin A and its Analogs (Retinoids) in Cancer Prevention," in *Nutrition and Cancer*, Myron Winick, ed. (New York: John Wiley & Sons, 1977), pp. 119–30.

22. See the article by R. P. Heumer in the *Journal of the International Academy of Preventive Medicine*, vol. 5 (1978), p. 59.

23. See: Lesser, Michael. *Nutrition and Vitamin Therapy* (New York: Grove Press, 1980), p. 147.

24. See a preliminary report of ten cases treated with laetrile: Morrone, John A. "Chemotherapy of Inoperable Cancer," *Experimental Medicine and Surgery*, vol. 4 (1962). See also: Richardson, John, and Patricia Griffin. *Laetrile Case Histories* (New York: Bantam Books, 1977).

25. See: Moss, Ralph. *The Cancer Syndrome* (New York, Grove Press, 1980). See also: Manner, Harold, et al. *The Death of Cancer* (Chicago: Advanced Century Publishing, 1978).

26. See: Herbert, Victor. "The Nutritionally Unsound Nutritional and Metabolic Antineoplastic Diet of Laetrile Proponents," *Journal of the American Medical Association*, vol. 240, no. 11 (September 8, 1978), pp. 1139–40. See also: "Laetrile: The Cult of Cyanide Promoting Poison for Profit," *American Journal of Clinical Nutrition*, vol. 32, no. 5 (1979), pp. 1121–58.

27. Pinckney, Edward R., and Cathey Pinckney. *The Cholesterol Controversy* (Los Angeles: Sherbourne, 1973).
28. See: Winter, Ruth. *Cancer-Causing Agents* (New York: Herbert Michelman, Crown, 1979), p. 99. See also: Dayton, Seymour, and Morton L. Pearce. "Diet and Atherosclerosis," *Lancet* (February 28 1970), pp. 473–74.
29. See: Pritikin, Nathan. *The Pritikin Program for Diet and Exercise* (New York: Bantam Books, 1980). And: Fredericks, Carlton. *Breast Cancer: A Nutritional Approach* (New York, Grosset & Dunlap, 1979).
30. See: Harper, H. W., and W. J. Clifford. "The Immunostatus Differential—Early Detection of Cancer and the Pre-Cancer State," *Journal of the International Academy of Preventive Medicine,* vol. 6, no. 1 (1980), p. 71.

PART IV

Chapter 18

1. From the National Arthritis Foundation's Service Brochure (May 1980).
2. Martin, Eric. *Hazards of Medication* (Philadelphia: Lippincott, 1971).
3. Verrett, Jacqueline. *Eating May be Hazardous to Your Health* (Garden City, N.Y.: Doubleday, 1975).
4. See: Barton-Wright, E. C., and W. A. Elliot. "The pantothenic acid metabolism of rheumatoid arthritis," *Lancet* (Oct. 26, 1963), p. 863.
5. See the article about Eustace Barton-Wright in *Medical World News* (October 7, 1978).
6. See: Sahud, Mervyn, and Richard Cohen. "Effect of Aspirin Ingestion on Ascorbic Acid Levels in Rheumatoid Arthritis," *Lancet* (May 8, 1971), pp. 937–39.
7. See: Wilkins, E. S. and M. G. "Effect of aspirin and vitamins C and E on sinovial rheumatoid arthritic and other cells," *Experientia,* vol. 35 (1979), p. 244.
8. See: Klenner, Fred, in *A Physician's Handbook on Orthomolecular Medicine,* R. Williams and D. Kalita, eds. (Elmsford, N.Y.: Pergamon Press, 1977), p. 56.
9. See: Warter, Peter. "Seven Year Observations on Treatment of Arthritis with Hesperiden-Ascorbic Acid," *Journal of the American Geriatric Society,* vol. 4 (1956), pp. 592–98.
10. See: Ellis, John M., and James Presley. *Vitamin B_6: The Doctors Report* (New York: Harper & Row, 1973).
11. See: Kaufman, William. *The Common Form of Joint Dysfunction: Its Incidence and Treatment* (Vermont: E. L. Hildreth, 1949).
12. See: Labadarios, D., et al. "Metabolic abnormalities of tryptophan and nicotinic acid in patients with rheumatoid arthritis," *Rheumatology and Rehabilitation,* vol. 17 (1978), p. 17.
13. See: Kaijser, L., and A. Wennmalm, "Nicotinic acid stimulates prostaglandin synthesis in the rabbit heart without releasing noradrenaline," *Acta Physiologica Scandinavica,* vol. 102 (1978), p. 246.

14. See: Machley, I., and L. Ouakmine, "Tocopherol in osteoarthritis: a controlled pilot study," *Journal of the American Geriatric Society*, vol. 26 (1978), pp. 328–30.

15. See: Riley, A. J. "Peyronie's Disease: a report on a series of 18 patients treated with potassium p-Amino Benzoate," *British Journal of Sexual Medicine* (March 1979), pp. 29–31.

16. See: Salin, Marvin, and Joe McCord. "Free Radicals and Inflammation," *The Journal of Clinical Investigation*, vol. 56 (1975), pp. 1319–23.

17. See: Sorenson, J., et al. "Treatment of rheumatoid and degenerative diseases with copper complexes," *Inflammation*, vol. 2 (1977), pp. 217–38.

18. See: Rudolph, Charles, Jr. "Trace Element Patterning in Degenerative Disease," *Journal of the International Academy of Preventive Medicine*, vol. 4 (1977), p. 9.

19. Frank, Benjamin. "Nucleic Acid Therapy in Aging and Degenerative Disease," *Psychological Library*, no. 4 (1968).

20. See: Sorenson, John R. "Copper Chelates as Possible Active Metabolites of the Antiarthritic and Antiepileptic Drugs," *Journal of Applied Nutrition*, vol. 32, no. 1 (1980), pp. 4–26.

21. See: Niedermeier, W., and J. H. Griggs. "Trace metal composition of synovial fluid and blood serum of patients with rheumatoid arthritis," *Journal of Chronic Diseases*, vol. 23 (1971), p. 527.

22. See: Brusch, Charles, and Edwin Johnson. "A new dietary regimen for arthritis," *Journal of the National Medical Association* (July 1959).

23. See: Gough, K. R. "Folic acid deficiency in rheumatoid arthritis," *British Medical Journal*, vol. 1 (1964), p. 212.

24. See: Shatin, R. "Gluten, the small intestine, and rheumatoid arthritis," *Rheumatism*, vol. 22 (April 1966), pp. 48–52.

25. See: Childers, Norman, and Gerald Russo. *The Nightshades and Health* (Somerville, N. J.: Horticultural Publications, Somerset Press, 1977).

Chapter 19

1. See: Danowski, T. S., et al. "Insulin patterns in equivocal glucose tolerance tests (chemical diabetes)," *Diabetes*, vol. 22, no. 11 (November 1973), pp. 808–11.

2. See: Turkington, Roger, and Howard Weindling. "Insulin secretion in the diagnosis of adult onset diabetes mellitus," *Journal of the American Medical Association*, vol. 240, no. 9 (September 1, 1978), pp. 833–36.

3. See Special Report: Statement on Hypoglycemia, *Diabetes*, vol. 22 (1973).

4. See: University Group Diabetes Program. "A Study of the Effects of Hypoglycemia Agents on Vascular Complications in Patients with Adult-Onset Diabetes," *Diabetes*, vol. 19, Suppl. 2 (1970), pp. 747–832.

5. See the article about Peter Forsham in *Internal Medicine News* (February 15, 1979).

6. See: Stout, Robert. "Diabetes and Arteriosclerosis: The Role of Insulin," *Diabetologia*, vol. 16 (1979), p. 14.
7. See: Doisy, Richard. "Comparison and effects of material and synthetic glucose tolerance factor in normal and genetically diabetic mice," *Diabetes*, vol. 27, no. 1 (1978), pp. 49–56.
8. See: Pritikin, Nathan. *The Pritikin Program for Diet and Exercise* (New York: Bantam Books, 1980).
9. See: Crapo, Phyllis. "Plasma Glucose and Insulin Response to Orally Administered Simple and Complex Carbohydrates," *Diabetes*, vol. 25 (1976), p. 741.
10. See: Spellacy, W. N., et al. "Vitamin B_6 Treatment of Gestational Diabetes Mellitus," *American Journal of Obstetrics and Gynecology*, vol. 127 (1977), p. 599.
11. See: Philpott, William. *Brain Allergies: The Psycho-Nutrient Connection* (New Canaan, Ct.: Keats, 1980).
12. See the article about K. E. Sarji in *Internal Medicine News* (September 1, 1978), p. 12.
13. See: Shpirt, Y. Y. "The Use and Efficacy of Calcium Pangamate in the Treatment of Internal Diseases," in *Vitamin B_{15}*, E. D. Michlin, ed. (Moscow: Science Publishing House, 1965).
14. See: Salway, J. G., et al. "Effect of myoinositol on peripheral nerve function in diabetes," *Lancet* (December 1978), p. 1282.
15. See: Shute, Evan and Wilbur. *Complete Updated Vitamin E Book* (New Canaan, Ct.: Keats, 1975).
16. See: Rudolph, Charles, Jr. "Trace Element Patterning in Degenerative Diseases," *Journal of the International Academy of Preventive Medicine*, vol. 4 (1977), p. 9.
17. See: McNair, P. "Hypomagnesemia, a Risk Factor in Diabetic Retinopathy," *Diabetes*, vol. 27, no. 11 (1978), pp. 1075–77.
18. See: Mater, H. M., and G. E. Levin. "Magnesium Status in Diabetes." *Lancet* (April 28, 1979), p. 924.
19. See: Henzel, J. H., et al. *Trace Substances in Environmental Health*, Hemphill, ed., vol. 4, pp. 336–41.
20. See: Wren, Peter, et al. "Hyperzincuria of Diabetes Mellitus and Possible Genetical Implications of This Observation," *Diabetes*, vol. 19, no. 1 (1970), pp. 240–47.
21. See: Everson, G. I., and R. E. Shrader. "Abnormal glucose tolerance in manganese-deficient guinea pigs," *Journal of Nutrition*, vol. 94 (1968), pp. 89–94.
22. See: Mann, J. I., and H. C. R. Simpson. "Fibre, Diabetes, and Hyperlipidaemia," *Lancet* (January 5, 1980), p. 44.

PART V

Introduction

1. See: "Heart Disease Still No. 1 Killer," *American Medical Association News* (May 26, 1978).
2. See: Montgomery, Beverly. "High plasma insulin levels a prime risk

factor for heart disease," *Journal of the American Medical Association*, vol. 242, no. 16 (April 20, 1979), p. 1665. See also: Stout, Robert. "The relationship of abnormal circulating insulin levels to atherosclerosis," *Atherosclerosis*, vol. 27 (1977), pp. 1–13.

3. See: Sloan, I. M. "The Incidence of Plasma, Insulin, Blood Sugar and Serum Lipid Abnormalities in Patients with Atherosclerotic Disease," *Diabetologia*, vol. 7 (1971), pp. 431–33.

4. See: Ratts, Thomas. "Axioms on coronary heart disease," *Hospital Medicine* (March 1978), pp. 36–53.

5. See: Ahrens, E. H. "Dietary Fats and Coronary Heart Disease: Unfinished Business," *Lancet* (December 22/29, 1979), pp. 1345–48.

6. See: Silverstein, A. "Neurological Complications of Anti-Coagulation Therapy: A Neurologist's Review," *Archives of Internal Medicine*, vol. 139, no. 2 (February 1979), pp. 217–20. See also: Bill, B. A. "Iatrogenic Intramural Hemorrhage," *Journal of the Royal College of Surgeons, Edinburgh*, vol. 24, no. 2 (March 1979), pp. 104–6.

7. See: "Clofibrate: a final verdict?" *Lancet*, vol. 2 (1978), pp. 1131–32.

8. See: Aldersberg, D., and O. Porges. "Dehydration action of low carbohydrate diet and its therapeutic use," *Klin. Wochenschr.*, vol. 12 (1933), p. 1446.

Chapter 20

1. See: Coca, Arthur. *The Pulse Test* (New York: Lyle Stuart, 1967).

2. See: Markiewiez, W., et al. "Mitral valve prolapse in one hundred presumably healthy young females," *Circulation*, vol. 53 (1976), p. 464.

3. See: Boudoulas, H., et al. "Metabolic studies in mitral valve prolapse syndrome," *Circulation*, vol. 61, no. 6 (1980), p. 1200.

4. See: "Magnesium Deficiency May Cause Heart Rhythm Irregularities," *Internal Medical News* (August 1979), p. 7. See also: Moore, Michael. "Magnesium deficiency as a cause of serious arrhythmias," *Archives of Internal Medicine*, vol. 138 (1978), p. 825. And: Sullivan, James. "Magnesium in cardiac function," *Practical Cardiology* (March 1978), pp. 63–70.

5. Harrison, Tinsley. "Glucose deficiency as a factor in production of symptoms referable to cardiovascular system," *American Heart Journal*, vol. 26 (August 1943), pp. 147–63.

Chapter 21

1. Atkins, Robert, and Shirley Linde. *Dr. Atkins' Superenergy Diet* (New York: Crown, 1977).

2. See four studies which all confirm that eating eggs does *not* raise the cholesterol level: Slater, G., et al. "Plasma cholesterol and triglycerides in man with added eggs in the diet," *Nutrition Reports International*, vol. 14 (1976), p. 249. Also: Porter, M. W., et al. "Effect of dietary egg on serum cholesterol and triglyceride of human males," *American Journal of Clinical Nutrition*, vol. 30 (1977), p. 490. And: Kummerow, F. A., et al. "The influence of egg consumption on the serum cholesterol level in human subjects," *American Journal of Clinical Nutrition*, vol. 30 (1977), pp. 664–73. And finally: Flynn, M. A., G. B.

Nolph, and T. C. Flynn. "Effect of dietary egg on human serum cholesterol and triglycerides," *American Journal of Clinical Nutrition*, vol. 32 (May 1979), pp. 1051–57. For a review article containing 143 references on the egg and cholesterol question, see H. C. McGill, Jr.'s "The relationship of dietary cholesterol to serum cholesterol concentration and to atherosclerosis in man," *American Journal of Clinical Nutrition*, vol. 32, suppl. (1979), pp. 2664–702.

3. See: Reiser, Raymond. "Oversimplification of diet: coronary heart disease relationships and exaggerated recommendations," *American Journal of Clinical Nutrition*, vol. 31 (May 1978), pp. 865–75.

4. See: Macdonald, Ian. "The effects of dietary carbohydrate on high density lipoprotein levels in serum," *Nutrition Reports International*, vol. 17, no. 6 (1978), pp. 663–68.

5. Hall, Ross Hume. *Food for Nought* (New York: Harper & Row, 1974).

6. See: Hulley, Stephen B. "The high density lipoprotein: epidemiological and practical considerations," *Practical Cardiology* (May 1978), pp. 70–81.

7. For general cholesterol metabolism, see: Geyton, Arthur. *Textbook of Medical Physiology* (Philadelphia: W. B. Saunders, 1976), pp. 41–42. For the effect of diet and lipid metabolism, see: Kritchevsky, David. "Diet, Lipid Metabolism and Aging," *Federation Proceedings*, vol. 28, no. 6, pp. 2001–6.

8. See: *Practical Cardiology*, vol. 6, no. 6 (1980), p. 157.

9. See: Coronary Drug Project Research Group, "Clofibrate and niacin in coronary heart disease," *Journal of the American Medical Association*, vol. 231, no. 4 (January 27, 1978), pp. 360–81. See also: Gotto, Antonio Jr. "Drug treatment of hyperlipidemias," *Modern Medicine* (February 15, 1978), pp. 92–101.

10. See: Carlson, L. A., and E. E. Böttiger. "Ischemic heart disease in relation to fasting values of plasma triglycerides and cholesterol," *Lancet*, vol. 1 (1972), pp. 865–86. See also: Goldstein, J. L., et al. "Hyperlipidemia in coronary heart disease—lipid levels in 500 survivors of myocardial infarction," *Journal of Clinical Investigation*, vol. 52 (1933), pp. 1533–77.

11. See: Engelberg, Hyman, and H. F. Greenberg. *The Doctor's Modern Heart Attack Prevention Program* (New York: Funk & Wagnalls, 1974), p. 83.

12. For the Framingham study, see: Kannel, W., and T. Gordon. "Framingham Study, September 24, 1970, Diet and Regulation of Serum Cholesterol," Superintendent of Documents, class no. HE20.3002, F84, Sec. 24. For the Tecumseh study, see: Nichols, A. B., et al. "Daily nutritional intake and serum lipid levels: the Tecumseh study," *American Journal of Clinical Nutrition*, vol. 29 (1977), p. 1384. See also: Reiser, Raymond. "The three weak links in the diet-heart disease connection," *Nutrition Today* (July/August, 1979), pp. 18–26.

13. See: "Clofibrate increases gallstones," *Internal Medicine News* (July 11, 1979), p. 24.

14. See: Dayton, Seymour, and Morton Pearce. "Diet and Atherosclerosis," *Lancet* (February 28, 1970), pp. 473–74.

15. See: "The controversy over the relationship of animal fats to heart

disease," *Bio Science*, vol. 24, no. 3 (March 1974), p. 142. See also: McMichael, Sir John. "Fats and Atheroma: an Inquest," *British Medical Journal*, vol. 1 (1979), pp. 173–75.

16. See: Panwanesch, M. R., et al. "Efficacy of hypolipidemic treatment of experimental atherosclerosis: the effect of nicotinic acid and related compounds," *Atherosclerosis*, vol. 31, no. 4 (1978), pp. 395–461.

17. See: Coronary Drug Project Research Group. "Clofibrate and niacin in coronary heart disease," *Journal of the American Medical Association*, vol. 231, no. 4 (January 27, 1978), pp. 360–81.

18. See: Lecithin Helps Form Cholesterol Ester to Lower Lipid Levels," *Internal Medicine News* (November 15, 1977).

19. See: Kesten, H. D., and R. Silbowitz. "Experimental Atherosclerosis and Soya Lecithin," *Proceedings of the Society for Experimental Biology and Medicine, New York City*, vol. 49 (1942), p. 71. See also: Krumdieck, M. C., and C. E. Butterworth. "Ascorbate-cholesterol-lecithin interaction," *American Journal of Clinical Nutrition*, vol. 27 (1974), p. 866.

20. Ahrens, E. H. "Dietary Fats and Coronary Heart Disease: Unfinished Business," *Lancet*, vol. 2 (1979), pp. 1345–48.

21. See: Vessby, B. "PABA reduces cholesterol," *Internal Medicine News* (November 15, 1977).

22. See: Ginter, Emil. "The effect of ascorbic acid on plasma cholesterol on humans in a long-term experiment," *International Journal of Vitamin Nutrition Research*, vol. 47, no. 2 (1977), pp. 123–34.

23. See: Leslie, Constance. "Atherosclerosis and Vitamin C," *Lancet* (December 11, 1971), p. 1280.

24. See: Anisimov, V. E., and I. G. Salikov. "Use of pangamic acid for internal disease," *Vitamin B$_{15}$* (Montreal: McNaughton Foundation, 1967), p. 125. See also: Yakovleva, I. N. "Pangamic acid treatment for middle-aged and elderly people," ibid., p. 161.

25. See: "The herbs and the heart," *Nutrition Reviews*, vol. 34, no. 2 (February 1976), pp. 43–44. See also: Bordia, A., et al. "Effect of the essential oils of garlic and onion on alimentary hyperlipemia," *Atherosclerosis*, vol. 21 (1975), pp. 15–19.

26. See: Moncada, S., and R. J. Gryglewski. "Polyunsaturated fatty acids and thrombosis," *European Journal of Clinical Investigation*, vol. 9 (1979), pp. 1–2. See also: Reiser, Raymond. "Saturated fat in the diet and serum cholesterol concentrations, a critical examination of the literature," *American Journal of Clinical Nutrition*, vol. 26 (May 1973), pp. 524–55. And: Kaunitz, H. "Dietary lipids and arteriosclerosis," *Journal of the American Oil Chemists Society*, vol. 52, no. 8 (1975) pp. 293–97.

27. Hall, Ross Hume. *Food for Nought* (New York: Harper & Row, 1974).

28. See: Horrobin, David. "A new concept of lifestyle-related cardiovascular disease," *Medical Hypothesis*, vol. 6 (1980), pp. 785–800.

29. See: Passwater, Richard. *Cancer and Its Nutritional Therapies* (New Canaan, Ct.: Keats, 1973).

30. Stillman, I. M., and S. Baker. *The Doctor's Quick Weight Loss Diet* (New York: Dell, 1978). See also: Rickman, F., et al. "Changes in

Serum Cholesterol During the Stillman Diet," *Journal of the American Medical Association*, vol. 228 (1974), p. 54.

Chapter 22

1. See: Benditt, E. P., and J. M. Benditt. "Evidence for a monoclonal origin of atherosclerotic plaque," *Proceedings of the National Academy of Science*, vol. 70 (1973), pp. 1753–56.
2. See: Passwater, Richard. *Supernutrition for Healthy Hearts* (New York: Jove, 1978).
3. See: McCully, K. S. "Homocystine, atherosclerosis and thrombosis implications for oral contraceptives users," *American Journal of Clinical Nutrition*, vol. 28 (1977), p. 545.
4. See: Davignon, Jean. In *Hypertension*, J. Genest, ed. (New York: McGraw-Hill, 1977), p. 961.
5. See: Taylor, C. B., et al. "Spontaneously occurring angiotoxic derivatives of cholesterol," *American Journal of Clinical Nutrition*, vol. 32 (January 1979), pp. 40–57. See also: Kummerow, F. A. "Nutrition imbalance and angiotoxins as dietary risk factors in coronary heart disease," ibid, pp. 58–83.
6. See: "Atherogenic hormones," editorial, *Lancet*, vol. 1 (1977), pp 1347–48.
7. See: Stamler, J. "Hypertension, Blood Lipids and Cigarette Smoking as Cofactors for Coronary Heart Disease," *Annals of the New York Academy of Science*, vol. 304 (1978), pp. 140–46.
8. See: Steiner, Manfred, and John Anastase. "Vitamin E: An inhibitor of the platelet release reaction," *Journal of Clinical Investigation*, vol. 57 (March 1976), pp. 732–37.
9. See: Jain, R. C. "Effect of garlic oil in experimental cholesterol atherosclerosis," *Atherosclerosis*, vol. 29, no. 2 (1978), pp. 125–29.
10. See: Taussig, S. J., and H. Nieper. "Bromelain: Its Use in Prevention and Treatment of Cardiovascular Disease—Present Status," *Journal of the International Academy of Preventive Medicine*, vol. 6, no. 1 (1979), p. 139.
11. See: Moncada, S., and J. R. Vane. "Arachidonic acid metabolites and the interactions between platelets and blood-vessel walls," *New England Journal of Medicine*, vol. 300, no. 20 (May 17, 1979), pp. 1142–47. See also: "Does Eicosapentenoic Acid Prevent Thrombosis and Atherosclerosis?" *Nutrition Reviews*, vol. 37, no. 10 (October 1979). And: Marx, J. L. "Blood clotting: The role of prostaglandins," *Science*, vol. 106, no. 19, pp. 1072–75.
12. See: Sanders, T. A. B. "Cod Liver Oil, Platelet Fatty Acids, and Bleeding Time," *Lancet*, vol. 1 (May 31, 1980), p. 1189.
13. See: Horrobin, D. F., et al. "The Nutritional Regulation of T-Lymphocyte Function," *Medical Hypothesis*, vol. 5 (1979), pp. 969–85.
14. See: Burnett, William, and Robert Chahine. "Sexual dysfunction as a complication of propanolol therapy in men," *Cardiovascular Medicine* (July 1979), pp. 811–15.
15. See: Dollery, C. T., and C. George. "Propanolol, Ten Years from Introduction," *Cardiovascular Clinics*, vol. 6 (1974), p. 255.

16. See: "Spasm's role in heart disease spotlighted by drug successes," *Medical World News* (December 10, 1979), p. 43. See also: Temkin, L. P. "Calcium Blocking Agents—New Directions in the Treatment of Angina Pectoris," *Arizona Medicine*, vol. 37, no. 5 (1980), pp. 328–33.

17. See: Medical News, "Attrition rate disturbing after coronary artery bypass surgery," *Journal of the American Medical Association*, vol. 240, no. 25 (December 15, 1978), pp. 2709–10.

18. See: Mann, George. "Diet-Heart: End of an Era," *New England Journal of Medicine*, vol. 297 (September 22, 1977), pp. 644–49. See also: Reiser, R. "The Three Weak Links in the Diet-Heart Disease Connection," *Nutrition Today* (July 1979), p. 221. And: "In the Melting Pot," editorial, *Lancet*, vol. 1 (November 19, 1977), pp. 1061–62. And finally: McMichael, Sir J. "Fats and Atheroma: an Inquest," *British Medical Journal*, vol. 1 (1979), pp. 173–75.

19. See the four-part article "Nutrition's Own Mount St. Helens Erupts: Is the Link Between Diet and Heart Disease Shattered?" *Nutrition Today*, vol. 15 (1980), pp. 6–20. The Food and Nutrition Board report appears here in toto.

20. Pritikin, Nathan. *Pritikin Program for Diet and Exercise* (New York: Bantam Books, 1980).

21. See: Skyler, J. S. "Nutritional Management of Diabetes Mellitus," in *Diabetes, Obesity, and Vascular Disease*, H. Katzen and R. Mahler, eds. (New York: John Wiley and Sons, 1978). See also: Wall, J. R., et al. "Effect of carbohydrate restriction in obese diabetics: relationship of control to weight loss," *British Medical Journal*, vol. 1 (1973), pp. 577–78. And: Doar, J. W. H., et al. "Influence of treatment with diet alone on oral glucose tolerance test and plasma sugar and insulin levels in patients with maturity-onset diabetes mellitus," *Lancet*, vol. 1 (1975), pp. 1263–66. And finally: Hadden, D. R., et al. "Maturity onset diabetes mellitus: Response to intensive dietary management," *British Medical Journal*, vol. 3 (1975), pp. 276–78.

22. See: Williams, Roger. *Biochemical Individuality* (Austin: University of Texas, 1974).

Chapter 23

1. See: deWolfe, V. G. "Intermittent Claudication and After," *Emergency Medicine* (May 15, 1979), p. 204.

2. See: Haeger, Kurt. "The treatment of peripheral occlusive arterial disease with α tocopherol as compared with vasodilator agents and antiprothombin (Dicumerol)," *Vascular Disease*, vol. 5 (1968), pp. 199–213.

3. See: Oski, Frank A. "Metabolism and Physiologic Roles of Vitamin E," *Hospital Practice*, vol. 12, no. 10 (October 1977), pp. 79–85.

Chapter 24

1. See: Nieper, Hans, in *Electrolytes and Cardiovascular Diseases*, E. Bajusz, ed. (Baltimore: Williams & Wilkins, 1965).

2. See: Nieper, Hans. "Capillarographic criteria on the effect of magnesium orotate, EPL substances, and clofibrate on the elasticity of blood vessels," *Agressologie*, vol. 15, no. 1 (1974), pp. 73–78.

3. See: Frank, Benjamin. *The No Aging Diet* (New York: Dial, 1976).

4. See: Frank, Benjamin. "Nucleic Acid Therapy in Aging and Degenerative Disease," *Psychological Library*, no. 4 (1968).

Chapter 25

1. See: Walker, Morton. *Chelation Therapy* (Seal Beach, Cal.: '76 Press).

2. See: Halstead, Bruce W. *The Scientific Basis of EDTA Chelation Therapy* (Colton, Cal.: Golden Quill, 1979).

3. The figures come from a personal communication to the author from Garry Gordon, president of the American Academy of Medical Preventics.

4. See: Ross, Richard S. "Ischemic Heart Disease: An Overview," *American Journal of Cardiology*, vol. 36 (1975), p. 496.

5. Ibid.

Chapter 26

1. See: Ratts, Thomas. "Axioms on Coronary Artery Disease," *Hospital Medicine* (March 1978), pp. 36–53.

2. See: Gillum, Richard F. "Dietary control and prevention of essential hypertension," *Practical Cardiology* (June 1978), p. 27.

3. See: Morgan, T., et al. "Hypertension treated by salt restriction," *Lancet* (February 4, 1978), p. 227.

4. Gorlin, Richard. "Strict low salt diet: Is it necessary?" *Primary Cardiology* (March 1978), p. 7.

5. See: Swales, J. D. "Dietary salt and hypertension," *Lancet*, vol. 1 (1980), pp. 1177–79. See also: Murray, R. H., et al. "Blood pressure response to extremes of sodium intake in normal man," *Proceedings of the Society for Experimental Biology and Medicine*, vol. 159 (1978), pp. 432–36.

6. See: Bing, R. F., et al. "Salt Intake and Diuretic Treatment of Hypertension," *Lancet* (July 21, 1979), pp. 121–22.

7. See: Lewis, P. J. "Deterioration in Glucose Tolerance Following Prolonged Diuretic Treatment for Hypertension," *British Journal of Clinical Pharmacology*, vol. 2, no. 4 (August 1975), p. 375.

8. See: "Hypertension Outlook," *Primary Cardiology* (June 1978), p. 12. See also: "Weight reduction alone significantly lowers blood pressure," *Modern Medicine* (May 15, 1978), p. 81. And: Gillum, Richard. "Dietary control of hypertension," *Practical Cardiology* (June 1978), p. 29.

9. See Dr. Schnapper's article in *Internal Medicine News* (July 1, 1979).

10. See: Jackson, G., et al. "Inappropriate Antihypertension Therapy in the Elderly," *Lancet* (December 18, 1976).

11. Atkins, Robert *Dr. Atkins' Diet Revolution* (New York: McKay, 1972).

12. See: Nieper, Hans, in *Electrolytes and Cardiovascular Diseases*, E. Bajusz, ed. (Baltimore: Williams & Wilkins, 1965).

13. See: Hogan, William. "The Therapeutic Effect of Magnesium Orotate in Serum Lipid Reduction," *Journal of Manipulative and Physiological Therapies*, vol. 1 (1978), pp. 27–31. See also: Rutolo, David. "Orotic Acid and Its Salts: A Brief Review of Physiology, Pharmacology, Toxicology, and Therapeutic Nutritional Uses," *Journal of Manipulative and Physiological Therapies*, vol. 1, no. 3 (1978), 163–69.

14. See: Schroeder, Henry. *The Poisons Around Us* (Bloomington: Indiana University Press, 1974).

15. See the article about Gerald Berenson in *Medical Tribune* (March 15, 1978).

16. See: Ahrens, Richard. "Sucrose, hypertension and heart disease: an historical perspective," *American Journal of Clinical Nutrition*, vol. 27, no. 4 (1974), pp. 1403–22.

17. See: Yudkin, John. "Dietary factors in arteriosclerosis: sucrose," *Lipids*, vol. 13, no. 5 (1978), pp. 370–72. See also: Yudkin, John. "Sugar intake and myocardial infarction," *American Journal of Clinical Nutrition* (May 1967), p. 503.

18. See: Christlieb, A. R. "Diabetes and Hypertension," *Cardiovascular Reviews and Reports*, vol. 1 (November 1980), pp. 609–16.

BOOK THREE

Chapter 27

1. See: Randolph, Theron. "Stimulatory and withdrawal levels of the alternation allergic manifestation," in *Clinical Ecology*, L. D. Dickey, ed. (Springfield, Ill.: Charles C. Thomas, 1978), pp. 156–75.

2. See: Rippere, Vicky. "A little something between meals: Masked addiction, not low blood sugar," *Lancet* (June 23, 1979).

3. See: Crook, William. "Wheat-milk combination," *Medical World News* (March 6, 1978).

4. See: Philpott, William. *Brain Allergies: The Psycho-Nutrient Connection* (New Canaan, Ct.: Keats, 1980).

5. Sheinkin, David, and Michael Schachter. *The Food Connection* (Indianapolis: Bobbs-Merrill, 1976).

6. Mackarness, Richard. *Eating Dangerously* (New York: Harcourt, Brace, Jovanovich, 1976).

7. See: Mandell, Marshall, and Lynne Waller Scanlon. *Dr. Mandell's Five-Day Allergy Relief System* (New York: Thomas Y. Crowell, 1979).

8. See: Rinkel, H. J. "Food Allergy; role of food allergy in internal medicine," *Annals of Allergy*, vol. 2 (1944), pp. 115–24.

9. See *Dr. Mandell's Five-Day Allergy Relief System*, mentioned above in note 7.

10. See Sheinkin and Schachter's *The Food Connection*, mentioned above in note 5.

11. See: Coca, Arthur. *The Pulse Test* (New York: Lyle Stuart, 1967).
12. See: Westlake, Aubrey T. *The Pattern of Health: A Search for a Greater Understanding of the Life Force in Health and Disease* (Boulder, Col.: Shambhala Publications, 1973).
13. See Mackarness' *Eating Dangerously*, mentioned above in note 6.

Chapter 28

1. Atkins, Robert. *Dr. Atkins' Diet Revolution* (New York: McKay, 1972).
2. Atkins, Robert, and Shirley Linde. *Dr. Atkins' Superenergy Diet* (New York: Crown, 1977), p. 370.
3. See: Rabast, U. "Comparative Studies in Obese Subjects Fed Carbohydrate-Restricted and High Carbohydrate 1,000-Calorie Formula Diets," *Nutrition and Metabolism*, vol. 22, no. 5 (1978), pp. 269–77.
4. See: Young, Charlotte M., et al. "Effect on body composition and other parameters in obese young men of carbohydrate level of reduction diet," *American Journal of Clinical Nutrition*, vol. 24 (1971), p. 290.
5. See: Fujita, Y., et al. "Basal & Postprotein Insulin Levels During High and Low Carbohydrate Intake and Their Relationship to Plasma Triglycerides," *Diabetes*, vol. 24, no. 552 (1975).
6. Gare, Fran, and Helen Monica. *Dr. Atkins' Diet Cookbook* (New York: Bantam Books, 1979).
7. Gare, Fran, and Helen Monica. *Dr. Atkins' Superenergy Cookbook* (New York: New American Library, 1977).
8. See: Rinkel, Herbert J., and Theron G. Randolph, and Michael Zeller. *Food Allergy* (Springfield: C. C. Thomas, 1951). (Available from the NE Foundation for Allergic and Environmental Diseases, Norwalk, Ct. 06850.) See also: Mandell, Marshall, and Lynne Waller Scanlon. *Dr. Mandell's Five-Day Allergy Relief System* (New York: Thomas Y. Crowell, 1979). And: Randolph, Theron G., and Ralph W. Moss. *An Alternative Approach to Allergies* (New York: Lippincott & Crowell, 1980).

Chapter 29

1. See: Krumdieck, C. L. "Folic Acid," in Nutrition Reviews' *Present Knowledge in Nutrition*, 4th ed., Stanley N. Gershoff, ed. (New York: The Nutrition Foundation, 1976), pp. 175–87.
2. See: Gershoff, Stanley N. "Vitamin B$_6$," in Nutrition Reviews' *Present Knowledge in Nutrition*, 4th ed., Stanley N. Gershoff, ed. (New York: The Nutrition Foundation, 1976).
3. See: Thomsen, James. "Amino Acid May Help Angina Patients," *Current Prescribing* (May 1977), p. 11.
4. See: Maebashi, M., et al. "Lipid Lowering Effect of Carnitine in Patients with Type-IV Hyperlipoproteinaemia," *Lancet* (October 14, 1978), pp. 805–9.

5. See: Pfeiffer, Carl. "Observations on the therapy of the schizophrenic," *Journal of Applied Nutrition*, vol. 26, no. 4 (1974), pp. 29–36.

Chapter 30

1. See: Lamb, L. E. *Metabolics* (New York: Harper & Row, 1974).
2. See: Schroeder, Henry. *The Poisons Around Us: Toxic Metals in Food, Air and Water* (Bloomington: Indiana University Press, 1974).
3. See: Bland, Jeffrey. *Trace Elements in Human Health and Disease* (Hayward, Cal.: Mineral Lab Publications), p. 86.
4. "Lead and Mental Handicap," *Lancet* (February 18, 1978), pp. 365–67.
5. See the article by Charles Rudolph in the *Journal of the International Academy of Preventive Medicine*, vol. 4 (1977), p. 9.

Chapter 31

1. Proxmire Amendment, Public Law 94-278, April 22, 1976, Title V, Federal Food, Drug, and Cosmetic Act. Amendments, Section 411, Vitamins and Minerals.

Chapter 32

1. The eight studies cited are: 1) Kekwick, A., et al. "The effect of high fat and high carbohydrate diets on rates of weight loss in mice," *Metabolism*, vol. 13 (1964), p. 87. 2) Krehl, W. A., et al. "Some metabolic changes induced by low-carbohydrate diets," *American Journal of Clinical Nutrition*, vol. 20 (1967), p. 139. 3) Young, C. M. "Effect on body composition and other parameters in obese young men of carbohydrate level of reduction diet," *American Journal of Clinical Nutrition*, vol. 24 (1971), p. 290. 4) Piscatelli, R. L., et al. "The Ketogenic Diet in the Management of Obesity," in *Obesity*, N. L. Wilson, ed. (Philadelphia: F. A. Davis, 1969). 5) Kasper, H., et al. "Response of body weight to a low-carbohydrate, high-fat diet in normal and obese subjects," *American Journal of Clinical Nutrition*, vol. 26 (1973), p. 197. 6) Khurani, R. C. "Modified Ketogenic Diet for Obesity," *Current Medical Dialogue*, vol. 40 (1973), p. 528. 7) Wipping, F., et al. "Vergleichende untersuchengen uber die winkung einer relativ kohlenhydratreiche reduktionsdiat," *Verhandlung Deutsche Gesellschaft für Inner Medizin*, vol. 80 (1974), p. 1227. And 8) Bassøe, H. H., et al. "Reducing Diet with High Fat Content," *Tidsskrift Norwegia Laegeboren*, vol. 98 (1978), p. 957.
2. See: Reisell, P. K., et al. "Treatment of Hypertriglyceridemia," *American Journal of Clinical Nutrition*, vol. 19 (1966), p. 84.
3. Atkins, Robert C. "In Answer to 'Dietmania,'" *Medical Times*, vol. 107 (December 1979), pp. 69–72.
4. See: Owen, O. E., et al. "Brain metabolism during fasting," *Journal of Clinical Investigation*, vol. 46 (1967), p. 1589. See also: Page, M. A., and D. H. Williamson. "Enzymes of ketone body utilisation in human brain," *Lancet*, vol. 2 (1971), p. 66.

INDEX

NATIONAL NUTRITION STUDY
PARTICIPATION QUESTIONNAIRE

Those of us interested in nutrition would be greatly enlightened if we had an answer to the question: Can dietary change and vitamin/mineral therapy exert any significant effect on health when applied on a wide scale?

This book affords an opportunity to answer this question and to gather other health information that can be of great interest to scientists and policy makers.

By filling in the following questionnaire you will become a participant in a nationwide study that could involve tens of thousands of subjects. If you and *all* the readers of this book help in this study, it can have great statistical significance and perhaps be instrumental in forming national nutrition policy. Without your participation the study will have only limited significance.

I pledge to communicate with all participants to thank you for your cooperation and to keep you informed of some future developments in nutrition medicine.

Please note that the questionnaire comes in two parts. The first is to be filled out now (your registration in the study). The second is to be filled out after following one of the recommended diets and nutritional plans (or one of your own) *for eight weeks.*

REGISTRATION INFORMATION (To be filled out and mailed before you start the diet.) Please mail to: Dr. Robert C. Atkins, 400 East 56th Street, New York, N.Y. 10022.

Dr. Atkins: Yes, I want to participate in your nationwide test of a personalized nutrition program. Please register my name and "benchmark" information immediately. As I progress, I will fill in the questionnaire and complete and mail it to you in eight weeks.

BASIC DATA

Mr.
Mrs. ———————————— AGE ————————————
Ms.

ADDRESS ———————— SEX ————————————
                           A)
CITY ———————————— HEIGHT ——————————
                                      feet   inches
STATE ———— ZIP ———— WEIGHT ————————

B) Have you consulted your doctor? ☐ Yes ☐ No
    (If "no," skip next question)

C) Were laboratory tests done? ☐ Yes ☐ No

D) Are you currently taking medications? ☐ Yes ☐ No

E) Your weight goal: ☐ Lose ☐ Gain ☐ Stay the same

F) Your primary diagnosis, condition, or symptom ——— ————

G) Do you want me to arrange for a hair mineral analysis for you
    (at the standard laboratory rate)? ☐ Yes ☐ No

PARTICIPATION QUESTIONNAIRE

To participate in what may be the most comprehensive worldwide study of the effects of nutritional changes on illness and on health, fill in the following questionnaire. All participants will receive a progress report on the results of this study and information on the latest developments in nutrition.

The study comes in two parts. Part A should be filled in *before* you start the diet. Part B should be completed after eight or more weeks on your nutritional program.

PART A. **To be filled in *before* you begin the Nutrition Breakthrough program.**

1. AGE _____ SEX M F HEIGHT _____ WEIGHT _____
                                        ft. in.   lbs.

2. List any medications you take or have taken recently (specify dosage, if possible, and how often you take them).

   _____

   _____

3. List all vitamins you take regularly. If none, check here ☐
   Write total number of pills taken daily here _____

   _____

   _____

4. Your present diet in terms of the number of times per week you consume:
   Sugar or sweets (exclude saccharin) _____
   Meat, fish, or fowl _____.
   Refined starch carbohydrates (bread, flour, pasta, etc.) _____
   Coffee _____ Tea _____ Fruit or juice _____ Alcohol _____

5. Energy on a scale of 1 to 100 (100 being the best); write your estimate of your energy level: _____

6. Mood: Using the same scale, write your estimate of your mood level: _____

7. Symptoms: Identify your major symptoms, if any, up to three of them, and their scores. (In these, 100 is the *absence* of symptoms; 0 is the symptom *at its worst*):

_____ _____
score

_____ _____

_____ _____

8. Laboratory tests, if done, or if known:
   Cholesterol _____ Triglyceride _____
   Sugar _____ Blood pressure _____
   Any other tests: _____

9. Your weight goal: To maintain same ☐   To lose _____ lbs.
   To gain _____ lbs.

PART B. **To be filled in after being on new regimen for eight or more weeks.**

1. WEIGHT. Present weight _____ A gain of _____ lbs. A loss of _____ lbs. No change _____

2. List any medications you now take (specify dosage and frequency): _____
   _____
   _____

3. List your present vitamin regimen: _____
   _____
   _____

4. Your present diet in terms of the number of times per week you consume:

   Sugar or sweets (exclude saccharin) _____ __
   Meat, fish, or fowl _____
   Refined starch carbohydrates (bread, flour, pasta, etc.)
   _____
   Coffee _____ Tea _____ Fruit or juice _____ Alcohol _____

5. Diet you now follow: Atkins ☐ Meat and Millet ☐
   Vegetarian ☐ Balanced ☐ Other, specify _____

6. Energy on a scale of 1 to 100 (100 being the best); write your estimate of your energy level: _____

7. Mood: Using the same scale, write your estimate of your mood level: _____

8. Symptoms: Relist your major symptoms identified in Part A, and their current scores. (In these, 100 is the *absence* of symptom; 0 is the symptom *at its worst*):

   _____   _____
                                             score
   _____   _____
   _____   _____

9. Laboratory tests, if done, or if known:
   Cholesterol ———————————— Triglyceride ————————————
   Sugar ———————————— Blood pressure ————————————
   Any other tests: ————————————————————————————

10. Your future diet plans: Stay on same diet as #5, Always ☐
    For a limited time ☐   From time to time ☐
    Other ————————————————————————————————